The chemistry and biology of benz[a]anthracenes

Cambridge Monographs on Cancer Research

Scientific Editors
J. Ashby, Imperial Chemical Industries, Macclesfield, Cheshire
M. M. Coombs, Imperial Cancer Research Fund Laboratories, London

Executive Editor
H. Baxter, formerly at the Laboratory of the Government Chemist, London

Books in this Series
Martin R. Osborne and Neil T. Crosby. Benzopyrenes
Maurice M. Coombs and Tarlochan S. Bhatt. Cyclopenta[a]phenanthrenes

THE CHEMISTRY AND BIOLOGY OF

BENZ[A]ANTHRACENES

M.S.NEWMAN
Department of Chemistry, Ohio State University, Columbus, Ohio, USA

B.TIERNEY
Cambridge Life Sciences, Cambridge Science Park, Cambridge, UK

S.VEERARAGHAVAN
Chemsyn Science Laboratories, Lenexa, Kansas, USA

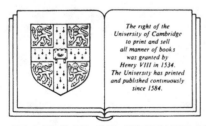

The right of the
University of Cambridge
to print and sell
all manner of books
was granted by
Henry VIII in 1534.
The University has printed
and published continuously
since 1584.

CAMBRIDGE UNIVERSITY PRESS
Cambridge
New York   New Rochelle   Melbourne   Sydney

CAMBRIDGE UNIVERSITY PRESS
Cambridge, New York, Melbourne, Madrid, Cape Town, Singapore, São Paulo, Delhi

Cambridge University Press
The Edinburgh Building, Cambridge CB2 8RU, UK

Published in the United States of America by Cambridge University Press, New York

www.cambridge.org
Information on this title: www.cambridge.org/9780521105897

First published 1988
This digitally printed version 2009

A catalogue record for this publication is available from the British Library

Library of Congress Cataloguing in Publication data
Newman, Melvin S. (Melvin Spencer), 1908–
   The chemistry and biology of benz[a]anthracenes.
   (Cambridge monographs on cancer research)
   Includes bibliographies and index.
   1. Benzanthracenes—Toxicology. 2. Benzanthracenes—
Metabolism. 3. Benzanthracenes—Synthesis.
4. Carcinogens. I. Tierney, B. II. Veeraraghavan, S.
III. Title. IV. Series
   RC268.7.B42N49 1987   616.99′4071   87-14692

ISBN 978-0-521-30544-0 hardback
ISBN 978-0-521-10589-7 paperback

Contents

Contents

Authors' preface

In Part 1 of this book the syntheses of benz[a]anthracenes are covered from the middle 1930s to the end of 1984. Prior to the middle 1930s almost all of the references are to quinones of possible use as dyestuff intermediates and are not covered here. Early syntheses were reviewed by Cook (1931). The synthetic procedures of interest in early studies of the carcinogenic activity of polycyclic aromatic hydrocarbons were reviewed by Fieser (1937). The present state of the synthetic approaches to benz[a]anthracenes is organized into several different categories. Advantages and difficulties in various synthetic routes are pointed out. Often the poor yields in certain steps should be capable of improvement by the use of alternate reagents and methods. Since many of the older methods have not been restudied, it is left to the reader to decide the best course of action in any chosen case.

The syntheses of arene oxides, dihydrodiols, quinones, phenols and diphenols in the benz[a]anthracene series will not be covered in depth and the reader is referred to the monograph *Polycyclic Hydrocarbons and Carcinogenesis* by Harvey (1985), which addresses these topics more fully.

In Part 2 the biological properties of benz[a]anthracene and its substituted derivatives (such as the highly active 7,12-dimethylbenz[a]anthracene) are discussed in relation to literature available up to the end of 1985. These types of compounds can be formed during the combustion of organic matter (such as coal or tobacco) and are widely distributed throughout the environment; being present in the air, in water and in the soil. Because of their occurrence in the environment and because certain benz[a]anthracene derivatives exhibit potent biological activity they have been the subject of intense study.

The text in Part 2 has been divided into four sections: metabolism, interactions with cellular macromolecules, mutagenicity and carcinogenicity. A brief, general, historical perspective has been given at the beginning of the metabolism section. I have tried to provide enough background information in each section so that the development and significance of ideas can be followed. Review articles have been cited wherever possible.

B.T. wishes to thank members of the Cancer Research Unit, York, for their understanding whilst this work was being prepared and his wife without whose support and encouragement this work would not have been possible.

M.S.N.
B.T.
S.V.

Abbreviations employed in this book

Journal titles

Acta Crystallogr. Acta Crystallographica
Acta Unio Int. Cancrum Acta Unio Internationalis contra Cancrum
Adv. Lipid Res. Advances in Lipid Research
Am. J. Cancer American Journal of Cancer
Am. J. Physiol. American Journal of Physiology
An. Assoc. Quim, Argent. Anales de la Associacion Quimica Argentina
Angew. Chem. Angewandte Chemie
Ann. Chim. App. Akad. Nauk SSSR Annalen Chemie Applicata Akad. Nauk. SSSR
Annalen Justus Liebigs Annalen der Chemie
Arch. Biochem. Biophys. Archives of Biochemistry and Biophysics
Arch. Geschwulstforsch. Archiv für Geselwulstforschung
Aust. J. Chem. Australian Journal of Chemistry
Ber. Berichte der Deutschen Chemischen Gesellschaft
Biochem. J. Biochemical Journal
Biochem. Pharmacol. Biochemical Pharmacology
Biochim. Biophys. Acta Biochimica et Biophysica Acta
Biomed. Mass Spectrum. Biomedical Mass Spectrometry
Br. J. Cancer British Journal of Cancer
Br. Med. J. British Medical Journal
Bull. Acad. Polon. Sci., Sér. Sci. Chim. Bulletin de l'Academie Polonaise de Sciences, Série des Sciences Chimique
Bull. Chem. Soc. Japan Bulletin of the Chemical Society of Japan
Bull. Int. Acad. Polonaise Bulletin International de l'Académie des Sciences
Bull. Soc. Chem. Japan Bulletin of the Society for Chemistry Japan
Bull. Soc. Chim. Belges Bulletin des Sociétés Chimiques Belges
Bull. Soc. Chim. France Bulletin de la Société Chimique de France
Cancer Biochem. Biophys. Cancer Biochemistry and Biophysics
Cancer Lett. Cancer Letters
Cancer Res. Cancer Research
Can. J. Chem. Canadian Journal of Chemistry
Can. J. Res. Canadian Journal of Research
Chem. Abst. Chemical Abstracts
Chem. Ber. Chemische Berichte
Chem. Biol. Interact. Chemistry and Biological Interactions
Chem. Ind. (London) Chemistry and Industry (London)

Chem. Lett. Chem. Soc. Japan   Chemistry Letters, The Chemical Society of Japan
Chi. Dai. Kog. Ken. Hok.   Chiba Daigaku Kogakubu Kenkyu Hokoku
Collect. Czeck Chem. Commun.   Collection of Czech Chemical Communications
C. R. Acad. Sci. URSS   Comptes rendus de l'Académie des Sciences, URSS
C. R. Hebd. Séances Acad. Sci.   Comptes rendus Hebdomadaires des Séances de l'Academie des Sciences
C. R. Hebd. Séances Acad. Sci. Sér. C   Comptes rendus Hebdomadaires des Séances de l'Academie des Sciences, Séries C, Séries Chimiques
Curr. Sci.   Current Science
Dokl. Akad. Nauk. SSSR   Doklady Akademii Nauk SSSR
Dokl. Bolg. Acad. Nauk   Doklady Bolgarshoi Akademii Nauk
Drug Met. Dispos.   Drug Metabolism and Disposal
Edinburgh Med. J.   Edinburgh Medical Journal
FEBS Lett.   Federation of European Biochemical Societies Letters
Fed. Proc.   Federation of American Societies for Experimental Biology Proceedings
Gazz. Chim. Ital.   Gazzetta Chimica Italíana
Geochim. Cosmochim. Acta   Geochimica et Cosmochimica Acta
Helv. Chim. Acta   Helvetica Chimica Acta
Heterocycles   Heterocycles
Indian J. Chem.   Indian Journal of Chemistry
Indian J. Phys.   Indian Journal of Physics.
Industr. Engng Chem.   Industrial and Engineering Chemistry
Int. Abst. Surg.   International Abstracts of Surgery
Int. J. Cancer   International Journal of Cancer
Izv. Akad. Nauk SSSR Otdel. Khim. Nauk.   Izvestiya Akademii Nauk SSSR Otdelenii Khimicheskikh Nauk
J. Am. Chem. Soc.   Journal of the American Chemical Society
J. Am. Med. Assoc.   Journal of the American Medical Association
J. Biol. Chem.   Journal of Biological Chemistry
J. Chem. Engng Data   Journal of Chemical and Engineering Data
J. Chem. Phys.   Journal of Chemical Physics
J. Chem. Res.   Journal of Chemical Research
J. Chem. Soc.   Journal of the Chemical Society
J. Chem. Soc., Chem. Commun.   Journal of the Chemical Society, Chemical Communications
J. Chem. Soc. Japan   Journal of the Chemical Society of Japan
J. Chem. Soc., Perkin Trans. I   Journal of the Chemical Society, Perkin Transactions I
J. Exp. Med.   Journal of Experimental Medicine
J. Gen. Chem. (USSR)   Journal of General Chemistry, USSR
J. Heterocyclic Chem.   Journal of Heterocyclic Chemistry
J. Indian Chem. Soc.   Journal of the Indian Chemical Society
J. Labelled Compd. Radiopharm.   Journal of Labelled Compounds and Radiopharmaceuticals
J. Math. Sci.   Journal of Mathematical Science
J. Med. Chem.   Journal of Medicinal Chemistry
J. Nat. Cancer Inst.   Journal of the National Cancer Institute
J. Org. Chem.   Journal of Organic Chemistry
J. Soc. Org. Syn. Chem., Japan   Journal of the Society of Organic Synthetic Chemistry, Japan
J. Prakt. Chem.   Journal für Praktische Chemie
J. Path. Bact.   Journal of Pathology and Bacteriology
Liebig's Annal. Chem.   Justus Liebig's Annalen der Chemie

Mitt. Geb. Lebensmittelunter. Hyg. Mitteilungen aus dem Gebeite der Lebensmittel-untersuchung und Hygiene
Monatsh. Chem. Monatshefte für Chemie
Mutation Res. Mutation Research
Nippon Kag. Kaishi Nippon Kagaku Kaishi (Continuation of Journal of the Chemical Society of Japan
Nucleic Acids Res. Nucleic Acids Research
Org. Prep. Proc. Int. Organic Preparations and Procedures International
Proc. Am. Pet. Inst. Proceedings, American Petroleum Institute
Proc. Nat. Acad. Sci. USA Proceedings of the National Academy of Sciences of the United States of America
Proc. Nat. Cancer Inst. Proceedings of the National Cancer Institute
Proc. R. Soc. (London), A Proceedings of the Royal Society of London, Series A
Proc. Soc. Exp. Biol. Med. Proceedings of the Society for Experimental Biology and Medicine
Prog. Exp. Tumor Res. Progress in Experimental Tumor Research
Rec. Trav. Chim. Recueil des Travaux Chimiques des Pays-Bas
Recerca Sci. Recerca Science
Roczniki Chem. Roczniki Chemii
Science Science (Washington, DC)
Science Cult. Science and Culture
Synthesis Synthesis
Synthetic Commun. Synthetic Communications
Tetrahedron Tetrahedron
Tetrahedron Lett. Tetrahedron Letters
Trans. Faraday Soc. Transactions of the Faraday Society
Yale J. Biol. Med. Yale Journal of Biology & Medicine
Z. Ernaehungswiss. Zeitschrift für Ernaehungswissenschaft
Z. Krebsforsch. Zeitschrift für Krebsforschung
Z. Kristallogr. Zeitschrift für Kristallographie
Z. Naturforsch. Zeitschrift für Naturforschung
Z. Physiol. Chem. Zeitschrift für Physiologische Chemie
Zh. Obshch. Khim. Zhurnal Obshchei Khimii

Other abbreviations
BA benz[a]anthracene
BAQ benzanthracene quinone (7,12-benz[a]anthraquinone)
DHBA dihydrobenz[a]anthracene
DMBA dimethylbenz[a]anthracene
EBA ethylbenz[a]anthracene
HOBA (OHBA) hydroxybenz[a]anthracene
MBA methylbenz[a]anthracene
PBA propylbenz[a]anthracene
i-PBA isopropylbenz[a]anthracene
TMBA trimethylbenz[a]anthracene
BrBA, ClBA, FBA halogenated benz[a]anthracene with Br, Cl or F, respectively
MeOBA, CH_3OBA methoxybenz[a]anthracene
PhBA phenylbenz[a]anthracene
TeMBA tetramethylbenz[a]anthracene
BA1,2-dihydrodiol *trans*-1,2-dihydro-1,2-dihydroxybenz[a]anthracene
BA1,2,-diol 3,4-epoxide 1,2-dihydro-1,2-dihydroxy-3,4-epoxybenz[a]anthracene
OHMBA hydroxymethylbenz[a]anthracene
3-MC 3-methylcholanthrene

7-OHM-12-MBA   7-hydroxymethyl-12-methylbenz[a]anthracene
7,12-DiOH-DMBA   7,12-dihydroxymethylbenz[a]anthracene
m-CPBA   m-chloroperoxybenzoic acid
B[a]P   benzo[a]pyrene
B[e]P   benzo[e]pyrene
NADPH   nicotinamide-adenine dinucleotide phosphate, reduced
PAH   polycyclic aromatic hydrocarbon
PB   phenobarbital
poly(A)   polyadenylic acid
poly(G)   polyguanylic acid
TCDD   2,3,7,8-tetrachlorodibenzo-p-dioxin
TPA   12-O-tetradecanoylphorbol-13-acetate
HPLC   high-pressure liquid chromatography
tlc   thin-layer chromatography

PART 1: CHEMISTRY

M. S. NEWMAN AND S. VEERARAGHAVAN

Nomenclature of BAs

Some confusion exists in the literature because of different names and numbering systems that have been used. In this book BA refers to benz[a]anthracene whose numbering system is shown and compared to that of 1:2-benzanthracene which is no longer in use. Older titles have been given modern nomenclature. The naming of different areas in BA is illustrated on the formula: K- and L-regions (Pullman and Pullman, 1954), and bay region (Jerina and Daly, 1976). Positions 7 and 12 are often referred to as the *meso* positions.

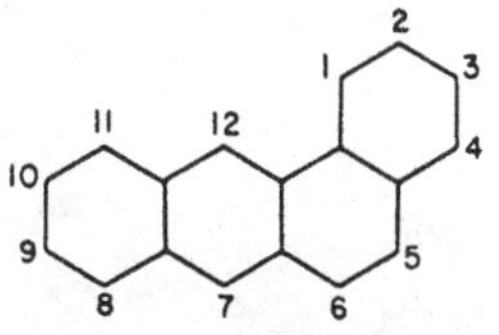

Benz[a]anthracene
(occasionally called
tetraphene with the
same numbering as for
BA)

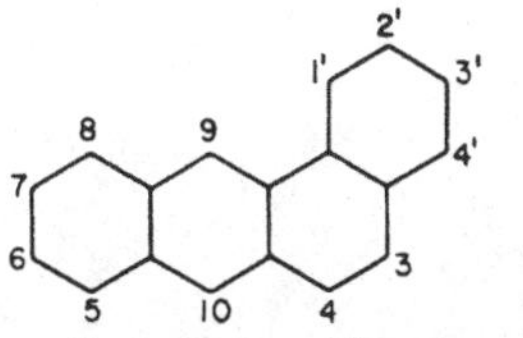

1:2-benzanthracene

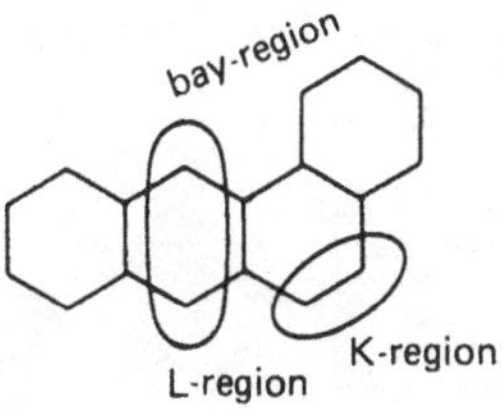

L-region   K-region

Purification of BAs

Reaction of most of the polynuclear aromatic hydrocarbons with compounds such as picric acid, 1,3,5-trinitrobenzene, and 2,4,7-trinitrofluorenone results in the formation of molecular complexes. These complexes have proved to be extremely useful for purposes of characterization and purification since the hydrocarbon portion of the complex can be readily recovered either by chromatography or by treating a solution of the complex with a base (Brass and Fanta, 1936; Orchin and Woolfolk, 1946).

1

Synthetic routes from benzenes and naphthalenes

1.1 The ketoacid route

The two most widely used routes to BA compounds having methyl groups in the 7-, 12- or 7,12-positions and other groups such as F, Cl, Br, OCH_3 in various positions involve condensation of a naphthylmagnesium bromide, **2**, with a phthalic anhydride, **1**, or a phenylmagnesium bromide **5**, with a 1,2-naphthalic anhydride, **6** (see Scheme I). The former reaction affords a mixture of acids, **3** and **4**,

Scheme I. Condensation of Anhydrides with Grignard Reagents

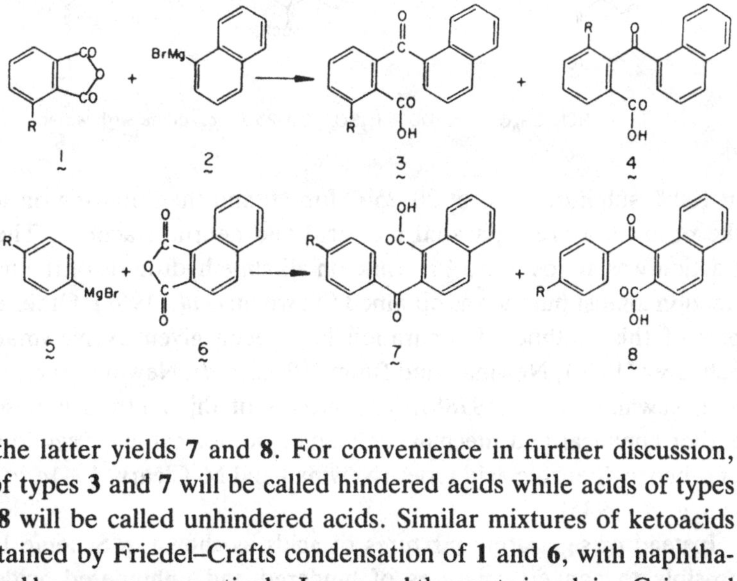

while the latter yields **7** and **8**. For convenience in further discussion, acids of types **3** and **7** will be called hindered acids while acids of types **4** and **8** will be called unhindered acids. Similar mixtures of ketoacids are obtained by Friedel–Crafts condensation of **1** and **6**, with naphthalenes and benzenes, respectively. In general the route involving Grignard reagents is preferable to that using Friedel–Crafts condensations. For example, when 3-fluorophthalic anhydride is condensed with naphthalene not only does reaction occur at each carbonyl group of the anhydride but also at the 1- and 2-positions of naphthalene (Newman and Blum, 1964d; Sheikh et al., 1979). Early studies on the reactions shown in Scheme I have been reviewed (Fieser, 1937).

In the early work leading to acids of types 3, 4, 7 and 8 separation into pure isomers was accomplished by fractional recrystallization. In later work, differences in chemical reactivity were used to simplify separation. For example, when the mixture of acids, 9 and 10, formed by the Friedel–Crafts reaction of 7-fluoro-1,2-naphthalic anhydride with benzene, was esterified a mixture of normal esters, 11 and 13, and pseudo ester, 12, was obtained (see Scheme II). After keeping this ester mixture

Scheme II Separation of Ketoacid Mixtures

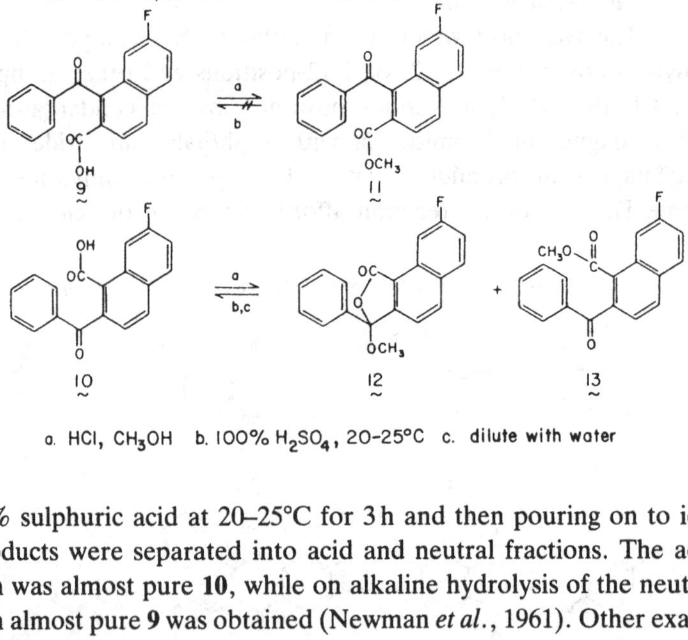

a. HCl, CH_3OH b. 100% H_2SO_4, 20–25°C   c. dilute with water

in 100% sulphuric acid at 20–25°C for 3 h and then pouring on to ice, the products were separated into acid and neutral fractions. The acid fraction was almost pure 10, while on alkaline hydrolysis of the neutral fraction almost pure 9 was obtained (Newman et al., 1961). Other examples of this method of separation have been given by Newman and Scheurer (1956), Newman and Blum (1964a,b,d), Newman et al. (1972) and Newman et al. (1978b). The success of this method is based on earlier chemical and mechanistic studies on normal and pseudo esters of o-benzoylbenzoic acid types (Newman and McCleary, 1941a,b; Newman et al., 1945).

Instead of separating mixtures of acids as shown in Scheme II it is possible to convert mixtures of hindered and unhindered acids into mainly hindered or unhindered acids. For example, when a mixture of **7** and **8** (where R = Cl) in 96% sulphuric acid was held at 120–125°C for 15 min and poured on to ice, an 83% yield of almost pure **7** was obtained when the alkali-soluble portion of the products was isolated (Newman *et al.*, 1986). Alternatively, when a mixture of **3** and **4** (R = CH₃, rich in **3**) was heated with 80% sulphuric acid at 85–90°C for 30 min, acid **4** was obtained in 75% yield on crystallization of the products (Newman, 1983). The latter method of isomerization to the unhindered acid was developed in the anthracene series by Cristol and Casper (1968). For explanations of the isomerization of **3** to **4** and of **8** to **7**, see a discussion of the Hayashi rearrangement (Section 1.4).

The yield of mixtures of acids, such as **3** and **4**, can often be increased if the 1-naphthylmagnesium bromides used are prepared from pure sub-limed magnesium activated by ethylene dibromide (Pearson *et al.*, 1959), and phthalic anhydride (Newman and Tuncay, 1980).

With pure ketoacids of desired structure the introduction of methyl groups at positions 7- and/or 12- can be accomplished in several ways. For example, reaction of **3** (R = CH₃) with methylmagnesium bromide gave the lactone **14** which on reduction yielded the acid **15**. Cyclization of **15** afforded the benzanthrone **16** which was immediately reduced and the resulting alcohol (not isolated) dehydrated to 8,12-DMBA (Newman, 1937), Scheme III.

Scheme III. Synthesis of 12-MBAs.

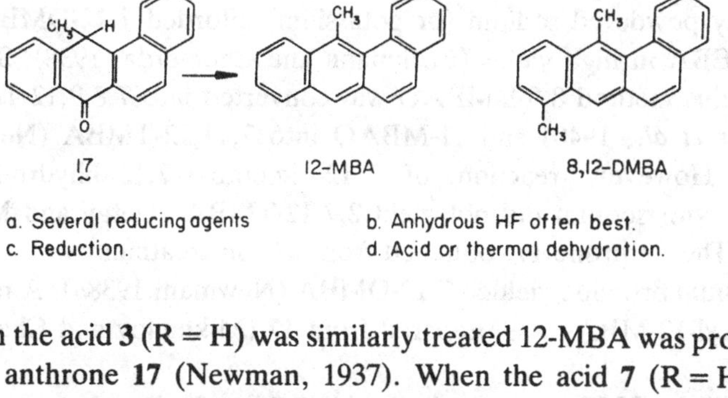

a. Several reducing agents   b. Anhydrous HF often best.
c. Reduction.   d. Acid or thermal dehydration.

When the acid **3** (R = H) was similarly treated 12-MBA was produced via the anthrone **17** (Newman, 1937). When the acid **7** (R = H) was reacted with methylmagnesium iodide the lactone **18** was obtained. Reduction furnished the acid **19**, which was cyclized to the benzanthrone and thence to 7-MBA (Fieser and Newman, 1936; Cook *et al.*, 1937). Use of ketoacid **20** in an identical sequence of reactions yielded 7,8-DMBA (Fieser and Newman, 1936), Scheme IV. An unusual base-pro-

Scheme Ⅳ. Synthesis of 7-MBAs

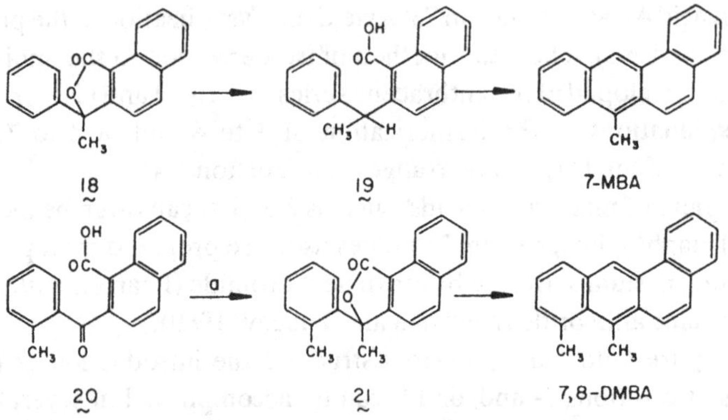

a. CH₃MgX.

moted cyclization occurred when *o*-(naphthylmethyl)benzoic acid was treated with phenyllithium to yield 7-PhBA (Bradsher and Webster, 1958). No other example of such a cyclization has been observed.

The syntheses of 7,12-DMBA types have been accomplished by a wide variety of methods. The reaction of benz[a]anthracene-7,12-dione, BAQ, **22**, with methylmagnesium bromide (or ethylmagnesium bromide) yielded **23** (or **24**). All early attempts to convert **23** to 7,12-DMBA with acid reagents failed (Bachmann and Chemerda, 1938). However, treatment of **23** with acidic methanol for a short time gave the dimethyl ethers **25** and **26**. Subsequent treatment of **25** and **26** with two equivalents of finely powdered sodium (or potassium) afforded 7,12-DMBA and 7,12-DEBA in high yields (Bachmann and Chemerda, 1938), Scheme V. By this method 8,9-DMBAQ was converted into 7,8,9,12-TeMBA (Badger *et al.*, 1940) and 11-MBAQ into 7,11,12-TMBA (Newman, 1983). However, reaction of 7,12-dimethoxy-7,12-dihydro-2,7,12-TMBA with sodium did not yield 2,7,12-TMBA (Defay and Martin, 1955). The anthrone **17**, obtained from **27**, on treatment with methylmagnesium bromide yielded 7,12-DMBA (Newman, 1938a). A number of 7-alkyl-12-MBAs was prepared from **17** (Mikhailov and Chernova, 1938).

Later 7,12-DMBA was synthesized by adding **23** directly to a solution of hydriodic acid in methanol to yield 7-iodomethyl-12-MBA, **28**, which

Scheme Ⅴ. Synthesis of 7,12-DMBAs.

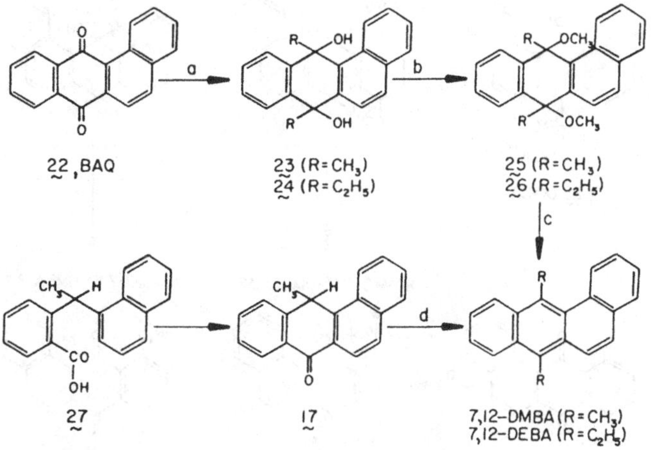

22 ,BAQ   23 (R=CH₃)   25 (R=CH₃)
           24 (R=C₂H₅)   26 (R=C₂H₅)

27   17   7,12-DMBA (R=CH₃)
           7,12-DEBA (R=C₂H₅)

a. RMgX or RLi   b. CH₃OH, trace H₂SO₄
c. Na (or K)   d CH₃MgBr, Δ

was immediately reduced in high yield to 7,12-DMBA by treating with stannous chloride and hydrochloric acid (Sandin and Fieser, 1940). Since the iodomethyl derivatives, **28**, are not too stable, syntheses of 7,12-DMBAs were improved by reacting **23** with dry HCl (instead of HI) to obtain the more stable **29** in high yields (Newman and Sankaran, 1977). Reduction of **29** by SnCl₂-HCl (Sandin and Fieser, 1940), was quantitative. However, when this two-step conversion of **23** to 7,12-DMBA was tried with **30** and **31** only tars resulted (Newman and Kanaka-rajan, 1980). Yet, when **30** and **31** were treated with a solution of SnCl₂ and HCl in ethyl acetate, high yields of 8-MeO-7,12-DMBA, **32**, and 11-MeO-7,12-DMBA, **33**, were produced (Newman and Kanakarajan, 1980). Interestingly, good yields of **30** and **31** could not be obtained by treating 8-MeO-BAQ, **34**, and 11-MeO-BAQ, **36**, with methyl-magnesium iodide or methyllithium. However, when **34** was treated with the methylene reagent formed from trimethylsulphonium iodide (Corey and Chaykovsky, 1965; McCarthy *et al.*, 1978; Newman and Kanakara-jan, 1980), an excellent yield of **35** was obtained. Subsequent reduction with LiAlH₄ led to **30** in high yield. Transformation of **36** into **33** via **31** was accomplished likewise with similar results (Newman and Kanakara-jan, 1980), Scheme VI.

Improvements on the ketoacid route to 7,12-DMBA (Newman, 1938*a*) have been made (Scheme VII). Reduction of the phthalide **37** with 90% formic acid and zinc dust gave **38** in 97% yield (Letsinger *et al.*, 1961). The fact that reduction of a lactone similar to **37** but having methoxy

Scheme VI. Synthesis of 8- and 11- Methoxy-7,12-DMBAs.

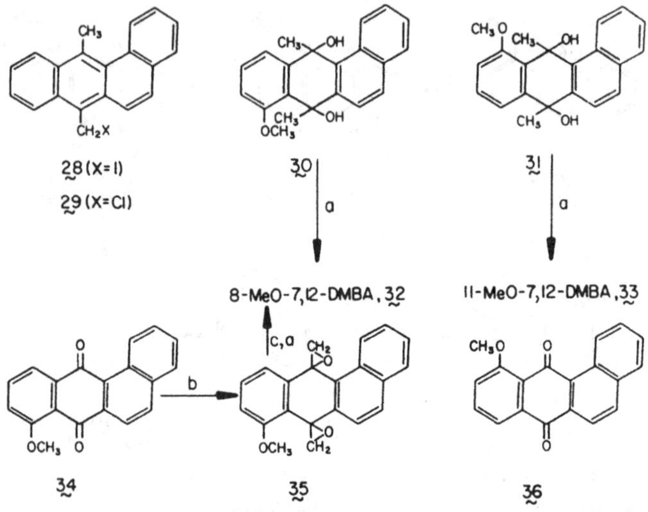

28 (X=I)
29 (X=Cl)

30

31

8-MeO-7,12-DMBA, 32   11-MeO-7,12-DMBA, 33

34   35   36

a. SnCl₂–HCl   b. (CH₃)₃S⁺O I⁻   c. LiAlH₄

Scheme VII. Synthesis of BAs.

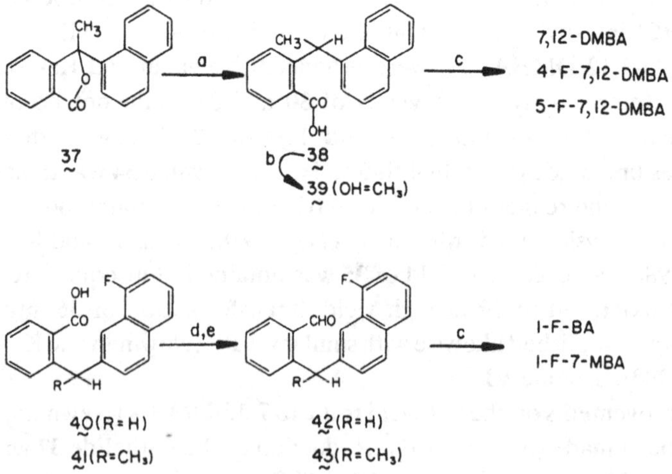

7,12-DMBA
4-F-7,12-DMBA
5-F-7,12-DMBA

37

38
39 (OH=CH₃)

40 (R=H)
41 (R=CH₃)

42 (R=H)
43 (R=CH₃)

1-F-BA
1-F-7-MBA

a. Zn, 90% HCOOH   b. CH₃Li   c. PPA   d. LiAlH₄   e. CrO₃,C₅H₅N

groups in the 3- and 4-positions of the naphthyl moiety went in almost quantitative yield (Newman and Davis, 1967), indicates that the formic acid method of reduction works well with compounds that are often sensitive to acid reagents. Conversion of **38** to the methyl ketone **39** was effected in 75% yield with methyllithium and ring closure to 7,12-DMBA was achieved in 87% yield by heating for 1 h at 95°C with polyphosphoric acid (PPA) (Newman and Naiki, 1962). Similarly 4-F- and 5-F-7,12-DMBAs were made from the appropriate fluorinated intermediates (Newman and Naiki, 1962).

Often in the conversion of acids such as **38** to methyl ketones by treatment with methyllithium the yields were higher if the methyllithium reagent was prepared from methyl iodide rather than methyl bromide (Newman and Cunico, 1972).

In a modification to avoid cyclization of an acid to a benz[a]anthrone followed by reduction and dehydration to a BA compound, the acids **40** and **41** were converted into the aldehydes **42** and **43** by first reducing the acids to primary alcohols with LiAlH$_4$ followed by oxidation with chromic oxide in pyridine at 20°C (Poos *et al.*, 1953). PPA cyclization of the aldehydes gave 1-FBA and 1-F-7-MBA in good overall yields (Newman and Seshadri, 1962). The oxidation of primary alcohols to aldehydes has also been accomplished (Newman *et al.*, 1983), by the N-chlorosuccinimide-dimethyl sulphide reagent (Corey and Kim, 1972). Similar uses of aldehydes were involved in the syntheses of 5-F-6,8-DMBA (Newman *et al.*, 1972), 5-FBA (Newman and Din, 1971), and 5-Br-12-MBA (Newman and Hussain, 1982).

Benz[a]anthrones have been made from acids such as **19** and **27** by treatment with acidic cyclization reagents. The use of anhydrous HF appears to be the best in that anthrones are easily isolated in high yields in the cases of **44**, **46** and **48** shown in Scheme VIII (Fieser and Hershberg, 1939, 1940; Newman and Blum, 1964*a,b*; Newman and Davis, 1967; Pataki and Balick, 1977).

1.2 Organometallic intermediates

Additional ways to convert BA into 7,12-DMBA, shown in Scheme IX, involved reaction of BA with lithium or sodium to yield 7,12-dimetallated derivatives, **50**, which were reacted with methylating agents to yield 7,12-dihydro-7,12-DMBA, **51**. These could then be aromatized to BA compounds (Mikhailov, 1946; Mikhailov and Kozminskaya, 1947; Mikhailov and Blokhina, 1949*a,b*; Mikhailov, 1950). When 7-BrBA, **52**, was treated with butyllithium, 7-lithioBA, **53**, was formed and on reaction with carbon dioxide, methyl iodide, and ethyl iodide,

Scheme VIII. Benzanthrone Route to BA Compounds.

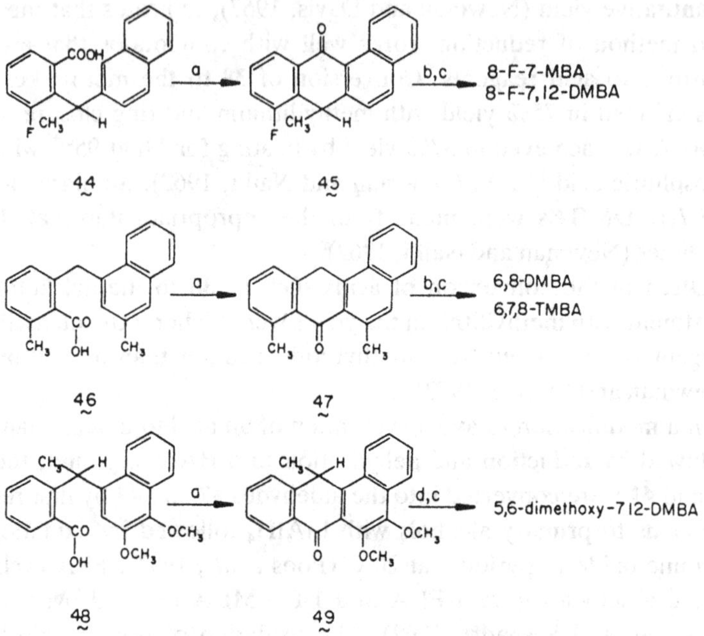

a HF   b. reduction or CH₃MgX   c. dehydration   d. CH₃MgX

Scheme IX. Lithiation of BA.

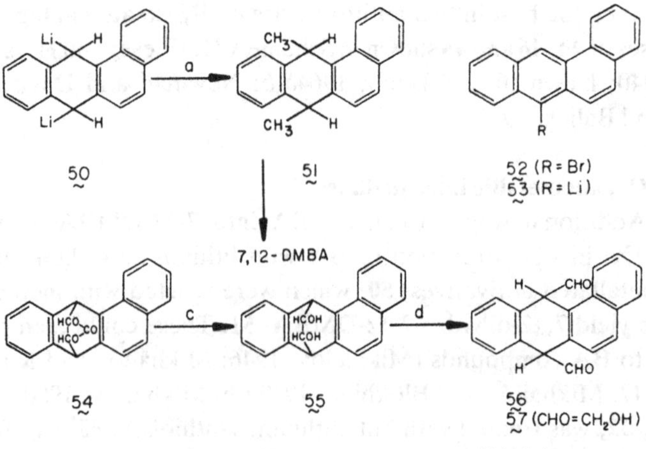

a. (CH₃)₂SO₄   b. aromatization   c. hydrolysis   d. Pb(OAc)₄

7-carboxyBA, 7-MBA and 7-EBA were obtained, respectively (Mikhailov and Kozminskaya, 1948, 1951).

When BA was reacted with vinylene carbonate (Newman and Addor, 1955), a good yield of adduct, **54**, was obtained. Hydrolysis gave the corresponding diol, **55**, which on treatment with lead tetraacetate furnished 7,12-dialdehydo-7,12-DHBA, **56**. Conversion of **56** into 7,12-bishydroxymethyl-7,12-DHBA, **57**, followed by reduction and dehydrogenation yielded 7,12-DMBA. Similarly, 5-FBA was converted into 5-F-7,12-DMBA (Newman and Din, 1971).

In the routes to BA derivatives outlined in Schemes I–VIII, the two carbons which end up in the meso positions of BA come from the two carbonyl groups in the phthalic anhydride or 1,2-naphthalic anhydride. The same is true of another route which starts with phthalaldehydic acid, **58**, or *o*-acetylbenzoic acid, **59**. The synthesis of the acid **48** began with the condensation of **59** with 1,2-dimethoxynaphthalene to yield 3-methyl-3-(3,4-dimethoxy-1-naphthyl)phthalide, **60**, which was then reduced to **48** (Newman and Davis, 1967), Scheme X. Later both **58**

Scheme X. Condensation of Phthalaldehydic and o-Acetylbenzoic Acids.

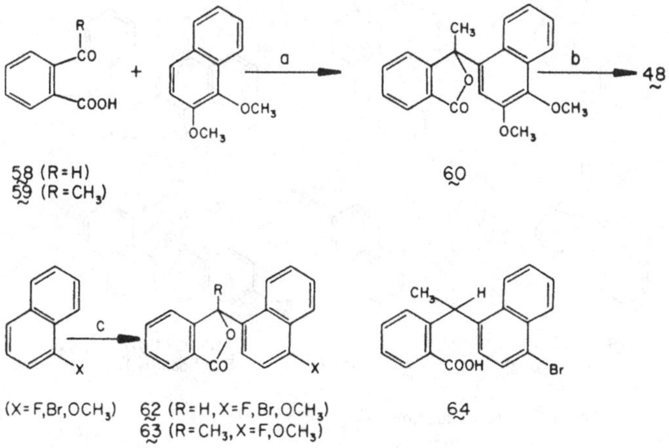
R
CO
COOH
+
OCH3
OCH3
a
CH3
O
CO
b
48
58 (R=H)
59 (R=CH3)
60
c
X
R
61 (X=F,Br,OCH3)
62 (R=H,X=F,Br,OCH3)
63 (R=CH3,X=F,OCH3)
CH3
H
COOH
Br
64

a. 90% CH_3SO_3H b. Zn, 90% HCOOH c 100% CH_3SO_3H ± sulfolane

and **59** were condensed with naphthalene and 1-substituted naphthalenes, **61**, to yield the substituted phthalides, **62**, **63** (Newman *et al.*, 1975). None of the expected phthalide was obtained when **59** was reacted with **61** (X = Br). However, the desired bromoacid, **64**, was made in high yield by bromination of **38** (Scheme VII) (Newman and Cunico, 1972).

The use of *o*-lithiated 2-aryl-4,4-dimethyl-2-oxazolines (Gschwend and Hamdan, 1975; Meyers *et al*., 1974) in BA syntheses has recently been exploited because the intermediates involved are often more easily obtained than the needed intermediates illustrated in Scheme I. For example, the lithiated derivative of **65** was condensed with 2-naphthalde-hyde to yield a product which was hydrolysed to the phthalide **66** (Scheme XI). Reduction of **66** to the corresponding substituted benzoic acid,

Scheme XI. Syntheses via Lithiated 4,4-Dimethyloxazolines.

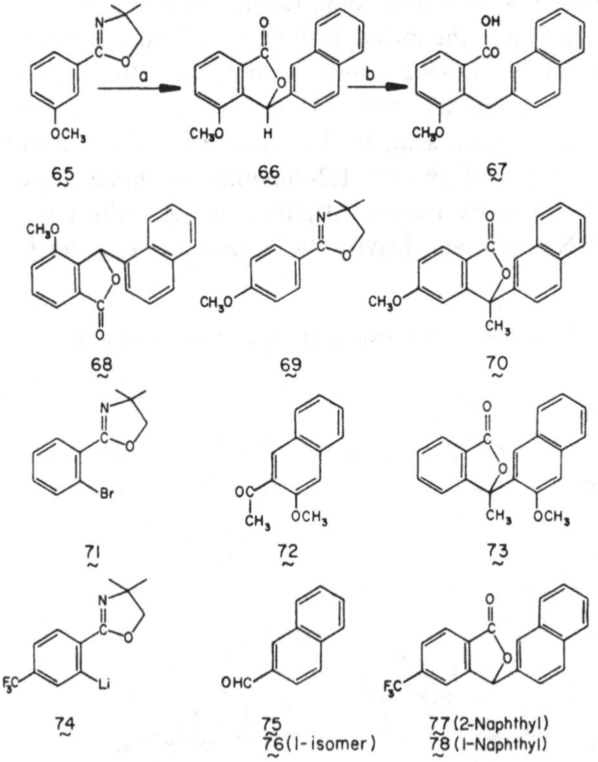

a. RLi   b. reduction

67, followed by cyclization to benzanthrone (not isolated) and oxidation afforded the quinone, **34** (Scheme VI), in high overall yield from **66**. Similarly, the use of 1-naphthaldehyde in this sequence yielded **36** (Scheme VI) via **68**. Both **34** and **36** were transformed into 8-MeO-7,12-DMBA and 11-MeO-7,12-DMBA as described (Newman and Kanakara-jan, 1980). Lithiated 2-(4-methoxyphenyl)-4,4-dimethyloxazoline, **69**, was condensed with methyl 2-naphthyl ketone to yield the phthalide,

70, which was converted to 9-MeO-7,12-DMBA. Analogous treatment of methyl 1-naphthyl ketone with lithiated **69** afforded 10-MeO-7,12-DMBA (Newman and Kumar, 1978).

The Grignard reagent formed from 2-(2-bromophenyl)-4,4-dimethyloxazoline, **71** (Meyers *et al.*, 1974), was condensed with methyl 3-methoxy-2-naphthyl ketone, **72**, to give the lactone **73**, which provided 6-MeO-7,12-DMBA via 6-MeO-BAQ (Newman *et al.*, 1978*b*, see also Sheikh *et al.*, 1982). Likewise, condensation of lithiated (2-phenyl)-4,4-dimethyloxazoline with 7-bromo-1-naphthaldehyde and 6-bromo-1-naphthaldehyde yielded 2-BrBAQ and 3-BrBAQ, respectively. These quinones were converted into the 7,12-dimethyl-7,12-diols, similar to **23**, which were treated with the HCl-SnCl$_2$ reagent (Newman and Kanakarajan, 1980), to obtain 2-Br-7,12-DMBA and 3-Br-7,12-DMBA, respectively (Newman *et al.*, 1983). In similar ways, lithiated 2-(4-trifluoromethylphenyl)-4,4-dimethyloxazoline, **74**, reacted with 2-naphthaldehyde, **75**, and 1-napthaldehyde, **76**, to give the lactones **77** and **78**, which then afforded 9-CF$_3$-7,12-DMBA and 10-CF$_3$-7,12-DMBA, respectively (Newman and Veeraraghavan, 1983).

Although lithiated N,N-diethylbenzamides and N,N-diethylnaphthamides undergo similar condensations with the appropriate carbonyl derivatives to yield BA compounds (Watanabe and Snieckus, 1980; Doadt *et al.*, 1982; Jacobs and Harvey, 1981; Harvey *et al.*, 1982), lithiation of naphthyloxazolines results in addition of alkyllithium to furnish 1,2-dihydronaphthyloxazolines (Barner and Meyers, 1984).

1.3 The Elbs reaction

Perhaps the simplest route to benz[a]anthracenes and other PAH involves the Elbs reaction (Elbs and Larsen, 1884). Reaction of benzoyl chloride with *p*-xylene yielded 2,5-dimethylbenzophenone, **79**, which on heating for two days at its boiling point, 303°C, gave a small yield of 2-methylanthracene, **80** (Scheme XII). This route was first used in the BA series to prepare 9-PhBA from **81** (Cook, 1930). Later, 2-, 3-, and 9-MBAs as well as 5-i-PBA and 2,9-, 2,10-, 3,9-, and 3,10-DMBAs and 7-arylBAs were obtained by this route (Cook, 1932; Vingiello and Thornton, 1966). In general, the yields are low in the Elbs reaction and the purification tedious but the starting ketones are readily made.

3-Methylcholanthrene, **83**, was synthesized in 49% yield by pyrolysis of 4-methyl-7-(1-naphthoyl)hydrindene, **82** (Fieser and Seligman, 1936). In a similar way, heating fluorinated derivatives of **82** at 405–410°C gave

Scheme XII. The Elbs Reaction.

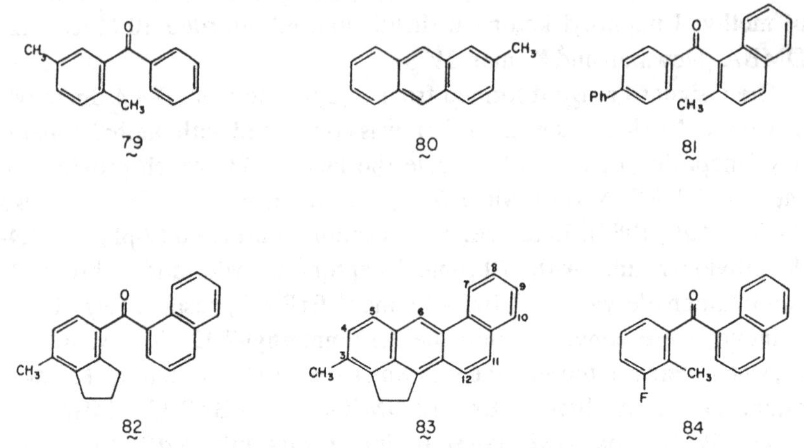

79   80   81

82   83   84

8-fluoro-3-methylcholanthrene and 10-fluoro-3-methylcholanthrene in fair yields, but attempts to prepare the 11-fluoro- and 12-fluoro-3-methyl-cholanthrenes failed (Newman and Khanna, 1980). The loss of a fluorine atom when *para* to the ketonic function has also been noted (Bergmann and Blum, 1960). If the fluorine is *meta* to the ketonic function it may or may not be lost in the Elbs reaction (Bergmann and Blum, 1961).

The Elbs procedure was successful when applied to the preparation of 8-methoxy-3-methylcholanthrene (Fieser and Desreux, 1938), and 9-methoxy-3-methylcholanthrene (Cook and deWorms, 1939), whereas it failed on attempted synthesis of 10- and 11-methoxy derivatives (Newman and Khanna, 1980). The pyrolysis of 1-(2-methyl-3-fluorobenzoyl) naphthalene, **84** at 405–410°C did not give 8-FBA (Newman and Wiseman, 1961), yet when the pyrolysis was carried out at 365–385°C a fair yield of 8-FBA was obtained (Newman and Blum, 1964a). The synthesis of 7-PhBA and 12-PhBA (Vingiello *et al.*, 1958; Vingiello and Thornton, 1966), as well as that of deuterated BAs (Buu-Hoi and Lavit, 1960), by an Elbs reaction has been reported.

1.4   BAQs and the Hayashi rearrangement

The importance of BAQs in the synthesis of 7,12-DMBAs has been illustrated in Schemes V and VI. BAQs have been prepared from ketoacids such as **3, 4, 7** and **8** (Scheme I) under quite a few acidic conditions.

A study (Groggins and Newton, 1930), showed that sulphuric acid is very useful for the formation of BAQ from 2-(1-naphthoyl)benzoic acid, **3** (R = H), (see also Fieser, 1933; Fieser and Fieser, 1933; Ahmed *et al.*, 1975; Marschalk and Dassigny, 1948, 1952; Weizmann and Bergmann, 1936). Polyphosphoric acid, PPA, although quite viscous, is another useful reagent for cyclization (Snyder and Werber, 1950). A mixture of sodium chloride and aluminium chloride has also been used, but side products are formed in small quantities with this reagent (Fieser and Peters, 1932). Cyclization has also been effected by heating a mixture of ketoacid and benzoyl chloride with a small amount of sulphuric acid (Badger and Cook, 1939; Martin, 1943). Attempted cyclization of *o*-(4-fluoro-1-naphthoyl)benzoic acid with benzoyl chloride and sulphuric acid, however, resulted in an unusual halogen exchange to afford 5-chloro-7,12-BAQ (Bergmann *et al.*, 1961). Treatment of 1-(1-naphthoyl)-2-naphthoic acid (an unhindered acid) with phosphorus pentoxide in nitrobenzene at 150°C yielded 7,14-dibenzo[a,h]anthraquinone, a result which undoubtedly involves a Hayashi rearrangement to 2-(1-naphthoyl)-1-naphthoic acid (a hindered acid) before ring closure to the quinone (Cook, 1932).

The Hayashi rearrangement is quite general. Hayashi discovered this rearrangement on treating 2-(5-chloro-2-hydroxybenzoyl)-3-methylbenzoic acid, **85**, and 2-(5-chloro-2-hydroxybenzoyl)-6-methylbenzoic acid, **86**, with concentrated sulphuric acid. Surprisingly, mainly 4-chloro-1-hydroxy-5-methylanthraquinone, **87**, was produced. Thus, quinone formation must have been preceded by rearrangement of **85** to **86**, the hindered acid. The spirocyclic intermediate **88** was suggested (Hayashi, 1927), as being involved in the rearrangement, Scheme XIII.

Later work in this area (Hayashi, 1930*a,b,c*; Hayashi *et al.*, 1936), gave more examples but many were beclouded because of uncertainty as to the structures of the ketoacids used, most of which had a hydroxy group *ortho* to the ketonic function. However, some work with 2-benzoyl-3-methylbenzoic acid, **89**, and 2-benzoyl-6-methylbenzoic acid, **90**, in sulphuric acid showed that the adjacent hydroxy group was not necessary for the rearrangement of **89** to **90** to occur (Hayashi and Turuoka, 1935; Cook, 1932), but no alternative to structure of type **88** was formulated. The structures postulated for **89** and **90** were later confirmed (Newman and McCleary, 1941*b*). When either **91** or **92**, prepared by condensation of 4-methylphthalic anhydride with naphthalene followed by separation into pure isomers (Rivett *et al.*, 1949), was treated with sulphuric acid a mixture of 9-MBAQ and 10-MBAQ was obtained. Hence the spirocyclic cation, **93**, involved in interconversion has no preference in cleavage of bonds a or b to an acyclic cation and a mixture of quinones results (Scheme XIV). It is noteworthy that no spirocyclic

Scheme XIII. The Hayashi Rearrangement.

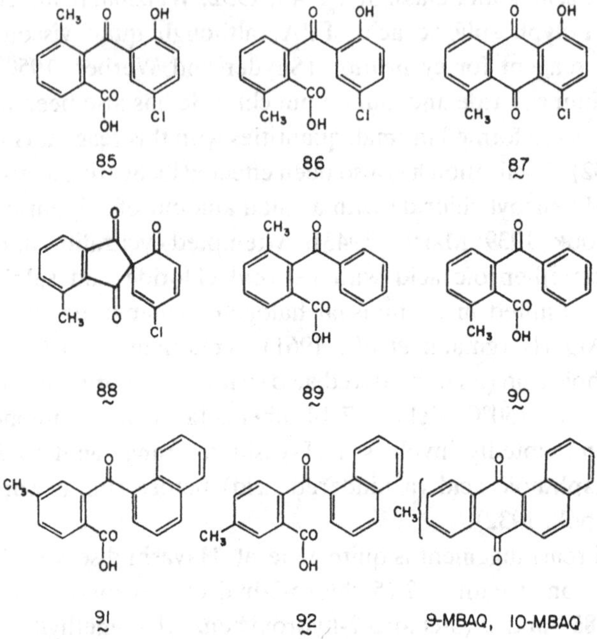

85   86   87

88   89   90

91   92   9-MBAQ, 10-MBAQ

intermediate, **88**, or cation, **93**, can be the immediate precursor to a quinone because the atom adjacent to the spiro carbon cannot approach within bond-forming distance to either of the carbonyl carbons regardless of the appearance of such spirocyclic species. Hence opening to an acyclic cation, as shown in Scheme XIV, must occur before ring closure to a quinone can take place. The acyclic cations are in equilibrium with the lactonic-type cations shown (Newman and McCleary, 1941*a,b*).

The conversion of an unhindered ketoacid, **8** (R = Cl), to a hindered ketoacid, **7** (R = Cl), by heating with concentrated sulphuric acid at a temperature lower than that needed to produce 10-ClBAQ has been noted (Newman *et al.*, 1986). Wood and Fieser (1951) deal with the case when R = Br. Conversely the conversion of a hindered ketoacid, **3**, to an unhindered ketoacid, **4**, by heating with 80% sulphuric acid has also been accomplished (Newman, 1983; Cristol and Caspar, 1968). Such interconversions undoubtedly take place through the spirocyclic cations, **94** and **95**. When heated in concentrated sulphuric acid to temperatures high enough to form a BAQ the **7, 8** mixture (R = Cl, Scheme I) yields mainly **96**, via the cation that is preferentially formed by breaking bond a in **94**. The **3, 4** mixture (R = CH₃, Scheme I) yields mainly **98** via the preferential breaking of bond b in **95** to form the open-chain

Scheme XIV. Cationic Intermediates.

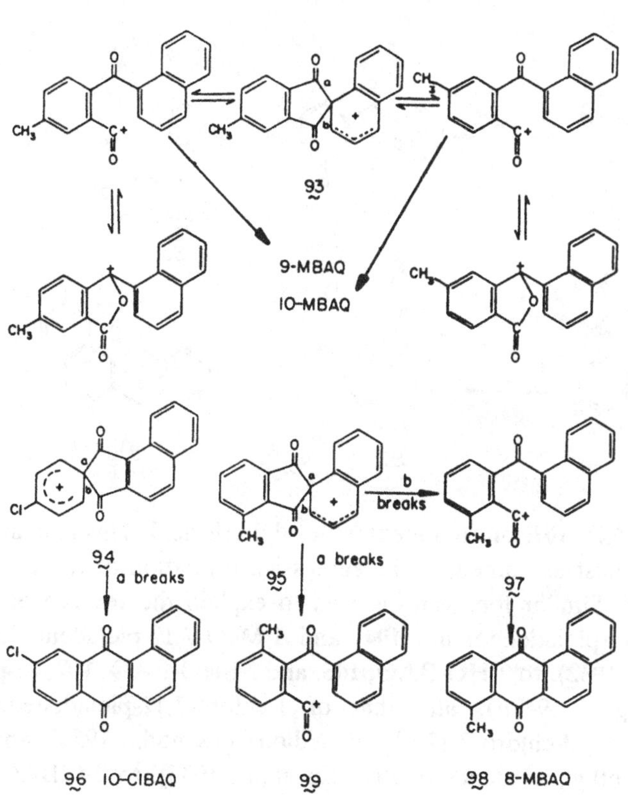

93

9-MBAQ
IO-MBAQ

94
a breaks

95
a breaks

b
breaks

97

96 IO-CIBAQ

99

98 8-MBAQ

cation, **97**, which must be the immediate precursor of **98**. In each case the open-chain cation stemming from the hindered acid is formed preferentially and closes to the BAQs noted. As yet there is no adequate explanation of the fact that the **3**, **4** mixture yields mainly the acyclic cation **97** when heated in concentrated sulphuric acid to form **98** whereas when 80% sulphuric acid is used cation **99** is preferred as demonstrated by the isolation of the ketoacid **4** (Newman, 1983). The most complete study of the species involved in the Hayashi rearrangement has been made on a number of substituted nitro-2-thienoylbenzoic acids (Newman and Ihrman, 1958), but since these acids are not involved in BA synthesis no further discussion will be given.

A Hayashi-type rearrangement may be the best explanation of the rearrangement of 7,12-pleiadenediones to BAQs. One such example is shown in Scheme XV. The condensation of phthalic anhydride with 2,6-dimethylnaphthalene yielded 1,5-dimethyl-7,12-pleiadenedione, **100** (Fieser and Peters, 1932; Fieser and Fieser, 1933), which rearranged

18   *Chemistry*

Scheme XV Synthesis of 7,12-BAQs from 7,12-Pleiadenediones

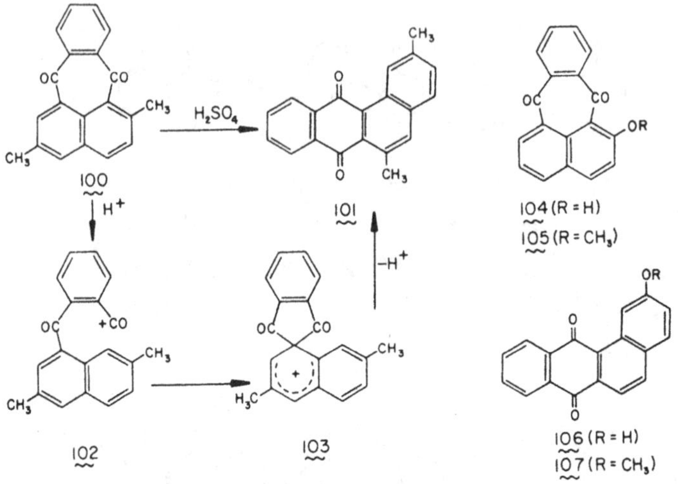

to 2,6-DMBAQ, **101**, on treatment with sulphuric acid. This rearrangement seems best explained by the successive formation of the cations **102** and **103**. Similar ions can be used to explain the rearrangement of 1-HO-7,12-pleiadenedione, **104**, and 1-MeO-7,12-pleiadenedione, **105** (Knapp, 1932), to 2-HO-BAQ, **106**, and 2-MeO-BAQ, **107**, respectively (Badger, 1947*b*), and that of 1-chloro-7,12-pleiadenedione (Badger, 1948), 3-chloro-7,12-pleiadenedione (Tsunoda, 1953), and 1-hydroxy-5-methylpleiadenedione (Fieser *et al.*, 1936), to 2-ClBAQ, 4-ClBAQ, and 2-HO-6-MBAQ, respectively.

Finally, it should be emphasized that to avoid the Hayashi rearrangement, ketoacids capable of undergoing the rearrangement, such as **4**, **7** and **8**, should have the keto group reduced to a methylene group. Such reduced acids are cyclized to benzanthrones without rearrangement and the latter can be oxidized to BAQs in high yield. This approach has been used by numerous investigators, e.g. Cook (1932).

1.5   Chemical reactivity of BA

It has long been known that the 7-position of BA is very susceptible to attack by electrophilic reagents. For example, the following compounds not containing an added carbon have been obtained from BA: Br (Badger and Cook, 1940; Mikhailov and Kozminskaya, 1948, 1951; Newman and Hussain, 1982); Cl (Muller and Hanke, 1949); F (Newman and Lilje, 1979; O'Malley *et al.*, 1981); NO_2 (Fieser and Hershberg, 1938); NH_2 and NCO (Fieser and Creech, 1939); SH (Wood and Fieser, 1940). Treatment of BA with osmium tetroxide yields 5,6-dihydroxy-5,6-

DHBA (Cook and Schoental, 1948). Other 5,6-dihydroxy-5,6-DHBAs have been prepared similarly (Hadler and Kryger, 1960; Tada and Takitani, 1961; Newman and Blum, 1964c; Newman and Davis, 1967). The introduction of fluorine at the meso carbons of BA has been difficult. Small amounts of 7-FBA and 7,12-diFBA have been obtained from BA either by electrophilic fluorination (O'Malley *et al.*, 1981), or by reaction with xenon fluoride (Agranat *et al.*, 1977). Reduction of 7-nitroBA, prepared from BA by an improved method, furnished 7-aminoBA. Only when 7-aminoBA was diazotized by successive treatments with nitric oxide and nitrogen dioxide (Rigaudy *et al.*, 1969), could a 7-diazoniumBA tetrafluoroborate be obtained which would yield 7-FBA on pyrolysis (Newman and Lilje, 1979). When 5,6-epoxy-7,12-DMBA was treated with sodium azide and the resulting azido alcohols were reacted with tributylphosphine, 5,6-imino-7,12-DMBA was produced (Blum *et al.*, 1979). Similar treatment of 5,6-epoxyBA yielded the 5,6-imine of BA (Weitzberg *et al.*, 1980). The synthesis of 12-F-7-MBA and 7-F-12-MBA by reaction of 7,12-dihydroxy-7,12-dihydro-7-MBA and 7,12-dihydroxy-7,12-dihydro-12-MBA with diethylaminosulphurtrifluoride (DAST), (Middleton, 1975), has been described (Newman and Khanna, 1979). Treatment of 5-MeO-7,12-DMBA with CF_3OF yielded 5,6-dihydro-6-F-5-keto-7,12-DMBA (Patrick *et al.*, 1976).

On reduction of BA with lithium in liquid ammonia 7,12-DHBA and 1,4,7,12-TeHBA as well as hexahydro- and dodecahydroBAs have been obtained (Harvey and Urberg, 1968). Addition of sodium, potassium or lithium occurs at the 7,12-positions in BAs and treatment of these derivatives with proton sources yields 7,12-DHBAs (Bachmann, 1936; Bachmann and Pence, 1937). When the dimetallic intermediates are reacted with alkylating agents, alkylated BAs result (Mikhailov, 1946; Mikhailov and Kozminskaya, 1947; Mikhailov and Blokhina, 1949a,b; Mikhailov, 1950; Lee and Harvey, 1979). When sodium in i-amyl alcohol was the reducing agent 1,2,3,4,7,12-hexahydroBA was obtained (Harvey and Urberg, 1968). Both *cis*- and *trans*-7,12-dihydroDMBAs have been isolated (Mikhailov, 1946; Harvey and Arzadon, 1969; Harvey *et al.*, 1969) when metals were used as reducing agents. Catalytic reduction of BA under several conditions led to a variety of reduced compounds (Fu *et al.*, 1980). The basicities of all of the MBAs towards HF and CF_3CO_2D have been measured and discussed by Mackor *et al.* (1956) and by Dallinga *et al.* (1958).

As far as carbon-containing reactants, the condensation of BA with formaldehyde, or chlorodimethyl ether, in acetic and hydrochloric acids yielded 7-chloromethylBA (Badger and Cook, 1939; Sangaiah *et al.*,

1983). Condensation of N-methylformanilide with BA and 11-MBA afforded 7-aldehydoBA (Fieser and Hartwell, 1938), and 7-aldehydo-11-MBA (Fieser and Johnson, 1939b), respectively. With oxalyl chloride, 7-carboxyBA was obtained (Dansi, 1937; Badger and Gibb, 1949; Hauptmann and Hartig, 1963). With acetyl chloride a small yield of 7-acetylBA (Cook and Hewett, 1933), and with stearoyl chloride 7-stearoylBA (Kloetzel et al., 1961) have been reported.

Treatment of BA, 7-MBA and 12-MBA and other alkylated BAs with oxygen in the presence of light affords 7,12-epidioxyBA, 7,12-epidioxy-7-MBA and 7,12-epidioxy-12-MBA (Cook and Martin, 1940; Wood et al., 1979), as well as other epidioxy compounds. The photochemical and thermal decomposition of 7,12-epidioxyDMBA has been studied (Lopp and Gubergrits, 1981). Other reagents which add across the 7,12-positions are maleic anhydride (Clar, 1932; Bachmann and Chemerda, 1938; Jones et al., 1948), and vinylene carbonate (Newman and Addor, 1955). The vinylene carbonate adducts allowed for the conversion of BA and 5-FBA to 7,12-DMBA and 5-F-7,12-DMBA, respectively, in high yield, see Scheme IX (Newman and Din, 1971). BAQs have been obtained from BAs and benz[a]anthrones by a variety of oxidizing agents. For example, chromic acid oxidation of 5,6-dihydroxy-5,6-DHBA and 5,6-dihydro-5,6-dihydroxy-7,12-DMBA yielded 5,6-diketoBA (Collins et al., 1951) and 5,6-diketo-7,12-DMBA (Newman and Davis, 1967), respectively. By the use of Fremy's salt, 1-hydroxy- and 3-hydroxy-7,12-DMBAs yielded 1,4-BAQ and 3,4-BAQ (Newman et al., 1979a; Sukumaran and Harvey, 1980).

The synthesis of a large number of BAQs by conventional routes has been carried out but will not be discussed in detail, because in the following references none were converted into BAs (Baddar et al., 1959; Johnson et al., 1932; Krohn and Baltus, 1982; Larner and Peters, 1952; Manning, 1981; Manning et al., 1977, 1979; Manning and Wilbur, 1980; Matsuoka et al., 1973; Scholl and Neuberger, 1912; Scholl et al., 1921; Scholl and Tritsch, 1911; Sempronj, 1939; Tada et al., 1968; Tanaka, 1935; Tanaka and Morikawa, 1930; Tsunoda, 1951a,b, 1952, 1953, 1954, 1956; Waldmann, 1931; Waldmann and Steskal, 1930).

2

Synthetic routes from anthracenes (A-ring formation)

2.1 Friedel–Crafts reactions

The Friedel–Crafts condensation of anthracene with succinic anhydride in nitrobenzene afforded γ-(2-anthryl)-γ-ketobutyric acid, **108**, in 18% yield (Cook and Robinson, 1938). Clemmensen reduction to γ-(2-anthryl)butyric acid, **109**, followed by ring closure of the acid chloride with stannic chloride yielded 1-keto-1,2,3,4-tetrahydroBA, **110**, an important intermediate for other BA syntheses, Scheme XVI. Reaction of **110** with methylmagnesium iodide followed by dehydration of

Scheme XVI. Friedel–Crafts Condensations of Anthracene.

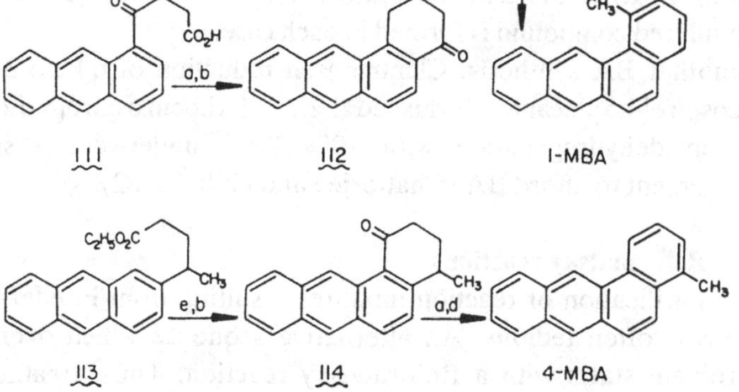

a. reduction   b. cyclization   c. CH₃MgX   d. aromatization   e. hydrolysis

the resulting alcohol and aromatization by heating with platinum black furnished 1-MBA. An alternate synthesis of **109**, starting from phthalic anhydride and γ-phenylbutyric acid has been accomplished (Fieser and Heymann, 1941).

If the condensation of anthracene with succinic anhydride was carried out in methylene chloride the main product was γ-(1-anthryl)-γ-keto-butyric acid, **111** (Schoental, 1952). Reduction to γ-(1-anthryl)butyric acid followed by ring closure of the acid chloride yielded 4-keto-1,2,3,4-tetrahydroBA, **112**, aromatization of which with palladium black led to 4-hydroxyBA in unstated yield.

Friedel–Crafts condensation of anthracene with ethyl allylacetate produced ethyl 4-(2-anthryl)pentanoate, **113**, in 50% yield (Mukherji and Dabas, 1971*a*). By conventional methods **113** was converted into 1-keto-4-methyl-1,2,3,4-tetrahydroBA, **114**, in 72% yield. Clemmensen reduction of **114** and aromatization of the resulting THBA gave 4-MBA in 71% yield.

2.2   Rearrangement of spiro compounds

By alkylation of 1-keto-1,2,3,4,5,6,7,8-octahydroanthracene, **115** (Turner, 1954), with 1,4-dibromobutane there was obtained the ketone **116**. On reduction to the alcohol followed by dehydration and aromatization, first with selenium dioxide and then by heating with Pd-C there was formed BA (Christol *et al.*, 1960), Scheme XVII. Similarly, substituted spiranes, **120–122** (Gupta and Chatterjee, 1954; Chatterjee and Chakravorty, 1972; Chatterjee and Bhattacharjee, 1974; Chatterjee and Chakravorty, 1976), have been aromatized by heating with Pt-C to yield 4-MBA, 3,4-DMBA and 4-E-3-MBA, respectively. Interestingly **120** gave only 4-MBA as rearrangement did not form the more sterically hindered 1-MBA. Evidently steric factors play a role in the mechanisms by which 4-MBA, 3,4-DMBA and 4-E-3-MBA are formed since the least-hindered compound is formed in each case.

In another BA synthesis, Clemmensen reduction of 6-keto-2,3:7,8-dibenzospiro[4,5]decane furnished 2,3:7,8-dibenzospiro[4,5]decane which on dehydrogenation with 10% Pd-C underwent a smooth rearrangement to afford BA (Chatterjee and Guha, 1982).

2.3   Reformatsky reactions

Purification of reaction mixtures resulting from Friedel–Crafts reactions is often tedious. An alternative sequence which overcomes this problem starts with a Reformatsky reaction. Thus, treatment of **115** with methyl bromoacetate and methyl α-bromopropionate yielded

Scheme XVII. Spiro Compound Rearrangements and Reformatsky Reactions.

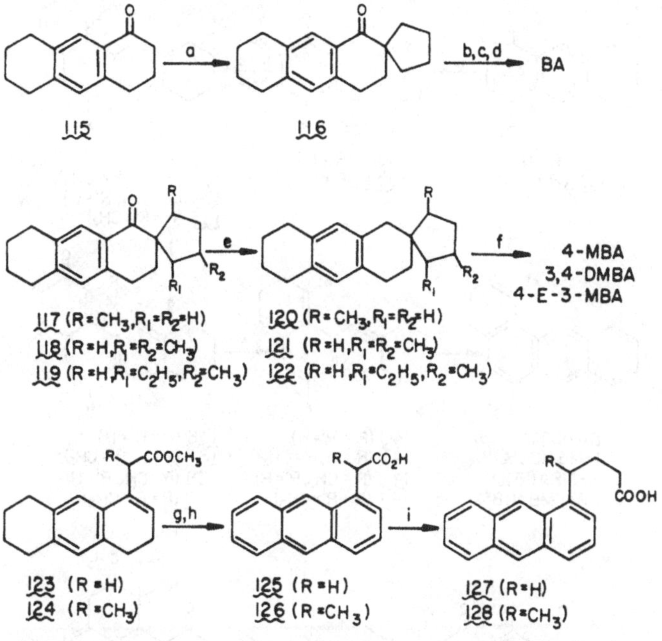
a
b,c,d
BA
115
116
e
f
4-MBA
3,4-DMBA
4-E-3-MBA
117 (R=CH3,R1=R2=H)
118 (R=H,R1=R2=CH3)
119 (R=H,R1=C2H5,R2=CH3)
120 (R=CH3,R1=R2=H)
121 (R=H,R1=R2=CH3)
122 (R=H,R1=C2H5,R2=CH3)
COOCH3
CO2H
COOH
g,h
i
123 (R=H)
124 (R=CH3)
125 (R=H)
126 (R=CH3)
127 (R=H)
128 (R=CH3)

a. $Br(CH_2)_4Br$, base b. reduction to alcohol c. dehydration
d. Δ, Pd-C e. Clemmensen reduction f. Δ, Pt-C
g. Δ in $(C_6H_5)_2O$, Pd-C h. alkaline hydrolysis
i. standard chain lengthening steps

methyl α-(3,4,5,6,7,8-hexahydro-1-anthryl)acetate, **123**, and methyl α-(3,4,5,6,7,8-hexahydro-1-anthryl)propionate, **124**, respectively, after dehydration of the first-formed hydroxyesters (Newman and Otsuka, 1958), Scheme XVII. After conversion to **125** and **126**, conventional chain-lengthening steps produced **127** and **128**. From **127** 4-MBA was prepared via **112**. Cyclization of **128** gave 1-methyl-4-keto-1,2,3,4-THBA (**112** with a methyl group in the 1-position) from which 1-MBA was obtained by reduction to the alcohol, dehydration and aromatization.

2.4 Robinson–Mannich synthesis and Michael reactions

Formylation of **115** and 4-methyl-1-keto-1,2,3,4,5,6,7,8-octahydroanthracene, **129** (Vig *et al.*, 1955), yielded **130** and **131**, respectively, Scheme XVIII. Condensation of **130** and **131** with the Mannich bases 1-N-piperidino-3-butanone methiodide or 1-diethylamino-3-pentanone methiodide led to the diketones, **132–135**, which on cyclization with acetic acid–hydrochloric acid afforded the enones, **136–139**.

Scheme XVIII. BAs via Robinson-Mannich and Michael Reactions.

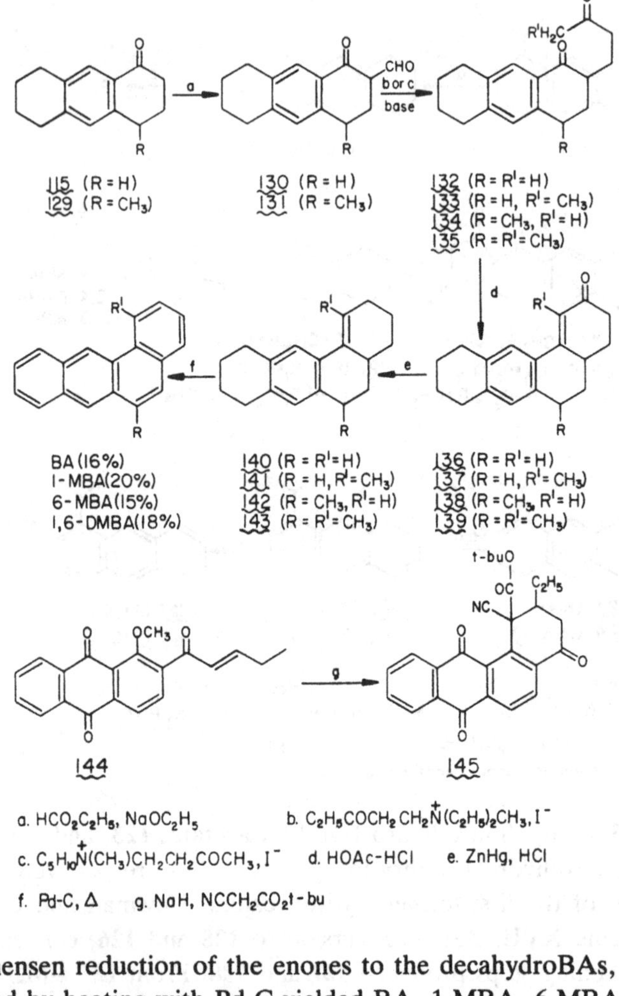

115 (R = H)
129 (R = CH₃)

130 (R = H)
131 (R = CH₃)

132 (R = R¹= H)
133 (R = H, R¹= CH₃)
134 (R = CH₃, R¹= H)
135 (R = R¹= CH₃)

BA (16%)
1- MBA (20%)
6- MBA (15%)
1,6-DMBA (18%)

140 (R = R¹= H)
141 (R = H, R¹= CH₃)
142 (R = CH₃, R¹= H)
143 (R = R¹= CH₃)

136 (R = R¹= H)
137 (R = H, R¹= CH₃)
138 (R = CH₃, R¹= H)
139 (R = R¹= CH₃)

144   145

a. HCO₂C₂H₅, NaOC₂H₅   b. C₂H₅COCH₂CH₂N⁺(C₂H₅)₂CH₃, I⁻

c. C₅H₁₀N⁺(CH₃)CH₂CH₂COCH₃, I⁻   d. HOAc-HCl   e. ZnHg, HCl

f. Pd-C, Δ   g. NaH, NCCH₂CO₂t-bu

Clemmensen reduction of the enones to the decahydroBAs, **140–143**, followed by heating with Pd-C yielded BA, 1-MBA, 6-MBA and 1,6-DMBA, respectively in the indicated overall yields from **115** and **129** (Mukherjee *et al.*, 1966, 1967, 1970*a*,*b*). By using methyl vinyl ketone instead of the Mannich bases above a better yield (33%) of BA has been reported (Buchta and Zoellner, 1968). A novel multistep BAQ synthesis which involved a Michael reaction among many others was effected by the ring closure of **144** to **145** (Ahmed and Cava, 1981).

2.5   Dienone–phenol rearrangement

An alternative BA synthesis, starting from 2-formyl-1-keto-2-methyl-1,2,3,4,5,6,7,8-octahydroanthracene, **146**, is shown in Scheme

XIX. Reaction of **146** with acetone yielded **147** which, on heating with

Scheme **XIX**. Dienone-Phenol Rearrangement.

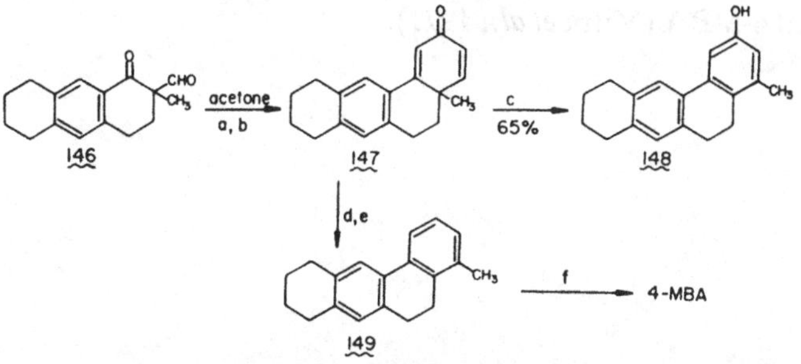

a. piperidine, HOAc   b. KOH, methanol   c. HOAc, HCl, H$_2$O   d. LiAlH$_4$ e. HCl   f. Δ, Pd-C

acetic acid–hydrochloric acid, rearranged to 2-hydroxy-4-methyl-5,6,8,9,10,11-hexahydroBA, **148**. Reduction of **147** to the corresponding alcohol followed by treatment with HCl caused rearrangement to **149** which on aromatization afforded 4-MBA (Mukherji *et al.*, 1970c). The utility of these reactions is limited by the poor yield of **147** from **146**.

2.6   Dieckmann cyclization

On alkylation of diethyl β-ketopimelate with 2-(2-naphthyl) ethyl bromide the ketoester diethyl β-(keto-α-[2-(2-naphthyl)ethyl] pimelate, **150**, was obtained. Ring closure of **150** with cold concentrated sulphuric acid followed by hydrolysis afforded the diacid, **151**. Dieckmann cyclization of the ester of **151** with sodium in benzene led to 4-keto-

Scheme **XX**. Dieckmann Cyclization.

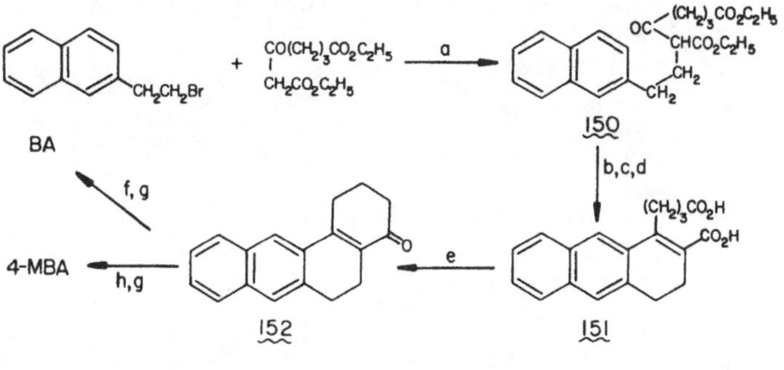

a. KOtbu   b. H$_2$SO$_4$, -10°C   c. KOH, H$_2$O   d. HCl   e. Na, C$_6$H$_6$ on the dimethyl ester, hydrolysis, -CO$_2$ f. LiAlH$_4$ g. Pd-C   h. CH$_3$MgI

1,2,3,4,5,6-hexahydroBA, **152**, Scheme XX. Reaction of **152** with LiAlH₄ followed by aromatization over Pd-C yielded BA. Treatment of **152** with methylmagnesium iodide followed by heating with Pd-C produced 4-MBA (Mitra *et al.*, 1971).

3

Synthetic routes from phenanthrenes (D-ring formation)

3.1 Friedel–Crafts reactions

The four carbons needed to convert phenanthrenes into BAs have been introduced by succinoylation, which takes place at the 3-position of phenanthrene and at the 2-position of 9,10-dihydrophenan threne, Scheme XXI. With succinic anhydride was produced **153** and with α-methylsuccinic anhydride **156** was formed. Reduction, usually by the Clemmensen route afforded the acids, **154** and **157**, which on ring closure yielded the 8-keto-8,9,10,11-tetrahydroBAs **155** (Haworth and Mavin, 1933), and **158** (Cook and Haslewood, 1934), respectively. Although ring closures to ketones **155** and **158** are most often effected by conversion of acids to acid chlorides followed by AlCl$_3$ or SnCl$_4$ promoted cyclizations, the use of trifluoromethanesulphonic acid anhydride (Hulin and Koreeda, 1984), and methanesulphonic acid (Premasagar *et al.*, 1981), for such closures has also been reported. By reduction of **155** and aromatization, BA was obtained. Similarly **158** yielded 9-MBA and by reaction of **158** with methylmagnesium iodide followed by aromatization, 8,9-DMBA was produced. The latter hydrocarbon was of interest in establishing the structure of methylcholanthrene (Cook and Haslewood, 1934). The condensation of succinic anhydride with 3-methylphenanthrene afforded β-[6-(3-methylphenanthroyl)]-propionic acid, **159**, from which 2-MBA was synthesized by conventional steps (Bachmann and Cortes, 1943). Similar reaction of succinic anhydride with 9,10-dihydrophenanthrene yielded β-(9,10-dihydro-2-phenanthroyl)propionic acid, **160**, which was converted into BA by reduction of the keto group, cyclization to 11-keto-5,6,8,9,10,11-hexahydroBA, **161**, further reduction to 5,6,8,9,10,11-hexahydroBA and aromatization by heating with selenium (Burger and Mosettig, 1937). From **161** the syntheses of 11-HOBA, 11-NH$_2$BA, 11-MBA, and

Scheme XXI. Friedel-Crafts Condensations of Phenanthrenes

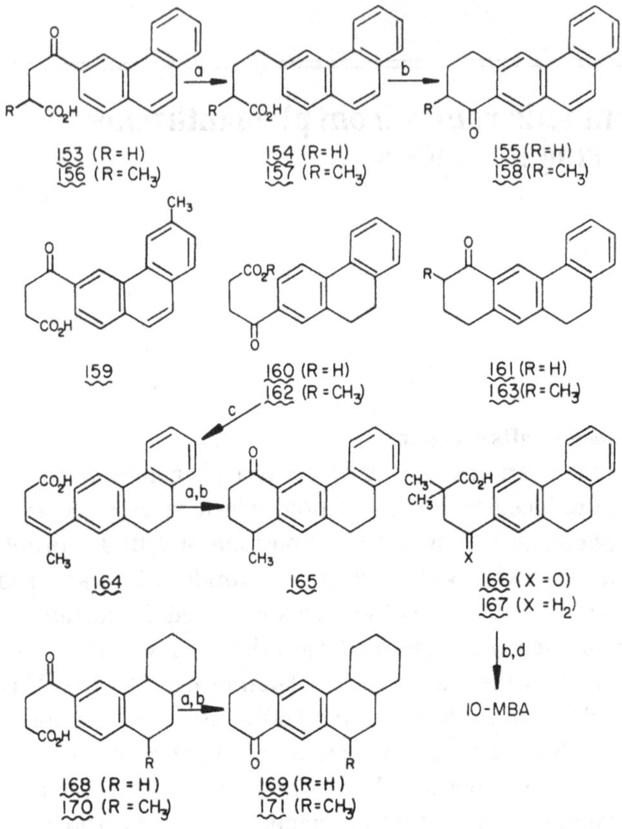

153 (R = H)   154 (R = H)   155 (R = H)
156 (R = CH₃)   157 (R = CH₃)   158 (R = CH₃)

159   160 (R = H)   161 (R = H)
         162 (R = CH₃)   163 (R = CH₃)

164   165   166 (X = O)
                  167 (X = H₂)

168 (R = H)   169 (R = H)
170 (R = CH₃)   171 (R = CH₃)

IO-MBA

a. reduction   b. cyclization   c. CH₃MgI   d. Se, 340°

11-EBA were readily accomplished (Fieser and Johnson, 1939*a,b*). In
this work the earlier synthesis of 11-MBA (Cook and Robinson, 1938),
was questioned because of differences in the melting point of pure 11-
MBA in the two syntheses. Reaction of 11-MBA with N-methylformanilide yielded 7-formyl-11-MBA, which was then converted into
7,11-DMBA (Fieser and Johnson, 1939*b*). In another use of **160** in BA
synthesis, the methyl ester **162** was treated with methylmagnesium iodide
to yield the acid **164**, after hydrolysis (Fieser and Johnson, 1939*a*). From
this acid 8,11-DMBA was obtained via 11-keto-5,6,8,9,10,11-hexahydro-
8-MBA, **165**. Alternatively, **161** was methylated to yield 11-keto-
5,6,8,9,10,11-hexahydro-10-MBA, **163**, from which 10-MBA was readily
synthesized (Bachmann and Chemerda, 1941). When α,α-dimethyl-
succinic anhydride was condensed with 9,10-dihydrophenanthrene the
ketoacid **166** resulted. Wolff–Kishner reduction of **166** gave γ-2-(9,10-

dihydrophenanthryl)-α,α-dimethylbutyric acid, **167**, which was cyclized and heated with selenium at 340°C to yield 10-MBA (Carruthers and Watkins, 1964). Succinoylation of 1,2,3,4,4a,9,10,10a-octahydrophenanthrene afforded β-[6-(1,2,3,4,4a,9,10,10a-octahydrophenanthroyl)]propionic acid, **168**, which was reduced and cyclized to 8-keto-1,2,3,4,4a,4b,5,6,8,9,10,11-dodecahydroBA, **169** (Cook and Haslewood, 1935). Later Mukherji *et al.* (1970*a*), treated 9-methyl-1,2,3,4,4a,9,10,10a-octahydrophenanthrene similarly to obtain **170** and **171**. From the latter, 6-MBA was produced by conventional methods.

If acetyl chloride and propionyl chloride were used instead of succinic anhydride in the above-mentioned Friedel–Crafts reactions, substituted BAs could be obtained by appropriate synthetic extensions. Thus, bromination of 3-propionylphenanthrene, **172**, followed by reaction with sodio diethyl malonate, hydrolysis of the resulting ester and decarboxylation afforded β-(3-phenanthroyl)butyric acid, **173**, Scheme XXII. Reduction

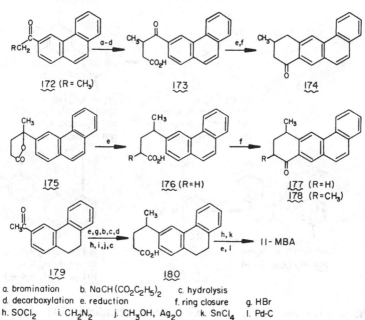

Scheme XXII. Acylation of Phenanthrenes.

a. bromination   b. NaCH(CO$_2$C$_2$H$_5$)$_2$ c. hydrolysis
d. decarboxylation   e. reduction   f. ring closure   g. HBr
h. SOCl$_2$ i. CH$_2$N$_2$ j. CH$_3$OH, Ag$_2$O   k. SnCl$_4$ l. Pd-C

of the keto group and ring closure led to 8-keto-8,9,10,11-tetrahydro-10-MBA, **174**, and from it 10-MBA and 8,10-DMBA were synthesized (Bachmann and Chemerda, 1938). Starting from the condensation product of 3-acetylphenanthrene with diethyl succinate and treatment of the first formed half-ester with hydrobromic acid there was obtained the lactone **175**. The lactone was reduced to γ-(3-phenanthryl)valeric acid, **176**, which was then cyclized to **177**. Methylation of **177** produced **178**. From **178**, 9,11-DMBA and 8,9,11-TMBA were synthesized (Riegel and Burr, 1948). In a similar manner, 2-acetylphenanthrene was converted into 8-MBA (Burr *et al.*, 1950). From 3-acetyl-9,10-dihydro-phenanthrene, **179** (Mosettig and Kamp, 1930), there was obtained γ-(9,10-dihydro-3-phenanthryl)valeric acid, **180** which was converted into 11-MBA (Bachmann and Chemerda, 1941), Scheme XXII.

3.2   1,4-Phenanthraquinone reactions

The phenanthraquinones, **185–188**, were made by reacting the appropriately substituted styrenes, **181–184**, with quinone (Rosen and Weber, 1977). Reaction of **185–188** with 1,3-butadiene yielded BAQ, 2-methoxy-, 3-methoxy- and 4-methoxyBAQs, **189**, **190** and **191**, respectively (Wunderly and Weber, 1978), as shown in Scheme XXIII. When

Scheme XXIII. Diels-Alder Reactions of 1,4-Phenanthraquinones.

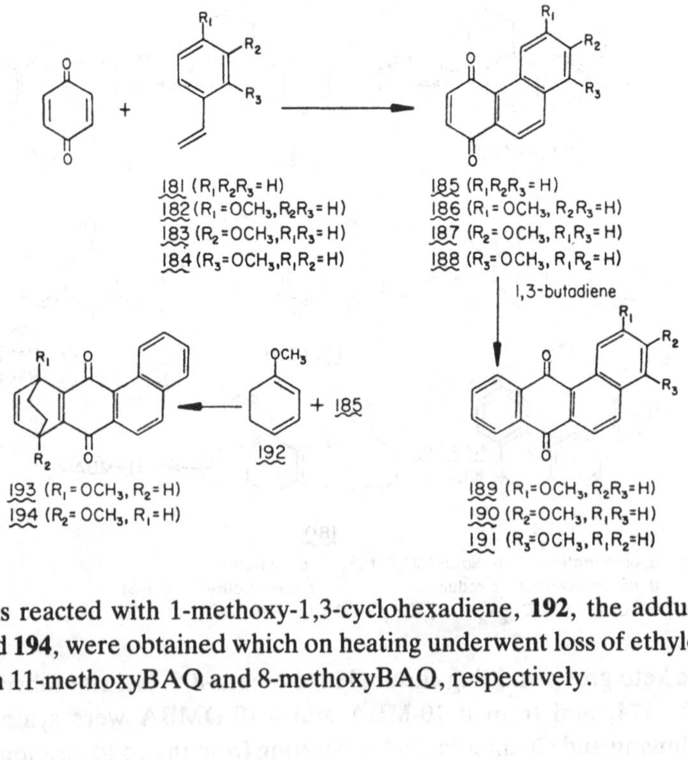

181 ($R_1R_2R_3$ = H)
182 (R_1 = OCH$_3$, R_2R_3 = H)
183 (R_2 = OCH$_3$, R_1R_3 = H)
184 (R_3 = OCH$_3$, R_1R_2 = H)

185 ($R_1R_2R_3$ = H)
186 (R_1 = OCH$_3$, R_2R_3 = H)
187 (R_2 = OCH$_3$, R_1R_3 = H)
188 (R_3 = OCH$_3$, R_1R_2 = H)

1,3-butadiene

193 (R_1 = OCH$_3$, R_2 = H)
194 (R_2 = OCH$_3$, R_1 = H)

189 (R_1 = OCH$_3$, R_2R_3 = H)
190 (R_2 = OCH$_3$, R_1R_3 = H)
191 (R_3 = OCH$_3$, R_1R_2 = H)

185 was reacted with 1-methoxy-1,3-cyclohexadiene, **192**, the adducts, **193** and **194**, were obtained which on heating underwent loss of ethylene to form 11-methoxyBAQ and 8-methoxyBAQ, respectively.

4

Synthetic Diels–Alder routes to rings B and C

4.1 Additions to 1,4-naphthoquinones

1-Vinylcyclohexene, **195**, has been reacted with 1,4-naphthoquinone, **196**, to give 1,2,3,4,6,6a,12a,12b-octahydroBAQ, **197**, in high yield (Backer and Bij, 1943; Azerbaev, 1945), Scheme XXIV. On air oxidation **197** was converted into 1,2,3,4-tetrahydroBAQ, **198** (Fieser and Hershberg, 1937*b*), which was reduced to 1,2,3,4-tetrahydroBA. With the exception of two other examples (Inbasekaran *et al.*, 1980; Carothers and Coffman, 1932), no further work with the use of vinylcyclohexenes in BA synthesis has been reported.

Rather, the addition of styrenes, **199**, to **196**, has been studied and well developed. When the reactions were carried out in refluxing toluene containing chloranil and trichloroacetic acid, the following nine BAQs, **200**, were obtained: 4-Br-, 1-, 2-, 3-, 4-Cl-, 4-F-, 4-methoxy-, 2-methyl-, and 1,4-dimethyl- (Manning *et al.*, 1977). Subsequently, 3,4-dimethoxy-BAQ, **201**, was synthesized (Manning and Wilbur, 1980) by a similar route. When 5-hydroxy-1,4-naphthoquinone, **202**, and 5-methoxy-1,4-naphthoquinone, **203**, were used, mixtures of 8-hydroxy- and 11-hydroxyBAQs, **204** and **206**, and 8-methoxy- and 11-methoxyBAQs, **205** and **207**, resulted (Manning, 1979). By the use of 6-hydroxy- and 6-methoxy-1,4-naphthoquinones, **208** and **209**, there were obtained mixtures of 9-hydroxy- and 10-hydroxyBAQs, **210** and **212**, and 9-methoxy- and 10-methoxyBAQs, **211** and **213**, respectively (Manning, 1979; Manning *et al.*, 1979; Manning, 1981). The conversion of many of the BAQs into BAs and 7,12-DMBAs by conventional methods has been described (Muschik *et al.*, 1979). However, difficulties were encountered in the synthesis of BAs bearing the 1-methoxy group because of steric factors. When α-arylstyrenes were used instead of styrenes the BAQs **214–216** were obtained (Awad *et al.*, 1979; Gates, 1982).

Scheme XXIV. Diels-Alder Reactions of 1,4-Naphthoquinone.

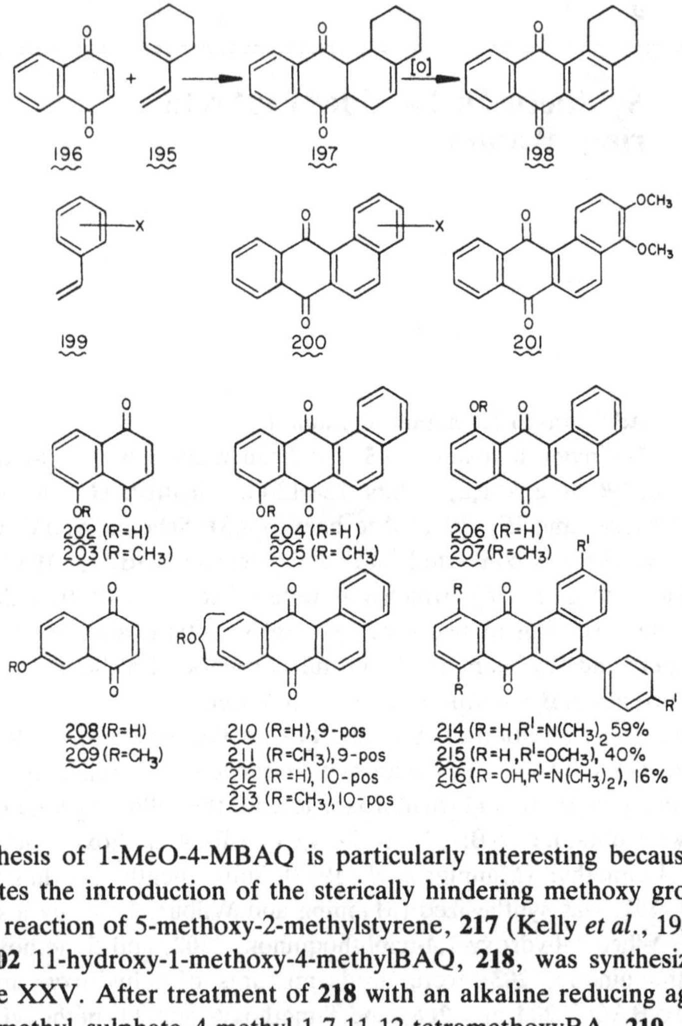

Synthesis of 1-MeO-4-MBAQ is particularly interesting because it illustrates the introduction of the sterically hindering methoxy group. By the reaction of 5-methoxy-2-methylstyrene, **217** (Kelly *et al.*, 1980), with **202** 11-hydroxy-1-methoxy-4-methylBAQ, **218**, was synthesized, Scheme XXV. After treatment of **218** with an alkaline reducing agent and dimethyl sulphate 4-methyl-1,7,11,12-tetramethoxyBA, **219**, was

Scheme XXV. Synthesis of a Polymethoxy BA.

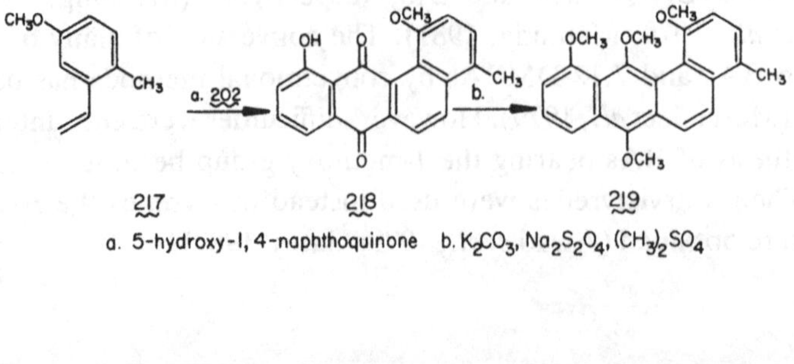

a. 5-hydroxy-1,4-naphthoquinone   b. K_2CO_3, $Na_2S_2O_4$, $(CH_3)_2SO_4$

produced. This compound was useful in determining the structure of the aglycone of chartreusin.

4.2   Route from substituted furans

The condensation of benzyne, formed by reaction of anthranilic acid with i-amyl nitrite, with dimethyl 2-benzyl-3,4-furan dicarboxylate, **220**, gave **221** in unstated yield. Treatment of **221** with PPA at 130–140°C produced **222**, also in unstated yield (Gomes, 1974). If the double bond in **221** was reduced to afford **223** then PPA treatment resulted in the lactone **224**. An improvement in this route was effected by Smith *et al.* (1981) who reacted transient benzyl isobenzofurans, **225–228**, with dimethyl maleate to form the diesters, **223, 229–231**. On subjecting these diesters to the action of PPA **224, 232–234** were obtained in high yields (92%, 78%, 94% and 95%, respectively). If methyl acrylate was used with **225** types instead of dimethyl maleate, a mixture of esters, **235–238** and **239–242**, was produced. Such mixtures contained exo- and endo-forms which did not need separation because on heating with *p*-toluene-sulphonic acid, water was eliminated to afford the B-ring aromatic esters which yielded the corresponding acids, **243–246**, on alkaline hydrolysis. PPA cyclization of these acids led to the 7-AcOBAs, **247–250**. Since the isomeric acids (not shown) formed from **235–238** are not cyclizable, separation could be effected by extraction of the reaction mixture with alkali, Scheme XXVI.

Another route involved the trapping of 1,3-dimethylisobenzofuran, **251** (Fieser and Haddadin, 1965; Priestly and Warrener, 1972), with methyl cinnamates, **252, 253**, to yield the adducts **254, 255** (Levy and Kumar, 1983). After dehydration with *p*-toluenesulphonic acid in benzene the esters, **256, 257**, were obtained. These esters were reduced to primary alcohols by LiAlH$_4$, converted successively to the corresponding chlorides with HCl, into nitriles with NaCN, and into acids, **258, 259**, by hydrolysis with sulphuric acid. Ring closure with HF afforded the ketones, **260, 261**, which were reduced to alcohols. Dehydration of these yielded 7,12-DMBA and 1,7,12-TMBA, respectively, Scheme XXVII.

The reaction of the substituted furans, **262, 263**, with 2-naphthyne afforded the adducts, **264, 265**, in low yields. Reduction of the double bond in **264** followed by acid hydrolysis gave 4-keto-1,2,3,4-tetra-hydroBA, **112**, Scheme XVI. When **263** was reacted with 1,4-dihydro-1,4-epoxynaphthalene (Fieser and Haddadin, 1965), the BA derivative **266** was formed. The approaches from **262** and **263** do not seem promising

Scheme XXVI. Route from 2-Benzylfurans.

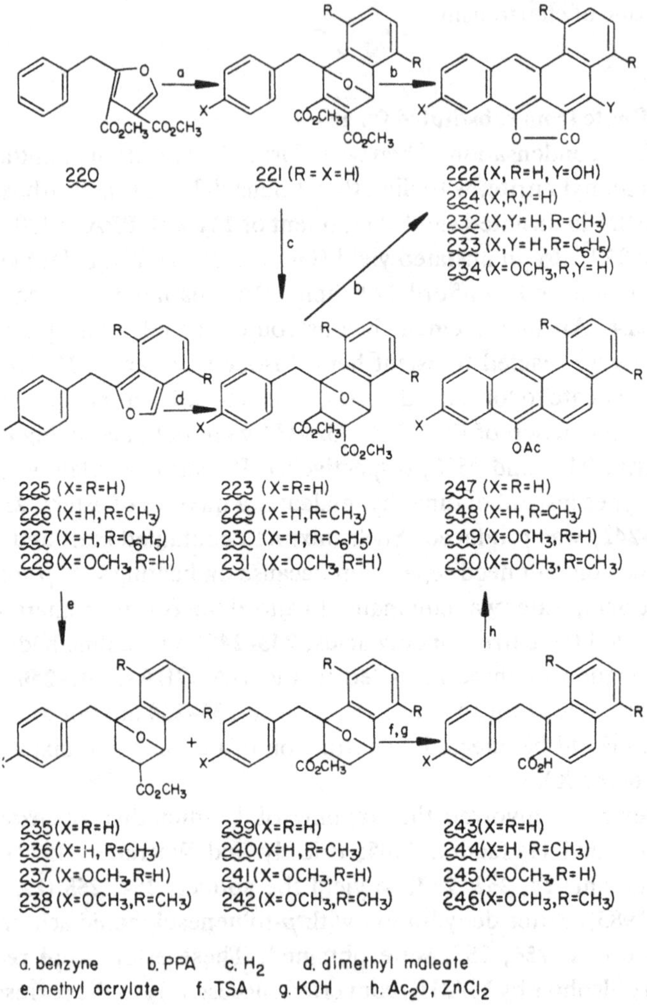

220   221 (R = X = H)   222 (X, R=H, Y=OH)
224 (X,R,Y=H)
232 (X,Y= H, R=CH₃)
233 (X,Y= H, R=C₆H₅)
234 (X=OCH₃,R,Y= H)

225 (X=R=H)   223 (X=R=H)   247 (X=R=H)
226 (X=H,R=CH₃)   229 (X=H,R=CH₃)   248 (X=H, R=CH₃)
227 (X=H, R=C₆H₅)   230 (X=H,R=C₆H₅)   249 (X=OCH₃,R=H)
228 (X=OCH₃ R=H)   231 (X=OCH₃,R=H)   250 (X=OCH₃,R=CH₃)

235 (X=R=H)   239 (X=R=H)   243 (X=R=H)
236 (X=H, R=CH₃)   240 (X=H,R=CH₃)   244 (X=H, R=CH₃)
237 (X=OCH₃,R=H)   241 (X=OCH₃,R=H)   245 (X=OCH₃,R=H)
238 (X=OCH₃,R=CH₃)   242 (X=OCH₃,R=CH₃)   246 (X=OCH₃,R=CH₃)

a. benzyne   b. PPA   c. H_2 d. dimethyl maleate
e. methyl acrylate   f. TSA   g. KOH   h. Ac_2O, $ZnCl_2$

for further development because the starting materials are not readily preparable and the yields are often low (Tochtermann *et al.*, 1978).

4.3   Photochemical cyclizations

Irradiation of 1-fluoro-2-(*o*-iodostyryl)naphthalenes, **267, 268,** prepared by the Wittig–Arbusov reaction of 2-naphthylmethyl bromides with *o*-iodobenzaldehyde, in cyclohexane with sixteen 75-W UV lamps afforded 52% and 11% yields, respectively, of **269** and **270** (Blum *et al.*, 1969), Scheme XXVIII. When one 450-W bulb was used instead of the sixteen lamps the fluorine atom was lost in the irradiation step.

Scheme XXVII. Route Involving Furan Intermediates

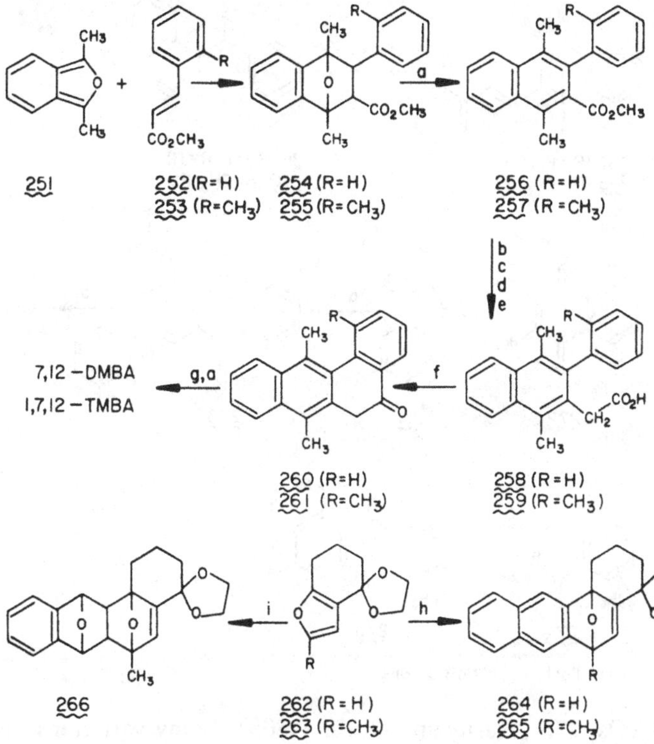

a. TSA b. LiAlH$_4$ c. HCl d. NaCN e. H$_2$SO$_4$, H$_2$O
f. HF g. NaBH$_4$ h. 2-naphthyne i. 1,4-dihydro-1, 4-epoxynaphthalene

If 1-fluoro-2-styrylnaphthalene was irradiated in the presence of iodine, no BA derivative was formed.

A large number of 1,1-diarylethylenes, **271**, has been condensed with 3-bromo-2-methoxy-1,4-naphthoquinone, **272**, to yield 5-aryl-BAQs, **273** (Maruyama and Otsuki, 1975; Maruyama *et al.*, 1976). Use of other 1,4-naphthoquinones containing 2,3-dichloro-, 2,3-dibromo-, and 2,3-diacetoxy- groups gave about the same yields of BAQs (Maruyama *et al.*, 1976). When the two aryl groups in **271** were different, mixtures of isomeric BAQs resulted, the amounts of which were estimated by NMR studies. Often no further work was carried out with the BAQs but in a few cases reduction of the BAQ with sodium borohydride and boron trifluoride produced the corresponding BAs (Maruyama and Otsuki, 1975). Condensation of 1,1-diphenylethylene with 3-bromo-2-methoxy-1,4-naphthoquinones, **274**, containing methoxy groups in the 5-, 6-, 7-, 8-positions and the 6,8-positions yielded the corresponding

36   *Chemistry*

Scheme XXVIII. Photochemical Cyclizations.

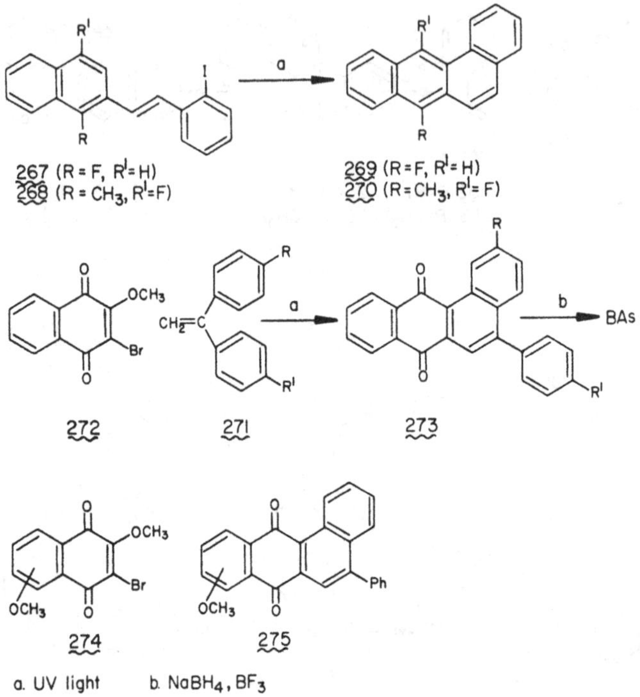

267 (R = F, R¹= H)
268 (R = CH₃, R¹=F)

269 (R = F, R¹= H)
270 (R = CH₃, R¹= F)

272   271   273

274   275

a. UV light   b. NaBH₄, BF₃

5-Ph-BAQs, **275** (Maruyama *et al.*, 1980*b*). Many variations involving the photo-cycloaddition of a variety of symmetrically substituted 1,1-diphenylethylenes, **271**, to **272**, have been reported (Maruyama *et al.*, 1980*a*), Scheme XXVIII. When 1-methyl-1-phenylethylene and 1-cyclohexyl-1-phenylethylene were condensed with **272**, 5-MBAQ and 5-cyclohexylBAQ were formed (Maruyama *et al.*, 1980*a*). However, styrene itself did not undergo the photochemical condensation. Poor yields of BAQs were obtained in attempts to react the *t*-butyldimethylsilyl enol ethers of acetophenone, *p*-methylacetophenone and methyl 2-thienyl ketone with **272**, 2-bromo-3,5-dimethoxy-1,4-naphthoquinone and 2-bromo-3,8-dimethoxy-1,4-naphthoquinone (Maruyama *et al.*, 1981).

5

Miscellaneous synthetic routes

5.1 Diels–Alder reactions and Stobbe condensations

On reaction of *trans*-decahydro-2-keto-naphthalene, **276**, with phenylmagnesium bromide and dehydration of the resulting alcohol there was produced the substituted styrene analogue, **277**. Treatment with maleic anhydride followed by dehydrogenation by heating with sulphur yielded 5,6-dicarboxyBA anhydride, **278** (Szmuszkovicz and Modest, 1950). Heating **278** with barium hydroxide furnished BA. No further work on this route has been published, Scheme XXIX.

Scheme XXIX. Diels–Alder Reactions.

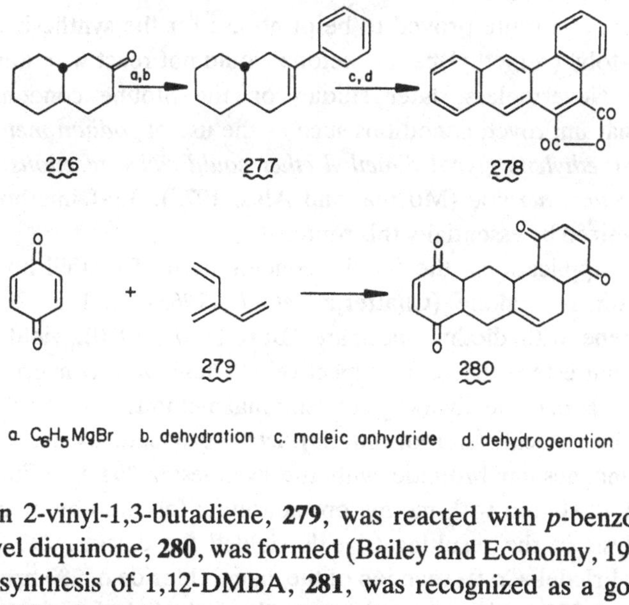

a. C6H5MgBr   b. dehydration   c. maleic anhydride   d. dehydrogenation

When 2-vinyl-1,3-butadiene, **279**, was reacted with *p*-benzoquinone the novel diquinone, **280**, was formed (Bailey and Economy, 1955).

The synthesis of 1,12-DMBA, **281**, was recognized as a goal in the middle 1930s in Fieser's group and elsewhere because of its resemblance to the powerful carcinogen, benzo[a]pyrene, **282**. Early attempts at the preparation of **281** by routes which were successful for the syntheses of 1-MBA and 1,7-DMBA (Fieser and Seligman, 1938) as well as 5,12-DMBA (Fieser and Seligman, 1939), failed mainly because of the large steric effects of the two methyl groups. A later attempt, by Cason and Wordie (1950), also failed as conditions for the cyclization of 1-(o-carboxyphenyl)-1-(8-methyl-1-naphthyl)ethane, **283**, to a benzanthrone could not be found. However, the first successful synthesis of **281** was accomplished (Cason and Phillips, 1952), by the cyclization of **284**, the tetrahydro analogue of **283**, to the benzanthrone **285**. Reduction of **285**, followed by dehydration and dehydrogenation over Pd-C at 330°C yielded **281**, described as 'brilliant yellow crystals which changed at 123.0°C to an opalescent melt which cleared sharply at 131.5–132.0°C', Scheme XXX.

The development of an entirely different route to **281** (Newman and Hart, 1947) commenced with the Stobbe condensation of benzyl phenyl ketone with dimethyl succinate (Hewett, 1942), to yield a mixture of esters which on alkaline hydrolysis, acidification and reduction afforded the diacid **286**. On ring closure with hydrogen fluoride, the diketone **287** was obtained. Reaction of **287** with methylmagnesium bromide, then dehydration and dehydrogenation yielded 5,7-DMBA. By this method 3-M-, 9-M- and 11-MBAs were prepared in relatively large yields (Newman and Gaertner, 1950).

However, this route proved to be of no use for the synthesis of **281** because o-tolyl (α-methyl)benzyl ketone would not react with dimethyl succinate. Nevertheless, later studies on the Stobbe condensation stressed that improved conditions such as the use of *sodium methoxide in refluxing ethylene glycol dimethyl ether could cause reactions which did not occur otherwise* (Morreal and Alks, 1975). 3,9-DimethoxyBA was synthesized by essentially this route.

In other applications, the Stobbe condensation of diethyl homophthalate with 1-tetralone (Chatterjea *et al.*, 1963), and of 2-acetylphenanthrene with diethyl succinate (Burr *et al.*, 1950), yielded the expected half-esters **288**, **289**, respectively. These were converted into **290** and 8-MBA, respectively by conventional methods.

The desired diacids (stereoisomeric), **293**, were made by the reaction of o-tolylmagnesium bromide with the cyanoester **291** to afford **292** which, on alkylation with methyl bromoacetate followed by hydrolysis and pyrolysis of the resulting triacids yielded the diacids, **293**. Intramolecular Friedel–Crafts reaction of the diacid chloride of **293** produced the diketone **294**, which was reduced to the dialcohol, dehydrated and

Scheme XXX. Synthesis of I, I2-DMBA and Stobbe Condensations.

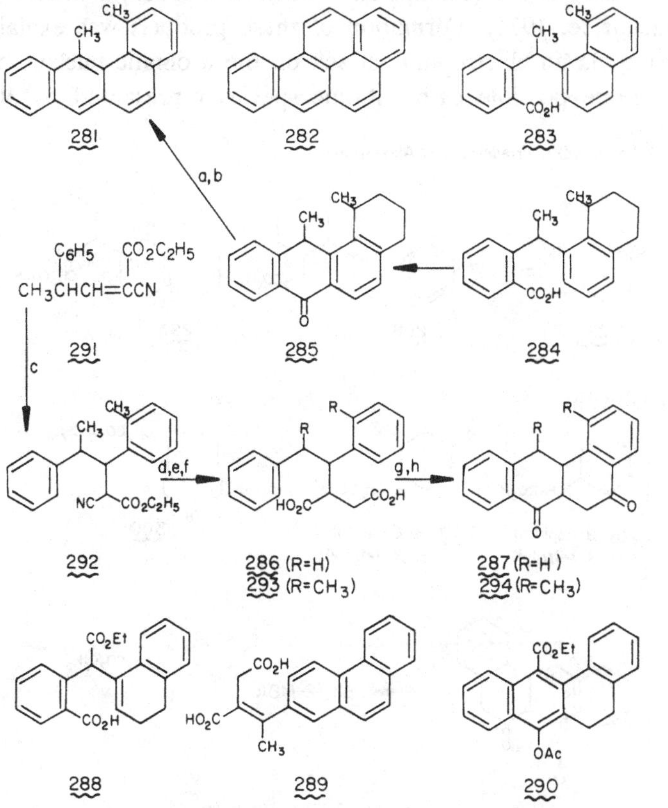

281   282   283

a, b

C_6H_5 $CO_2C_2H_5$
$CH_3CHCH{=}CCN$

291   285   284

c

292   286 (R=H)   287 (R=H)
      293 (R=CH$_3$)   294 (R=CH$_3$)

288   289   290

a. reduction   b. Δ, Pd-C, 330°   c. o-$CH_3C_6H_4MgBr$ d. $BrCH_2CO_2CH_3$, base
e. NaOH, H_2O f. HCl, Δ g. PCl_5 h. $AlCl_3$

heated with sulphur at 200°C to yield pure **281**, mp 135.5–136.5°C (Newman *et al.*, 1960). These crystals were shown to be 99+% pure by mass spectral analysis (Bailey, 1959). The difficulty in obtaining pure **281** by heating at 330°C with Pd-C (Cason and Phillips, 1952), could be explained as arising from the partial loss of methyl group to lead to the final product contaminated with 1- or 12-MBA. This explanation was supported by mass spectral analysis.

5.2   Friedel–Crafts alkylations

Friedel–Crafts condensation of **295** (R = H or CH$_3$) with naphthalene or tetralin afforded minor amounts of the expected 2-(β-naphthyl)- and 2-(β-tetralyl)cyclohexaneacetic acids, **296** and **297**, respectively (Scheme XXXI). The major products were the 3- and 4-isomers, **298** and **299** (Phillips and Chatterjee, 1958*a,b*; Chatterjee and Bhattacharjee, 1974). Formation of these products was explained as occurring via an electrophilic attack on the aromatic nucleus by each of the three possible carbocationic species represented by **300**. On

Scheme XXXI. Friedel-Crafts Alkylations.

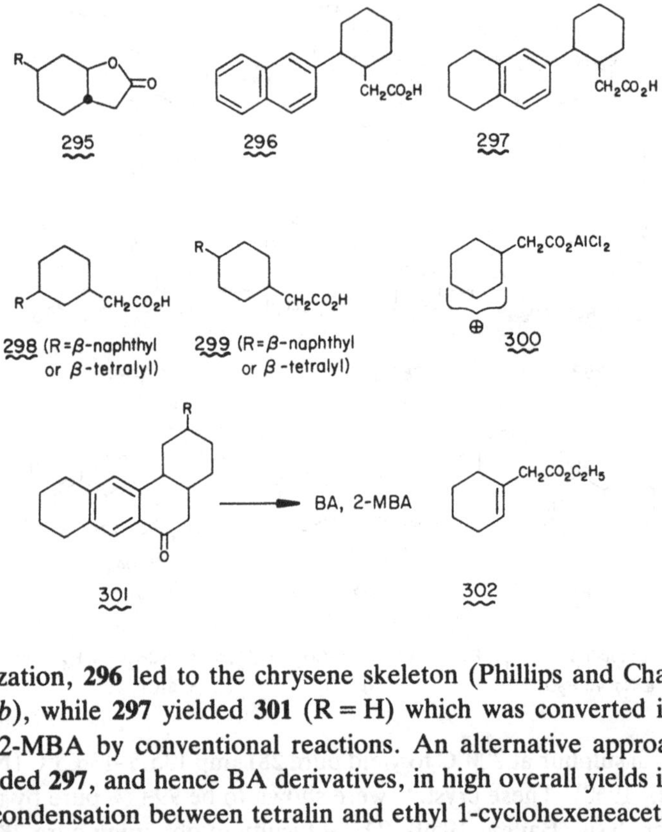

295   296   297

298 (R=β-naphthyl   299 (R=β-naphthyl   300
or β-tetralyl)   or β-tetralyl)

301 → BA, 2-MBA   302

cyclization, **296** led to the chrysene skeleton (Phillips and Chatterjee, 1958*b*), while **297** yielded **301** (R = H) which was converted into BA and 2-MBA by conventional reactions. An alternative approach that afforded **297**, and hence BA derivatives, in high overall yields involved the condensation between tetralin and ethyl 1-cyclohexeneacetate, **302** (Winternitz *et al.*, 1952).

Friedel–Crafts alkylation of tetralin with 2-allylcyclohexanones, **303**, gave **304**, which on reduction to **305**, followed by cyclization and aromatization furnished, via **306**, various 6-MBAs, **307**, in 15–40% overall yields, Scheme XXXII (Vig *et al.*, 1954, 1955; Gandhi *et al.*, 1957). An analogous reaction of naphthalene resulted in **308**. Conversion of **308** into BA derivatives was accomplished, in comparable yields, either by the reduction-cyclization-aromatization sequence as in the tetralin series or by a cyclodehydration-aromatization route via compounds of type **309** as shown in Scheme XXXII (Mukherji *et al.*, 1965; Sharma

Scheme XXXII. Friedel-Crafts Alkylation of Tetralins and
Naphthalenes with 2-Allylcyclohexanones.

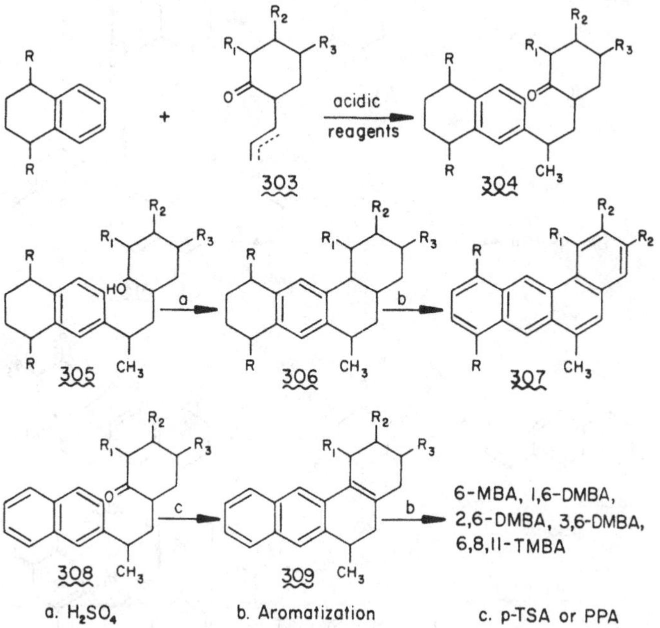

a. H_2SO_4 b. Aromatization   c. p-TSA or PPA

and Mukherji, 1966; Mukherji and Dabas, 1971a). Although cyclization of **308** (or the corresponding alcohol) could also result in benzo[c]-phenanthrene derivatives, the exclusive formation of BA compounds suggests the dominance of steric factors in the cyclization.

5.3   Grignard, Michael, Wittig and Vilsmeier reactions

Condensation of β-phenylethylmagnesium chloride, **310** (R = H), with *cis-* or *trans*-2-decalone, **311**, yielded 2-β-phenylethyldecalol, **312**, which on dehydration with $KHSO_4$ gave **313**. Aluminium chloride cyclization of **313** afforded **314** which was smoothly dehydrogenated by Se to BA and 4-MBA, Scheme XXXIII (Cook and Hewett, 1934; Cook *et al.*, 1937; Cook and Lawrence, 1937; Cook and Robinson, 1938).

A useful variation of Cook's Grignard route to BA compounds involved the reaction of β-(6-tetralyl)ethylmagnesium bromide, **315**, with cyclohexanones of type **316** to provide the alcohols **317**. Sulphuric acid treatment of **317** produced **319**, presumably via **318**. Heating with palladium on carbon converted **319** into BA, 2-MBA and 3-MBA in overall yields of 26–39%, Scheme XXXIII (Mukherji and Dabas, 1971b).

42   Chemistry

Scheme XXXIII. Grignard Reactions.

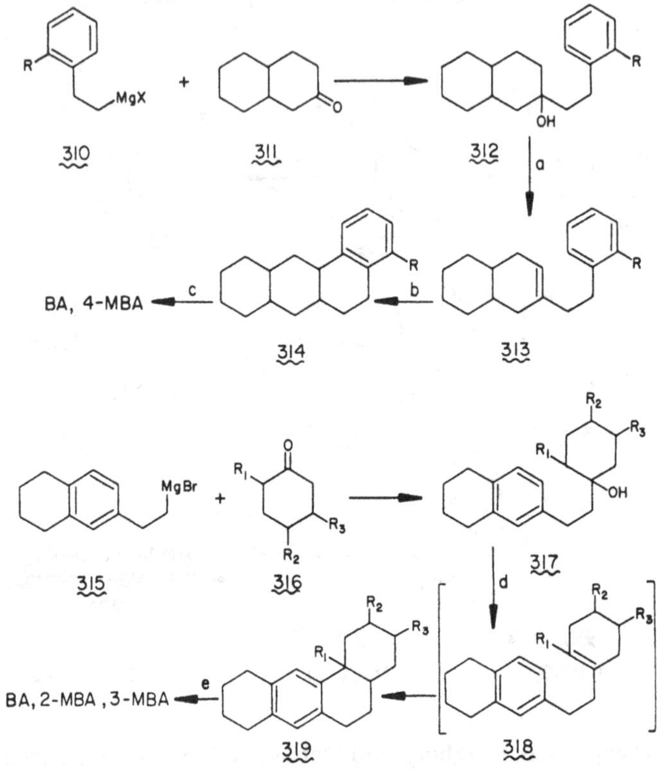

a KHSO$_4$ b. AlCl$_3$ c. Se, Δ d. H$_2$SO$_4$ e. Pd-C, Δ

Synthesis of 7-arylBAs has been accomplished by the reaction of appropriate aryl Grignard reagents with 2-(1-naphthylmethyl)benzonitrile followed by cyclodehydration under acidic conditions (Vingiello and Lewis, 1968).

Michael addition of sodio *cis*- and *trans*-2-decalone to acetyl-1-cyclohexene, **320**, gave the adduct **321**, ring closure of which to **322** followed by aromatization resulted in BA in unspecified yield (Cook and Lawrence, 1937), Scheme XXXIV.

The bis-ylide **324**, derived from *o*-xylenebis(triphenylphosphonium bromide), **323**, underwent a Wittig reaction with 1,2-naphthoquinone to afford BA in 20% yield (Nicolaides and Litinas, 1983), Scheme XXXIV.

Vilsmeier reaction of the tetralol **325** gave the dihydronaphthaldehyde **326** which on cyclodehydration provided **327**. Dehydrogenation of **327** produced 3-MeOBA in excellent yields (Reddy and Rao, 1981), Scheme XXXIV.

Scheme XXXIV. Michael, Wittig and Vilsmeier Reactions.

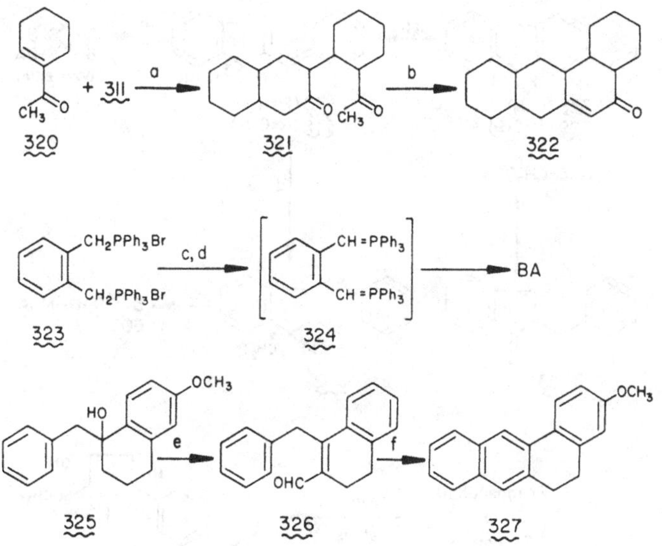

a. $NaNH_2$ b. H_2SO_4 c. LiOEt   d. 1,2-naphthoquinone   e. $POCl_3$, DMF
f. PPA

5.4   Wagner–Meerwein and anthrasteroid rearrangements

When 10-benz[b]fluorenylmethanol-11-^{14}C, **330**, obtained from
328 via carboxylation and reduction, was dehydrated with phosphorus
pentoxide, a ring expansion occurred leading to BA (49% overall from
328), in which the ^{14}C label was distributed between carbon atoms 5
and 6 in the ratio 48:52 (Collins *et al.*, 1951), Scheme XXXV. Similar
treatment of **331**, prepared from **329** via carboxylation and reduction,
afforded a 1:1 mixture of 5-MBA and 6-MBA, containing ^{14}C at the
5- and 6-positions (Anet and Bavin, 1960), which fact suggests equal
migratory aptitudes for the naphthalenic and benzenic groups. However,
when **332** was refluxed with 95% formic acid, 5-MBA was obtained
in 60% yield indicating the greater migratory power of the naphthalenic
moiety over the benzenic ring. These results were rationalized in terms
of the difference between the transition states leading to the rearrangement. The position of ^{14}C in the BAs was proved by appropriate oxidative
processes (Collins *et al.*, 1951). Reaction of 11*H*-benzo[b]fluorene-11-
one, **333**, with diazomethane gave a 38% yield of 5-MeOBA (Anet and
Bavin, 1960).

Prompted by a suggestion (Kennaway and Cook, 1932), that steroids
might be converted *in vivo* to PAHs, it was demonstrated (Nes and
Ford, 1962, 1963), for the first time that an aromatic hydrocarbon of

Scheme XXXV. Wagner-Meerwein and Anthrasteroid Rearrangements.

328 (R=H)
329 (R=CH₃)

330 (R=H)
331 (R=CH₃)

5-¹⁴C-BA
6-¹⁴C-BA
about equal

5-CH₃OBA

333

332

5-¹⁴C-6-MBA
60%

Pregnenolone
or
Ergosterol

several
steps

334

4,7-DMBA

336

335

a. Ph₃CNa, ¹⁴CO₂   b. LiAlH₄ on methyl ester   c. P₂O₅
d. tosylation   e. 95% HCO₂H   f. CH₂N₂
g. KOH, MeOH   h. LiAlH₄   i. Ac₂O   j. Pd-C, Δ

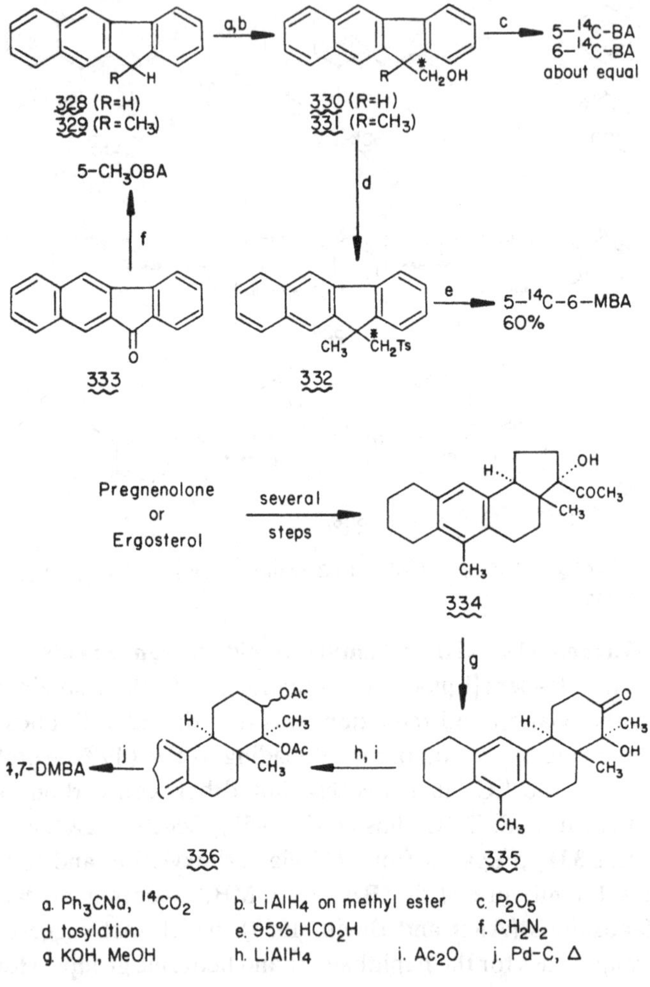

the BA class can indeed be obtained from either pregnenolone or ergo-sterol by successive anthrasteroid and D-homosteroid rearrangements. Thus, base-catalysed D-homosteroid rearrangement of **334** produced **335** which was transformed into 4,7-DMBA via **336** as shown, Scheme XXXV.

5.5   Reactions involving lithiated species

Reaction of the lithio phthalide **337** with naphthyne, generated *in situ* by treatment of 1-bromonaphthalene with lithium di-isopropyl-amide, gave **338**. Formation of **338** presumably occurs via a nucleophilic addition of **337** to naphthyne followed by intramolecular cyclization with concomitant opening of the lactone ring. Enolization to **339** and subsequent air-oxidation afforded 7,12-BAQs (Sammes and Dodsworth, 1979; Dodsworth *et al.*, 1981), Scheme XXXVI.

Scheme XXXVI. Reactions Involving Lithiated Species.

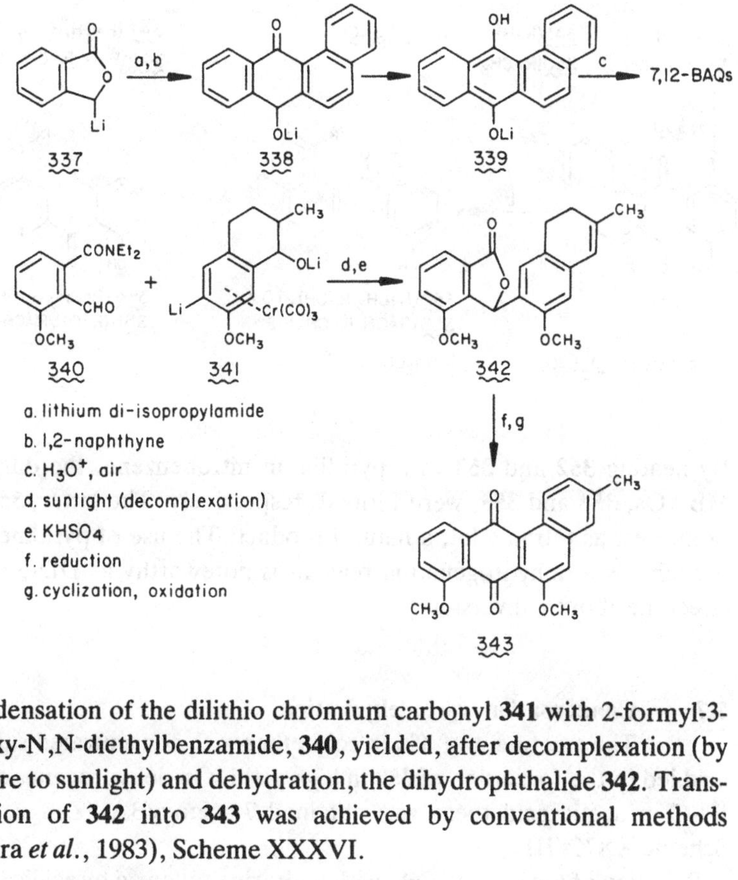

337   338   339   →   7,12-BAQs

340   +   341   d,e   →   342

a. lithium di-isopropylamide
b. 1,2-naphthyne
c. H_3O^+, air
d. sunlight (decomplexation)
e. $KHSO_4$
f. reduction
g. cyclization, oxidation

f,g

343

Condensation of the dilithio chromium carbonyl **341** with 2-formyl-3-methoxy-N,N-diethylbenzamide, **340**, yielded, after decomplexation (by exposure to sunlight) and dehydration, the dihydrophthalide **342**. Transformation of **342** into **343** was achieved by conventional methods (Uemura *et al.*, 1983), Scheme XXXVI.

5.6 Decarboxylative alkylation

On reaction of 2-chloro-1,4-naphthoquinone, **344**, with **345**, in the presence of silver nitrate and ammonium persulphate, a high yield of **346** was produced. Treatment of **346** with sodium carbonate on the steam bath formed a mixture of 4% of 1-hydroxyBAQ, **347**, and 26% of 3-hydroxyBAQ, **348**. When **349** and **350** were used, an 82% yield of **351** was obtained. This on treatment with sodium carbonate as above yielded 70% of 5,6-dihydro-1-MBAQ, **352**, plus small amounts of **353**, **355**, and other products (Brown and Thomson, 1976), Scheme XXXVII.

Scheme XXXVII. Decarboxylative Alkylation.

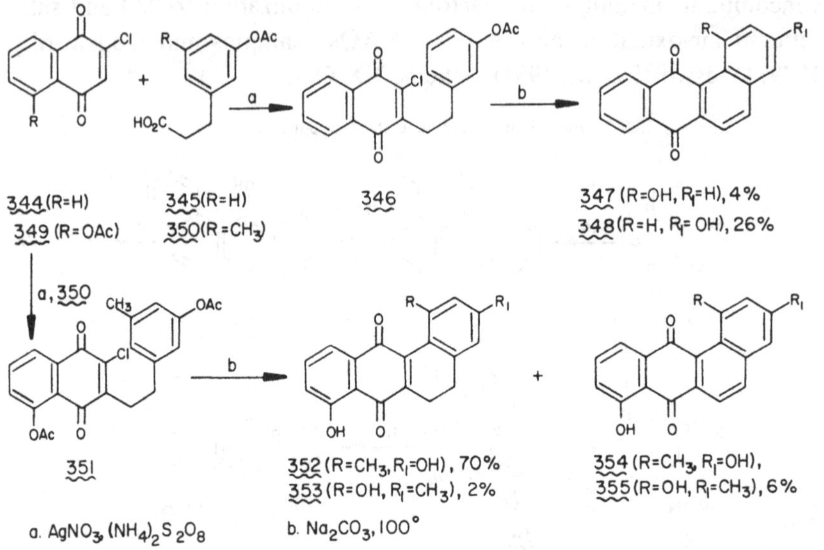

344 (R=H)   345 (R=H)   346   347 (R=OH, R$_1$=H), 4%
349 (R=OAc)   350 (R=CH$_3$)   348 (R=H, R$_1$= OH), 26%

a, 350

351

352 (R=CH$_3$, R$_1$=OH), 70%   354 (R=CH$_3$, R$_1$=OH),
353 (R=OH, R$_1$=CH$_3$), 2%   355 (R=OH, R$_1$=CH$_3$), 6%

a. AgNO$_3$, (NH$_4$)$_2$S$_2$O$_8$ b. Na$_2$CO$_3$, 100°

By heating **352** and **353** with pyridine in nitrobenzene, the dihydroxy MBAQs, **354** and **355**, were formed, respectively. The latter, **355**, was of interest as tetrangulol, a natural product. The use of pyridine-nitrobenzene as a dehydrogenation reagent is noteworthy as DDQ did not effect the above conversion.

5.7   Condensation, cyclodehydration

The treatment of **356** in cold ether with concentrated sulphuric acid led to the formation of **357** in high yield. On dehydrogenation over Pd-C in acetic acid there was obtained 7-acetoxyBA (Zaugg, 1946), Scheme XXXVIII.

Reaction of the nitriles, **358**, with hydrazine followed by acidic cyclization afforded high yields of BA (Zajac and Denk, 1962).

When the dialdehydes, **359–361**, were treated with tris-dimethyl-aminophosphine, the arene oxides, **362–364**, were formed (Newman and Blum, 1964c; Goh and Harvey, 1973), Scheme XXXVIII.

In another route the malonic ester **365** was treated with 1,3-dichloro-2-butene to yield the diester **366**. The latter was hydrolysed and decarboxylated to afford the acid **367**, which was cyclized with sulphuric acid to the ketone **368**. From **368**, BA, 2-MBA, 2-HOBA, and 2-PhBA were obtained in good yields by standard methods (Babayan *et al.*, 1953).

Scheme XXXVIII. Miscellaneous Cyclizations.

a H_2SO_4 b. N_2H_4 c. acid reagents   d. $(Me_2N)_3P$
e. alkylation with 1,3-dichloro-butene   f. hydrolysis, $-CO_2$

Cyclization of a number of ketones and acids of types **369**, **370**, and **371** yielded a variety of largely hydrogenated 7,12-DMBAs, none of which were aromatized (Pepin *et al.*, 1970), Scheme XXXIX.

When 1-(2-*trans*-decalenyl)-2-(1-cyclohexenyl)acetylene, obtained from 2-decalone, acetylene, and cyclohexanone, was stirred with a mixture of glacial acetic acid and sulphuric acid the polyhydrogenated BA **372** resulted. This was reduced and aromatized to BA (Marvel *et al.*, 1940).

Treatment of 3-benzyl-2,4-diphenyl-3-hydroxyglutaric acid, **373**, with sulphuric acid furnished 5,12-dihydroxy-6-phenylBA, **374** (Ivanov and Mladenova-Orlinova, 1964), Scheme XXXIX.

Reaction of benzylmagnesium chloride with phenyl 2-methoxy-1-naphthoate gave phenyl 2-benzyl-1-naphthoate which on treatment with sulphuric acid produced 12-HOBA (Fuson and Wassmundt, 1956).

5.8   Isotopically labelled BAs

The synthesis of BAs containing ^{14}C at one or more positions has been accomplished by the following: Anet and Bavin (1960), Catch

Scheme XXXIX. Miscellaneous Cyclizations.

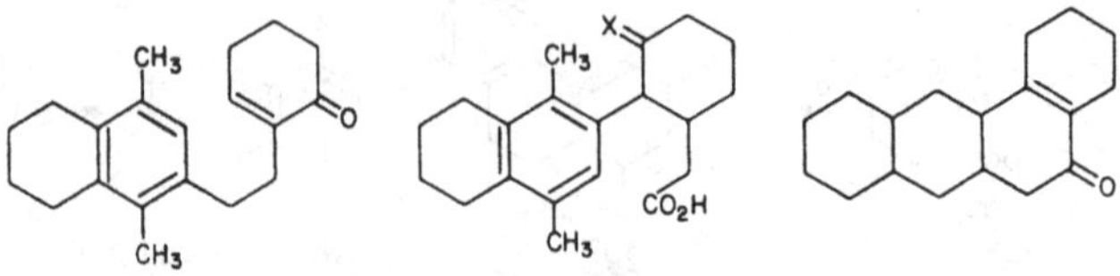

369   370(X=H₂)   372
          371(X=O)

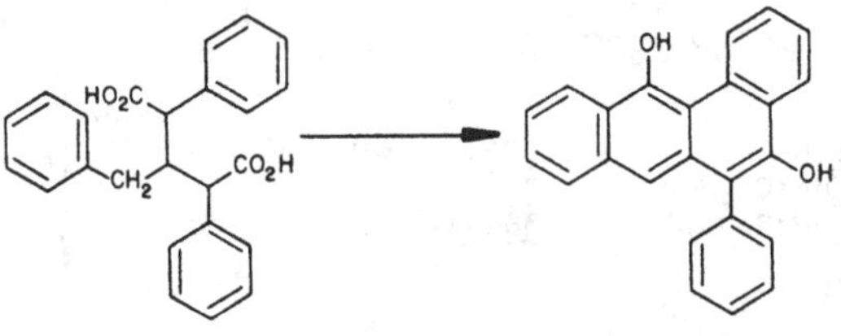

373   374

and Evans (1957), Collins *et al.* (1951), Evans (1957), Gaponenko *et al.* (1968), Hadler (1955), Hadler and Raha (1957) and Susan *et al.* (1981).

Syntheses involving the formation of deuterated BAs were carried out by Adapa *et al.* (1980), Buu-Hoi and Lavit (1960), and Cavalieri and Calvin (1976). The steric effects in the interaction of deutero trifluoroacetic acid with BA and the twelve MBAs were studied by Dallinga *et al.* (1958).

The syntheses of BAs containing tritium were described by Blackburn *et al.* (1981), Crowter *et al.* (1962), Emmerich and Schmialek (1966), Fu and Harvey (1977), Gaponenko *et al.* (1968), Lijinsky and Garcia (1963), Susan *et al.* (1981), and Susan and Wiley (1982).

6

Tables

Note: The numbers listed in the following Tables refer to bibliographic references on pages 63–81.

Table 6.1 *References to BA syntheses*

4, 8, 9, 25, 52, 53, 67, 68, 72, 75, 97, 99, 115c, 158, 170, 179, 185, 204, 219, 225, 227b, 229, 287, 301, 336, 364, 371

Table 6.2 *MBAs: references to methylBA syntheses*

Hydrocarbon	Position of methyl substituents	
BA	1-Methyl-	16, 83, 127, 232a, 273
	2-Methyl-	8, 14, 64, 75, 96, 227b, 250
	3-Methyl-	75, 97, 227b, 250
	4-Methyl-	85, 98, 146, 218, 219, 227a, 228, 273
	5-Methyl-	5, 73, 250, 252, 314, 336
	6-Methyl-	15, 76, 97, 123, 125, 229, 230, 231, 232b, 250, 345, 346
	7-Methyl-	48, 85, 95a, 113, 117, 124, 154, 170, 182, 209, 212b, 216, 217, 261
	8-Methyl-	19, 54, 76, 121b, 124, 250
	9-Methyl-	13, 75, 101, 250
	10-Methyl-	13, 57, 75, 250, 310
	11-Methyl-	13, 83, 88, 101, 121a,b, 250
	12-Methyl-	48, 59, 85, 118, 212b, 237, 250, 261

Table 6.3 *MonoalkylBAs: references to monoalkylBA syntheses*

Hydrocarbon	Position of substituents	
BA	7-Ethyl-	115*a*, 216, 217
	8-Ethyl-	12, 85
	11-Ethyl-	121*b*
	12-Ethyl-	211
	7-Allyl-	115*a*
	12-Allyl-	118
	7-Propyl-	115*a*, 217
	8-Propyl-	12, 78
	9-Propyl-	87
	5-Isopropyl-	75
	7-Isopropyl-	75, 115*a*
	8-Isopropyl-	88
	9-Isopropyl-	75
	10-Isopropyl-	75
	11-Isopropyl-	122
	7-*n*-Butyl-	115*a*, 217
	8-*n*-Butyl-	84
	7-*n*-Amyl-	115*a*
	8-*n*-Amyl-	84
	7-Isoamyl-	217
	8-Hexyl-	84
	7-Cyclohexyl-	351
	8-Heptyl-	84

Table 6.4 *DMBAs: references to dimethylBA syntheses*

Hydrocarbon	Position of methyl substituents	
BA	1,6-Dimethyl-	135, 227*a*, 232*a*
	1,7-Dimethyl-	127
	1,8-Dimethyl-	18
	1,9-Dimethyl-	166
	1,12-Dimethyl-	59, 275
	2,6-Dimethyl-	135, 227*a*
	2,9-Dimethyl-	75
	2,10-Dimethyl-	75
	3,4-Dimethyl-	65
	3,6-Dimethyl-	135, 320
	3,9-Dimethyl-	75, 251
	3,10-Dimethyl-	75
	4,7-Dimethyl-	218, 235, 236, 293
	4,12-Dimethyl-	293
	5,6-Dimethyl-	37
	5,7-Dimethyl-	252

Table 6.4 *(contd.)*

Hydrocarbon	Position of methyl substituents	
	5,12-Dimethyl-	128, 293
	6,7-Dimethyl-	123, 293
	6,8-Dimethyl-	241*b*
	6,11-Dimethyl-	15
	6,12-Dimethyl-	123, 293
	7,8-Dimethyl-	124
	7,11-Dimethyl-	121*b*
	7,12-Dimethyl-	11, 12, 30, 209, 210, 213, 214, 215, 238*a*, 247, 269, 313, 336
	8,9-Dimethyl-	13, 77
	8,10-Dimethyl-	13, 306
	8,11-Dimethyl-	13, 121*b*
	8,12-Dimethyl-	237
	9,10-Dimethyl-	75
	9,11-Dimethyl-	308

Table 6.5 *DialkylBAs: references to dialkylBA syntheses*

Hydrocarbon	Position of alkyl substituents	
BA	3-M-4-E-	66
	4-M-7-E-	218
	7-M-12-E-	211
	12-M-7-E-	213
	6,8-DE-	290
	7,8-DE-	290
	7,9-DE-	290
	7,12-DE-	11, 211, 212*a*
	8,12-DE-	290
	12-M-7-P-	213
	7,12-DP-	12
	7-M-3-i-P-	107
	12-M-7-butyl-	213
	12-M-7-i-butyl-	294

E, ethyl; DE, diethyl; M, methyl; P, propyl.

Table 6.6 *TMBAs: references to trimethylBA syntheses*

Hydrocarbon	Position of methyl substituents	
BA	1,7,12-Trimethyl-	184, 253
	1,8,9-Trimethyl-	166
	2,7,12-Trimethyl-	96, 253, 293
	3,4,7-Trimethyl-	236
	3,7,12-Trimethyl-	293
	4,7,12-Trimethyl-	98
	5,7,12-Trimethyl-	244, 293, 336
	6,7,8-Trimethyl-	241b
	6,7,12-Trimethyl-	293
	6,8,11-Trimethyl-	135
	6,8,12-Trimethyl-	293
	7,8,12-Trimethyl-	11
	7,9,12-Trimethyl-	27
	7,10,12-Trimethyl-	13, 293
	7,11,12-Trimethyl-	13, 239
	8,9,11-Trimethyl-	308

Table 6.7 *TrialkylBAs and TeMBAs: references to trialkylBA and tetramethylBA syntheses*

Hydrocarbon	Position of substituents	
BA	8-E-7,12-DMBA-	12
	8-P-7,12-DMBA-	12
	7,8,9,12-TeMBA-	27
	7,9,10,12-TeMBA-	198

Table 6.8 *ArylBAs: references to arylBA syntheses*

Hydrocarbon	Position of aryl substituents	
BA	1-Phenyl-	356
	2-Phenyl-	8
	7-Phenyl-	49, 349, 355
	8-Phenyl-	10
	9-Phenyl-	73, 353
	12-Phenyl-	71, 347b, 355
	7,12-Diphenyl-	69, 344
	1-(4-Methoxyphenyl)-	356
	5-Chloro-7,12-diphenyl-	31
	1-(4-Chlorophenyl)-	356
	7-(2-Chlorophenyl)-	354

Table 6.8 *(contd)*

Hydrocarbon	Position of aryl substituents	
	12-(2-Chlorophenyl)-	354
	1-(4-Fluorophenyl)-	356
	7-(2-Fluorophenyl)-	354
	12-(2-Fluorophenyl)-	354
	7-(3-Trifluoromethylphenyl)-	355
	12-(3-Trifluoromethylphenyl)-	355
	1-(4-Bromophenyl)-	356
	1-Tolyl- (2 isomers)	356
	7-Tolyl- (3 isomers)	349, 355
	12-Tolyl- (3 isomers)	347b, 355
	7-Benzyl-	73
	7-Xylyl- (6 isomers)	347a, 348b
	12-Xylyl- (6 isomers)	348a,b
	7-(2,4,6-Trimethylphenyl)-	348b
	7-(1-Naphthyl)-	350
	7-(2-Naphthyl)-	350
	12-(1-Naphthyl)-	350
	12-(2-Naphthyl)-	350
	7-[1-(4-Bromo)naphthyl]-	352
	7-[1-(4-Methyl)naphthyl]-	352

Table 6.9 *BromoBAs: references to brominated BA syntheses*

Hydrocarbon	Position of bromo substituents	
BA	4-Bromo-	29, 177, 218, 236
	7-Bromo-	26, 182
	4,7-Dibromo-	218
4-MBA	7-Bromo-	218
7-MBA	1-Bromo-	274
	2-Bromo-	254
	3-Bromo-	274
	4-Bromo-	218, 283
	5-Bromo-	254
	10-Bromo-	254
	11-Bromo-	254
9-MBA	7-Bromo-	26
12-MBA	5-Bromo-	254
	7-Bromo-	26, 254
7,12-DMBA	2-Bromo-	274
	3-Bromo-	274
	4-Bromo-	98, 254
	5-Bromo-	244
	8-Bromo-	368
	9-Bromo-	254

Table 6.10 *ChloroBAs: references to chlorinated BA syntheses*

Hydrocarbon	Position of chloro substituents	
BA	2-Chloro-	23
	3-Chloro-	23
	4-Chloro-	98, 177
	5-Chloro-	177
	7-Chloro-	233, 331
	9-Chloro-	272
	7,12-Dichloro-	233
7-MBA	4-Chloro-	283
	8-Chloro-	238b
	9-Chloro-	272
	10-Chloro-	271
7,12-DMBA	2-Chloro-	253
	10-Chloro-	246

Table 6.11 *FluoroBAs: references to fluorinated BA syntheses*

Hydrocarbon	Position of fluoro substituents	
BA	1-Fluoro-	279
	4-Fluoro-	33, 267
	5-Fluoro-	247, 267
	6-Fluoro-	140
	7-Fluoro-	2, 46, 266, 288
	8-Fluoro-	39
	12-Fluoro-	288
	9-Trifluoromethyl-	282
	7,12-Difluoro-	288
	8,9,10,11-Tetrafluoro-	143
7-MBA	1-Fluoro-	279
	2-Fluoro-	243
	3-Fluoro-	249
	4-Fluoro-	267
	5-Fluoro-	267
	6-Fluoro-	249
	8-Fluoro-	241a
	9-Fluoro-	280
	10-Fluoro-	280
	11-Fluoro-	286
	12-Fluoro-	46, 258
9-MBA	5-Fluoro-	42
12-MBA	5-Fluoro-	42, 44
	6-Fluoro-	140
	7-Fluoro-	258
	8-Fluoro-	39
	9-Fluoro-	257

Table 6.11 *(contd)*

Hydrocarbon	Position of fluoro substituents	
	10-Fluoro-	257
	11-Fluoro-	262
6,8-DMBA	5-Fluoro-	242
7,12-DMBA	2-Fluoro-	281, 321
	3-Fluoro-	321
	4-Fluoro-	269
	5-Fluoro-	42, 44, 247, 269
	6-Fluoro-	140
	8-Fluoro-	241a
	9-Fluoro-	257
	10-Fluoro-	257
	11-Fluoro-	241a
	9-Trifluoromethyl-	282
	10-Trifluoromethyl-	282

Table 6.12 *MethoxyBAs: references to methoxyBA syntheses*

Hydrocarbon	Position of methoxy substituents	
BA	1-Methoxy-	234, 315
	2-Methoxy-	22b, 185, 234
	3-Methoxy-	185, 234, 307, 323
	4-Methoxy-	185, 234, 315, 319
	5-Methoxy-	5, 86, 110, 119, 155, 277, 363
	6-Methoxy-	363
	7-Methoxy-	115a, 179, 372
	8-Methoxy-	87, 192
	9-Methoxy-	192
	10-Methoxy-	192
	11-Methoxy-	192
	3,9-Dimethoxy-	191, 220, 223
	3,10-Dimethoxy-	191
	5,7-Dimethoxy-	116
	7,12-Dimethoxy-	28
	2,7,12-Trimethoxy-	22b
1-MBA	5-Methoxy-	86
4-MBA	1,7,11,12-Tetramethoxy-	175
7-MBA	3-Methoxy-	182
	5-Methoxy-	115a, 241c, 277
	8-Methoxy-	285
	9-Methoxy-	280, 297
	10-Methoxy-	254
	11-Methoxy-	254
	12-Methoxy-	116
	3,9-Dimethoxy-	223

Table 6.12 *(contd)*

Hydrocarbon	Position of methoxy substituents	
	8,12-Dimethoxy-	285
7-EBA	5-Methoxy-	115*a*
7-PBA	5-Methoxy-	115*a*
12-MBA	5-Methoxy-	24, 277, 325
	6-Methoxy-	277
	7-Methoxy-	294
	3,9-Dimethoxy-	223
7,12-DMBA	1-Methoxy-	259
	2-Methoxy-	22*b*, 234, 259, 297
	3-Methoxy-	234, 259, 260, 327
	4-Methoxy-	129, 234, 259
	5-Methoxy-	86, 277, 325
	6-Methoxy-	259, 277
	8-Methoxy-	192, 221, 256
	9-Methoxy-	192, 265, 292
	10-Methoxy-	192, 221, 259, 265, 292, 297
	11-Methoxy-	192, 221, 256
	3,9-Dimethoxy-	191, 222
	3,10-Dimethoxy-	191
	5,6-Dimethoxy-	245
7,8,12-TMBA	5-Methoxy-	86
7,8,9,12-TeMBA	5-Methoxy-	86
12-M-7-EBA	5-Methoxy-	325
12-M-7-PhBA	5-Methoxy-	325

Table 6.13 *HydroxyBAs: references to hydroxyBA syntheses*

Hydrocarbon	Position of hydroxy substituents	
BA	1-Hydroxy-	130, 234, 315
	2-Hydroxy-	8, 130, 167, 234
	3-Hydroxy-	130, 234
	4-Hydroxy-	58, 168, 234, 315, 319
	5-Hydroxy-	110, 241*c*, 363
	6-Hydroxy-	363
	7-Hydroxy-	115*a*, 372
	8-Hydroxy-	87, 130
	9-Hydroxy-	130
	10-Hydroxy-	130
	11-Hydroxy-	121*b*, 130
	12-Hydroxy-	134
	3,9-Dihydroxy-	220, 223
7-MBA	2-Hydroxy-	182
	3-Hydroxy-	182

Table 6.13 *(contd)*

Hydrocarbon	Position of hydroxy substituents	
	5-Hydroxy-	115*a*, 241*c*
	10-Hydroxy-	254
	11-Hydroxy-	254
	3,9-Dihydroxy-	223
12-MBA	3,9-Dihydroxy-	223
7,12-DMBA	1-Hydroxy-	259
	2-Hydroxy-	234, 259
	3-Hydroxy-	234, 259, 327
	4-Hydroxy-	129, 234, 259
	8-Hydroxy-	256
	9-Hydroxy-	259
	10-Hydroxy-	221, 259
	11-Hydroxy-	256
	1,4-Dihydroxy-	260
	3,4-Dihydroxy-	260
	3,9-Dihydroxy-	222
6-PhBA	5,12-Dihydroxy-	169

Table 6.14 *AcetoxyBAs: references to acetoxyBA syntheses*

Hydrocarbon	Position of acetoxy substituents	
BA	2-Acetoxy-	130, 167
	3-Acetoxy-	130
	4-Acetoxy-	58, 168, 319
	5-Acetoxy-	110, 155, 241*c*
	6-Acetoxy-	155
	7-Acetoxy-	73, 115*a*, 324, 372
	8-Acetoxy-	130
	9-Acetoxy-	130
	11-Acetoxy-	121*b*, 130
	3,9-Diacetoxy-	220
	5,6-Diacetoxy-	110
	3-MeO-12-AcO-	323
	5-MeO-7-AcO-	116
	9-MeO-7-AcO-	324
	10-MeO-12-AcO-	259
1-MBA	12-Acetoxy-	127
7-MBA	2-Acetoxy-	182
	3-Acetoxy-	182
	5-Acetoxy-	116
	12-Acetoxy-	116, 154
	3-MeO-12-AcO-	182

Table 6.14 *(contd)*

Hydrocarbon	Position of acetoxy substituents	
9-MBA	7-Acetoxy-	22*a*
	7,12-Diacetoxy-	310
10-MBA	7,12-Diacetoxy-	310
11-MBA	7-Acetoxy-	239
12-MBA	7-Acetoxy-	238*a*, 294
1,4-DMBA	7-Acetoxy-	324
	9-MeO-7-AcO-	324
1,7-DMBA	12-Acetoxy-	127
7,12-DMBA	4-Acetoxy-	129
	5-Acetoxy-	270
	6-Acetoxy-	259, 270
	8-Acetoxy-	221, 256
	9-Acetoxy-	292
	10-Acetoxy-	292
	11-Acetoxy-	221, 256
	3,4-Diacetoxy-	327
	3,9-Diacetoxy-	223
	3,10-Diacetoxy-	191

Table 6.15 *Amino BAs: references to amino BA syntheses*

Hydrocarbon	Position of amino substituents	
BA	2-Amino-	23
	4-Amino-	29
	5-Amino-	108, 119
	7-Amino-	29, 108, 116
	11-Amino-	121*b*
7-MBA	10-Amino-	254
	11-Amino-	254
12-MBA	5-Amino-	325
7,12-DMBA	5-Amino-	325
	9-Amino-	254
	10-Amino-	297

Table 6.16 *CyanoBAs: references to cyanoBA syntheses*

Hydrocarbon	Position of cyano substituents	
BA	3-Cyano-	23
	4-Cyano-	177
	5-Cyano-	177
	7-Cyano-	26, 113, 233, 331
	8-Cyano-	88, 238b
	9-Cyano-	272
	10-Cyano-	271
	7,12-Dicyano-	226, 293
9-MBA	7-Cyano-	26
12-MBA	7-Cyano-	26
7,12-DMBA	2-Cyano-	253
	5-Cyano-	244
	8-Cyano-	368
	10-Cyano-	246

Table 6.17 *Halomethyl- and cyanomethylBAs: references to syntheses of halomethylBAs and cyanomethylBAs*

Hydrocarbon	Position of substituents	
BA	7-CH_2Cl-	25, 298
	7,12-Bisbromomethyl-	25
	7-CH_2CN-	26
7-MBA	5-CH_2Br-	171
12-MBA	7-CH_2Cl-	248, 294, 298
	3-MeO-7-CH_2Cl-	259, 327
	5-F-7-CH_2Cl-	248
	10-Cl-7-CH_2Cl-	246
	7-CH_2Br-	294
	7-CH_2I-	298
	4-MeO-7-CH_2I-	129
5-FBA	12-CH_2Br-	42
	12-CH_2CN-	42
9-FBA	12-CH_2Br-	257
	12-CH_2CN-	257
10-FBA	12-CH_2Br-	257
	12-CH_2CN-	257
11-FBA	12-CH_2CN-	262

Table 6.18 *HydroxymethylBAs: references to hydroxymethylBA syntheses*

Hydrocarbon	Position of hydroxymethyl substituent	
BA	7-Hydroxymethyl-	25
	7-(CHO)-12-hydroxymethyl-	294
8-MBA	7,12-Diacetoxymethyl-	291
9-MBA	7-Hydroxymethyl-	26
12-MBA	7-Hydroxymethyl-	129
	5-F-7-hydroxymethyl-	248
	7-Methoxymethyl-	32, 129
	7-Acetoxymethyl-	129
7-EBA	12-Hydroxymethyl-	294
12-EBA	7-Hydroxymethyl-	294
4,12-DMBA	7-Hydroxymethyl-	293
5,12-DMBA	7-Hydroxymethyl-	293
7,12-DMBA	5-Hydroxymethyl-	244
	10-Hydroxymethyl-	246

Table 6.19 *BA Carboxaldehydes: references to BA carboxaldehyde syntheses*

Hydrocarbon	Position of carboxaldehyde substituents	
BA	7-Carboxaldehyde-	113
	7,12-Di(CHO)-	294
7-MBA	5-Carboxaldehyde-	171
	12-Carboxaldehyde-	171, 294
11-MBA	7-Carboxaldehyde-	121*b*
12-MBA	7-Carboxaldehyde-	26, 294
12-EBA	7-Carboxaldehyde-	294
4,12-DMBA	7-Carboxaldehyde-	293
5,12-DMBA	7-Carboxaldehyde-	293

Table 6.20 *BA acids and lactones: references to syntheses of BA acids and BA lactones*

Hydrocarbon	Position of substituents	
BA	4-CO_2H-	29, 218
	6-CO_2H-	74
	7-CO_2H-	29, 94, 157, 216, 217
	8-CO_2H-	88
	1-CH_2CO_2H-	120
	5-CH_2CO_2H-	314
	7-CH_2CO_2H-	95*a,b*, 314

Table 6.20 *(contd)*

Hydrocarbon	Position of substituents	
	8-CH$_2$CO$_2$H-	314
	11-CH$_2$CO$_2$H-	314
	7-OH-6-CO$_2$H-, lactone	142, 324
	5,7-Di(OH)-6-CO$_2$H-, lactone	142
	5,6-Di(OH)-7-CO$_2$H-, lactone	332
	5-AcO-7-OH-6-CO$_2$H-, lactone	142
	9-MeO-7-OH-6-CO$_2$H-, lactone	324
	12-(2-Phenylethyl)-5,7-di(OH)-6-	
	CO$_2$H-, lactone	142
4-MBA	7-CO$_2$H-	218
7-MBA	9-CO$_2$H-	272
	10-CO$_2$H-	271
12-MBA	7-CO$_2$H-	217
	7-CH$_2$CO$_2$H-	214
1,4-DMBA	7-OH-6-CO$_2$H-, lactone	324
7,12-DMBA	2-CO$_2$H-	253
	5-CO$_2$H-	244
	10-CO$_2$H-	246
1,4-DPhBA	7-OH-6-CO$_2$H-, lactone	324

Table 6.21 *Isotopically labelled BAs: references to syntheses of labelled BAs*

Labelling agent	
Deuterium	1, 55, 62, 133, 150
Tritium	45, 92, 103, 131, 133, 136, 139, 186, 328, 329
Carbon-14	61, 72, 104, 136, 147, 149, 328

Table 6.22 *Miscellaneous BAs: references to syntheses of miscellaneous BAs*

Hydrocarbon	Position of substituents	
BA	5-CONH$_2$-	177
	7-CONH$_2$-	26
	5,6-Dihydro-7-AcO-12-CO$_2$H-, ethyl ester	63
	5,6-Di(CO$_2$H)-, anhydride	330
	9-CH$_3$CO-	79
	10-CH$_3$CO-	79
	5-C$_6$H$_5$CO$_2$-	119
	7-C$_6$H$_5$CO$_2$-	73
	10-C$_6$H$_5$CO$_2$-	130
	12-C$_6$H$_5$CO$_2$-	134
	5,6-Dihydro-5,6-imine-	47, 360
	5,6-Dihydro-5,6-oxide-	241c, 155

62   *Chemistry*

Table 6.22 *(contd)*

Hydrocarbon	Position of substituents	
	1,2,3,4-Tetrahydro-3,4-di(OH)-1,2-oxide-	370
	7-NO$_2$-	33, 108, 116, 266
	5-Isocyanate-	108
	7-Isocyanate-	108
	7-Mercaptan-	366
	7-Methylmercaptan-	366
	7-Thiocyano-	367
	12-Thiocyano-	367
	7-Isothiocyanomethyl-	367
	7-Thiocyanomethyl-	367
	7-Acetylthio-	38
	5-Methylamino-	119
	2,7,12-Tri(MeO)-5-[4-(N,N-dimethyl-amino)phenyl]-	137
	2-(N,N-Dimethylamino)-7,12-di(MeO)-5[4(N,N-dimethylamino)phenyl]-	137
	7-Triphenyllead-	138
	2-Sulphonic acid-	167
	4-Sulphonic acid-	168
	5-Cyano-6-amino-	362
7-MBA	8-CONH$_2$-	238*b*
	5,6-Dihydro-5,6-imine-	47
	5,6-Dihydro-5,6-oxide-	241*c*
	12-Thiocyano-	367
9-MBA	5-F-7-OH-	42
12-MBA	5-Isocyanate-	325
	7-Thiocyano-	367
7,12-DMBA	5-Isocyanate	325
	5,6-Dihydro-5,6-oxide-	155
	5,6-Dihydro-	148
	5,6-Dihydro-5,6-di(OH)-	148
	3-MeO-5-F-	322
	3-OH-5-F-	322
	3-Hydroxy-5-ethylthio-	322

7

References to Part 1

The numbers at the beginning of each Reference refer to citations in the Tables.

1. Adapa, S. R., Sheikh, Y. M., Hart, R. W. & Witiak, D. T. (1980). Preparation of site specifically deuterated 7,12-dimethylbenz[a]anthracene derivatives: mechanism of hydrogenolysis of aryl halides with lithium aluminium hydride. *J. Org. Chem.*, **45**, 3343–4.
2. Agranat, I., Rabinovitz, M., Selig, H. & Lin, C. (1977). Fluorination capabilities of xenon fluoride/graphite intercalates: introduction of fluorine into carcinogenic polycyclic aromatic hydrocarbons. *Synthesis*, 267–8.
3. Ahmed, Z. & Cava, M. P. (1981). A novel anthraquinone annelation. A new approach to alkavinones. *Tetrahedron Lett.*, 5239–42.
4. Ahmed, F. U., Rangarajan, T., Eisenbraun, E. J., Keen, G. W. & Hamming, M. C. (1975). The synthesis of BA. *Org. Prep. Proc. Int.*, 7, 267–70.
5. Anet, F. A. L. & Bavin, P. M. G. (1960). Studies in the Wagner–Meerwein rearrangement. IV. Derivatives of benz[b]fluorene. *Can. J. Chem.*, **38**, 240–3.
6. Awad, S. B., Sakla, A. B., Abdul-Malik, N. F. & Ishak, N. (1979). Cycloaddition of some quinones to 1,1-diarylethylenes. *Indian J. Chem.*, **17B**, 219–21.
7. Azerbaev, I. N. (1945). Hydrogenation of 1-ethynylcyclohexanol and 1-ethynylcyclohexene. Synthesis of 1-vinylcyclohexene. *J. Gen. Chem. U.S.S.R.*, **15**, 412—20. *Chem. Abst.*, **40**, 4683[4].
8. Babayan, V. O., Zagorets, P. A. & Tatevosyan, G. T. (1953). Synthesis of hydrocarbons of the BA Series. *Zh. Obshch. Khim.*, **23**, 1214–20. *Chem. Abst.*, **47**, 12214d.
9. Bachmann, W. E. (1936). The reaction of alkali metals with polycyclic hydrocarbons: benz[a]anthracene, dibenz[a,h]anthracene and methylcholanthrene. *J. Org. Chem.*, **1**, 347–53.
10. Bachmann, W. E. & Bradbury, J. T. (1937). Synthesis of 8-phenyl-7,12-dialkyl-7,12-dihydro-7,12-dihydroxyBAs and related compounds. *J. Org. Chem.*, **2**, 175–82.
11. Bachmann, W. E. & Chemerda, J. M. (1938). The synthesis of 7,12-DMBA, 7,12-DEBA and 7,8,12-TMBA. *J. Am. Chem. Soc.*, **60**, 1023–6.
12. Bachmann, W. E. & Chemerda, J. M. (1939). Synthesis of 7,12-dialkylBAs. *J. Am. Chem. Soc.*, **61**, 2358–61.
13. Bachmann, W. E. & Chemerda, J. M. (1941). The synthesis of 7,10,12-TMBA and 7,11,12-TMBA. *J. Org. Chem.*, **6**, 36–49.

64   *Chemistry*

14. Bachmann, W. E. & Cortes, G. D. (1943). Phenanthrene derivatives. XI. Acetylation and succinoylation of 3-methylphenanthrene. *J. Am. Chem. Soc.*, **65**, 1329–34.
15. Bachmann, W. E., Cronyn, M. W. & Struve, W. S. (1947). Reactions of 1,2,3,4-tetrahydrophenanthrene and derivatives. III. Alkyl derivatives and antimalarials. *J. Org. Chem.*, **12**, 596–605.
16. Bachmann, W. E. & Edgerton, R. O. (1940). Synthesis of 1-MBA and 5-methylchrysene. *J. Am. Chem. Soc.*, **62**, 2550–3.
17. Bachmann, W. E. & Pence, L. H. (1937). Reaction of alkali metals with polycyclic hydrocarbons. *J. Am. Chem. Soc.*, **59**, 2339–42.
18. Bachmann, W. E. & Safir, S. R. (1941). 7-Methylcholanthrene and 1,8-DMBA. *J. Am. Chem. Soc.*, **63**, 855–7.
19. Bachmann, W. E. & Wilds, A. L. (1938). Phenanthrene derivatives. IX. 1-Alkyl-1-hydroxytetrahydrophenanthrenes and related compounds. *J. Am. Chem. Soc.*, **60**, 624–7.
20. Backer, H. J. & Bij, J. R. (1943). Semicyclic dienes and their application to the synthesis of polynuclear compounds. *Rec. Trav. Chim.*, **62**, 561–79. *Chem. Abst.*, **39**, 3529[6].
21. Baddar, F. G., Dwidar, I. M. & Gindy, M. (1959). β-Aroylpropionic acids. Part IX. Their conversion into benz[a]anthraquinones. *J. Chem. Soc.*, 1002–9.
22. Badger, G. M. (1947a,b). (a) Oxidations and dehydrogenations with selenium dioxide. *J. Chem. Soc.*, 764–6. (b) PAH, XXXII, 2-methoxyBA and 2-methoxy-7,12-DMBA. *J. Chem. Soc.*, 940–3.
23. Badger, G. M. (1948). Polycyclic aromatic amines. Part I. *J. Chem. Soc.*, 1756–9.
24. Badger, G. M. (1949). An interpretation of some elimination reactions in disubstituted dihydro-derivatives of aromatic compounds. *J. Chem. Soc.*, 2497–501.
25. Badger, G. M. & Cook, J. W. (1939). The synthesis of growth-inhibitory polycyclic compounds. Part I. *J. Chem. Soc.*, 802–6.
26. Badger, G. M. & Cook, J. W. (1940). The synthesis of growth-inhibitory polycyclic compounds. Part II. *J. Chem. Soc.*, 409–12.
27. Badger, G. M., Cook, J. W. & Goulden, F. (1940). Polycyclic aromatic hydrocarbons. Part XXI. *J. Chem. Soc.*, 16–18.
28. Badger, G. M., Cook, J. W. & Ongley, P. A. (1950). The chemistry of the mitragyna genus. Part I. *J. Chem. Soc.*, 867–73.
29. Badger, G. M. & Gibb, A. R. M. (1949). Polycyclic aromatic amines. Part II. *J. Chem. Soc.*, 799–803.
30. Badger, G. M., Goulden, F. & Warren, F. L. (1941). Polycyclic aromatic hydrocarbons. Part XXVII. *J. Chem. Soc.*, 18–20.
31. Badger, G. M. & Mitchell, M. E. (1965). A 1,5-anionotropic rearrangement in a substituted benz[a]anthracene. *Aust. J. Chem.*, **18**, 919–21.
32. Badger, G. M. & Pearce, R. S. (1950). Substituted anthracene derivatives. Part II. An example of 1:5-anionotropic rearrangement. *J. Chem. Soc.*, 2311–14.
33. Badger, G. M. & Stephens, J. F. (1956). Fluorine-substituted polycyclic compounds. *J. Chem. Soc.*, 3637–40.
34. Bailey, W. (1959). Shell Development Corp., Private communication.
35. Bailey, W. J. & Economy, J. (1955). Pyrolysis of esters. III. Synthesis of 2-vinylbutadiene. *J. Am. Chem. Soc.*, **77**, 1133–6.
36. Barner, B. A. & Meyers, A. I. (1984). Asymmetric addition to chiral naphthyloxazolines. *J. Am. Chem. Soc.*, **106**, 1506–7.

37. Bavin, P. M. G. (1962). 5,6-Dimethylbenz[a]anthracene and 5,6-dimethyl-benzo[c]phenanthrene. *Can. J. Chem.*, **40**, 1399–402.
38. Beckwith, A. L. J. & See, L. B. (1964). Some reactions of anthracene, benz[a]anthracene and benzo[a]pyrene with thiols and oxygen. *Aust. J. Chem.*, **17**, 109–18.
39. Bentov, M. & Bergmann, E. D. (1963). Synthesis of some fluorinated benz[a]anthracenes. *Bull. Soc. Chim. France*, 963–6.
40. Bergmann, E. D. & Blum, J. (1960). Dehalogenation in the Elbs reaction. *J. Org. Chem.*, **25**, 474–5.
41. Bergmann, E. D. & Blum, J. (1961). Further observations on the Elbs reaction. *J. Org. Chem.*, **26**, 3214–16.
42. Bergmann, E. D. & Blum, J. (1962). Fluorine substituted benz[a]anthracene and benzo[c]phenanthrene derivatives and related compounds. *J. Org. Chem.*, **27**, 527–33.
43. Bergmann, E. D., Blum, J. & Butanaro, S. (1961). An unusual halogen exchange reaction. *J. Org. Chem.*, **26**, 3211–14.
44. Bergmann, E. D., Blum, J., Butanaro, S. & Heller, A. (1959). Fluoro derivatives of polycyclic carcinogenic compounds. *Tetrahedron Lett.*, 15–18.
45. Blackburn, G. M., Flavell, A. J., Orgee, L., Will, J. P. & Williams, G. M. (1981). The preparation of some specifically tritium labelled carcinogenic hydrocarbons and their covalent binding to DNA. *J. Chem. Soc., Perkin Trans.* I, 3196–204.
46. Blum, J., Grauer, F. & Bergmann, E. D. (1969). Synthesis of 12-F-7-MBA and 7-FBA. *Tetrahedron*, **25**, 3501–7.
47. Blum, J., Yona, I., Tsaroom, S. & Sasson, Y. (1979). K-Region imines of some carcinogenic aromatic hydrocarbons. *J. Org. Chem.*, **44**, 4178–82.
48. Bradsher, C. K. (1940). 7-Methyl- and 12-methylbenz[a]anthracenes. *J. Am. Chem. Soc.*, **62**, 1077–8.
49. Bradsher, C. K. & Webster, S. T. (1958). Further extension of the base-catalyzed cyclization. *J. Org. Chem.*, **23**, 482–3.
50. Brass, K. & Fanta, K. (1936). Molecular compounds of polycyclic hydrocarbons and their quinones with polynitro compounds and with metal salts. *Ber.*, **69B**, 1–11. *Chem. Abst.*, **30**, 2959[2,3].
51. Brown, P. M. & Thomson, R. H. (1976). A synthesis of tetrangulol(1,8-dihydroxy-3-methylBAQ. *J. Chem. Soc., Perkin Trans.* I, 997–1000.
52. Buchta, E. & Zoellner, R. (1968). Benzo[a]pyrene and BA. *Annalen*, **716**, 102–5.
53. Burger, A. & Mosettig, E. (1937). Studies in phenanthrene series XV. Observations on substitution in 9,10-dihydrophenanthrene: tetracyclic compounds derived from it. *J. Am. Chem. Soc.*, **59**, 1302–7.
54. Burr, J. G. Jr., Holton, W. F. & Webb, C. N. (1950). Some compounds of interest in cancer chemotherapy. *J. Am. Chem. Soc.*, **72**, 4903–6.
55. Buu-Hoi, N. P. & Lavit, D. (1960). Synthesis and properties of benz[a]anthracene-d_6 and dibenzo[a,h]anthracene-d_6. *Bull. Soc. Chim. France*, **2**, 346–8.
56. Carothers, W. H. & Coffman, D. D. (1932). Homologs of chloroprene and their polymers. *J. Am. Chem. Soc.*, **54**, 4071–6.
57. Carruthers, W. & Watkins, D. A. M. (1964). The constituents of high-boiling petroleum distillates. VIII. Identification of 1,2,3,4-tetrahydro-2,2,9-trimethyl-picene in American crude oil. *J. Chem. Soc.*, 724–9.
58. Cason, J. & Fieser, L. F. (1940). Synthesis of 4,11-dihydroxydibenzo[a,h]-anthracene and its relation to products of metabolism of the hydrocarbon. *J. Am. Chem. Soc.*, **62**, 2681–7.

59. Cason, J. & Phillips, D. D. (1952). The synthesis of 1,12-dimethylbenz[a]-anthracene. *J. Org. Chem.*, **17**, 298–312.

60. Cason, J. & Wordie, J. D. (1950). Syntheses in the peri substituted naphthalene series. *J. Org. Chem.*, **15**, 617–26.

61. Catch, J. R. & Evans, E. A. (1957). ^{14}C-Labelled polycyclic aromatic hydrocarbons. *Chem. Ind. (London)*, 78–9.

62. Cavalieri, E. & Calvin, M. (1976). Charge localization in the carbonium ions of MBAs. *J. Org. Chem*, **41**, 2676–9.

63. Chatterjea, J. N., Banerji, K. D. & Mukherjee, H. (1963). Stobbe reactions with diethyl homophthalate. *J. Indian Chem. Soc.*, **40**, 45–52.

64. Chatterjee, D. N. & Bhattacharjee, S. P. (1974). Friedel–Crafts condensation of the lactone of 4-methyl-2-hydroxycyclohexylacetic acid with aromatic hydrocarbons. II. Condensation with *p*-xylene and tetralin. *Indian J. Chem.*, **12**, 958–61.

65. Chatterjee, D. N. & Chakravorty, S. R. (1972). Synthesis and rearrangement of disubstituted spiranes. *Curr. Sci.*, **41**, 526–7.

66. Chatterjee, D. N. & Chakravorty, S. R. (1976). Studies in the rearrangement of spiranes. IV. *J. Indian Chem. Soc.*, **53**, 610–16.

67. Chatterjee, D. N. & Guha, J. (1982). Synthesis of a tetrahydronaphthalene-2,2-spirocyclopentane derivative and its rearrangement on catalytic dehydrogenation. *Curr. Sci.*, **51**, 233–4.

68. Christol, H., Koulodo, D. D., Mousseron, M. & Plenat, F. (1960). Polycyclic compounds. II. Ketones and hydrocarbons derived from 6,7-cyclenotetralones. *Bull. Soc. Chim. France*, 1576–81.

69. Clar, E. (1930). PAHs and their derivatives. VI. Synthesis of dibenzo[a,l]pyrene and its derivatives. *Ber.*, **63B**, 112–20.

70. Clar, E. (1932). Distribution of the double bonds in condensed aromatic hydrocarbons. *Ber.*, **65B**, 503–19.

71. Clar, E. & Stewart, D. G. (1951). Aromatic hydrocarbons. Part LIX. Dibenzo[a,l]pyrene. *J. Chem. Soc.*, 687–90.

72. Collins, C. J., Burr, J. G., Jr. & Hess, D. N. (1951). Studies on the Wagner rearrangement. II. The synthesis and structure determination of benz[a]anthracene-5,6-C[14]. *J. Am. Chem. Soc.*, **73**, 5176–8.

73. Cook, J. W. (1930). PAH. Part I. 1- and 2-Phenylanthracenes and derivatives of BA. *J. Chem. Soc.*, 1087–95.

74. Cook, J. W. (1931). Polycyclic aromatic hydrocarbons. Part VI. Benzo[c]phenanthrene and its quinone. *J. Chem. Soc.*, 2524–8.

75. Cook, J. W. (1932). PAH. IX. The synthesis of methyl and isopropyl homologs of BA. *J. Chem. Soc.*, 456–72.

76. Cook, J. W. (1933). PAH. Part XII. The orientation of derivatives of BA with notes on the preparation of some new homologs. *J. Chem. Soc.*, 1592–7.

77. Cook, J. W. & Haslewood, G. A. D. (1934). The synthesis of 8,9-dimethylBAQ, a degradation product of desoxychloic acid. *J. Chem. Soc.*, 428–33.

78. Cook, J. W. & Haslewood, G. A. D. (1935). Synthetic uses of as-octahydrophenanthrene. *J. Chem. Soc.*, 767–70.

79. Cook, J. W. & Hewett, C. L. (1933). Polycyclic aromatic hydrocarbons. Part XI. The acetylation of benz[a]anthracene. *J. Chem. Soc.*, 1408–10.

80. Cook, J. W. & Hewett, C. L. (1934). The synthesis of compounds related to the sterols, bile acids, and oestrus-producing hormones. Part II. The formation of some tetracyclic hydroaromatic compounds. *J. Chem. Soc.*, 365–77.

81. Cook, J. W. & Lawrence, C. A. (1937). The synthesis of polyterpenoid compounds. Part III. *J. Chem. Soc.*, 817–27.

82. Cook, J. W. & Martin, R. H. (1940). PAH. XXIV. *J. Chem. Soc.*, 1125–7.
83. Cook, J. W. & Robinson, A. M. (1938). PAH. XVII. Completion of the synthesis of the twelve MBAs. *J. Chem. Soc.*, 505–13.
84. Cook, J. W. & Robinson, A. M. (1940). PAH. XXIII. *J. Chem. Soc.*, 303–4.
85. Cook, J. W., Robinson, A. M. & Goulden, F. (1937). PAH. XV. New homologs of BA. *J. Chem. Soc.*, 393–6.
86. Cook, J. W. & Schoental, R. (1948). Oxidation of carcinogenic hydrocarbons by osmium tetroxide. *J. Chem. Soc.*, 170–3.
87. Cook, J. W. & Schoental, R. (1952). 8-HydroxyBA and 1-hydroxydibenz[a,h]-anthracene. *J. Chem. Soc.*, 9–11.
88. Cook, J. W. & deWorms, C. G. M. (1939). PAH. XX. *J. Chem. Soc.*, 268–71.
89. Corey, E. J. & Chaykovsky, M. (1965). Dimethyloxosulfonium methylide and dimethylsulfonium methylide. Formation and application to organic synthesis. *J. Am. Chem. Soc.*, **87**, 1353–64.
90. Corey, E. J. & Kim, C. U. (1972). A new and highly effective method for the oxidation of primary and secondary alcohols to carbonyl compounds. *J. Am. Chem. Soc.*, 7586–7.
91. Cristol, S. J. & Caspar, M. L. (1968). meso-Dihydroanthracene chemistry. II. The preparation of 1,5- and 1,8-dimethylanthraquinones. *J. Org. Chem.*, **33**, 2020–5.
92. Crowter, D. G., Evans, E. A. & Rasdell, R. (1962). Generally-labelled tritiated carcinogenic PAHs at high specific activity. *Chem. Ind. (London)*, 1622–3.
93. Dallinga, G., Smit, P. J. & Mackor, E. L. (1958). Steric effects in the interaction between protons and aromatic hydrocarbons. In *Steric Effects in Conjugated Systems*, ed. G. W. Gray, pp. 150–9. Butterworths Scientific Publications: London.
94. Dansi, A. (1937). The Friedel–Crafts reaction between oxalyl chloride and benz[a]anthracene. *Gazz. Chim. Ital.*, **67**, 85–88. *Chem. Abst.*, **31**, 6227s.
95. Dansi, A. & Ferri, C. (1939a,b). (a) The substitution reactions of benz[a]anthracene. *Gazz. Chim. Ital.*, **69**, 195–8. *Chem. Abst.*, **33**, 7296[1]. (b) Benz[a]anthralyl-7-acetic acid. *Ricerca Sci.*, **10**, 178. *Chem. Abst.*, **34**, 415[6].
96. Defay, N. & Martin, R. H. (1955). Syntheses in the field of carcinogenic hydrocarbons. XII. The carcinogenic activity of 4,7,12-trimethylbenz[a]-anthracene. *Bull. Soc. Chim. Belges*, **64**, 210–20.
97. Desai, N. B. & Venkataraman, K. (1959). Raney nickel reductions. VIII. Synthesis of BA and 3- and 6-MBAs. *Tetrahedron*, **5**, 305–10.
98. Descamps, C. & Martin, R. H. (1952). Carcinogenic hydrocarbons. V. 4-M- and 4,7,12-TMBAs. *Bull. Soc. Chim. Belges*, **61**, 223–33.
99. Doadt, E. G., Iwao, M., Reed, J. N. & Snieckus, V. (1982). Synthesis of PAHs and aza-PAHs using aromatic amide directed metallation strategy. In *PAH: Formation, Metabolism and Measurement*, eds M. Cooke & A. J. Dennis, pp. 413–25. Battelle Press (Pub. 1983): Columbus.
100. Dodsworth, D. J., Calcagno, M., Ehrmann, E. U., Devadas, B. & Sammes, P. G. (1981). A new route to anthraquinones. *J. Chem. Soc., Perkin Trans. I*, 2120–4.
101. Dziewonski, K. & Ritt, E. (1927). Synthesis of hydrocarbons of the benz[a]anthracene group. *Bull. Int. Acad. Polonaise*, 181–92. *Chem. Abst.*, **22**, 2561[7].

68   Chemistry

102. Elbs, K. & Larsen, E. (1884). Uber paraxylyl phenyl keton. *Ber.*, **17**, 2847–9.
103. Emmerich, H. & Schmialek, P. (1966). Eine Methode zur Darstellung Tritiummarkierter cancerogener polycyclischer Kohlenwasserstoffe mit extrem hoher spezifischer Aktivitat. *Z. Naturforsch.*, **21b**, 855–8.
104. Evans, E. A. (1957). ¹⁴C-Labelled PAHs. Part II. The synthesis of benz[a]anthracene and some methyl-substituted ¹⁴C-benz[a]anthracenes. *J. Chem. Soc.*, 2790–6.
105. Fieser, L. F. (1933). Some further derivatives of pleiadene. *J. Am. Chem. Soc.*, **55**, 4977–84.
106. Fieser, L. F. (1937). Cancer-producing hydrocarbons. In *Chemistry of Natural Products Related to Phenanthrene*, pp. 81–110. Reinhold: New York.
107. Fieser, L. F. & Clapp, R. C. (1941). Synthesis of 3-isopropyl-7-MBA from 9,10-dihydroretene. *J. Am. Chem. Soc.*, **63**, 319–23.
108. Fieser, L. F. & Creech, H. J. (1939). The conjugation of amino acids with isocyanates of the anthracene and benz[a]anthracene series. *J. Am. Chem. Soc.*, **61**, 3502–6.
109. Fieser, L. F. & Desreux, V. (1938). The synthesis of 2- and 6-substituted derivatives of 20-methylcholanthrene. *J. Am. Chem. Soc.*, **60**, 2255–62.
110. Fieser, L. F. & Dietz, E. M. (1929). 7,12-Benz[a]anthraquinone. *J. Am. Chem. Soc.*, **51**, 3141–8.
111. Fieser, L. F. & Fieser, M. (1933). The conversion of phthaloylnaphthalenes and naphthoyl-2-benzoic acids into benzathraquinones. *J. Am. Chem. Soc.*, **55**, 3342–52.
112. Fieser, L. F. & Haddadin, M. J. (1965). Isobenzofurane, a transient intermediate. *Can. J. Chem.*, **43**, 1599–606.
113. Fieser, L. F. & Hartwell, J. L. (1938). Meso aldehydes of anthracene and benz[a]anthracene. *J. Am. Chem. Soc.*, **60**, 2555–9.
114. Fieser, L. F., Hartwell, J. L. & Seligman, A. M. (1936). Concerning the mechanism of the Hooker oxidation. *J. Am. Chem. Soc.*, **58**, 1223–8.
115. Fieser, L. F. & Hershberg, E. B. (1937a,b,c). (a) 7-Substituted benz[a]anthracene derivatives. *J. Am. Chem. Soc.*, **59**, 1028–36. (b) 1,2,3,4-Tetrahydro-7-isopropyl-benz[a]anthracene. *Ibid.*, **59**, 2331–5. (c) Reduction and hydrogenation of compounds of the benz[a]anthracene series. *Ibid.*, **59**, 2502–9.
116. Fieser, L. F. & Hershberg, E. B. (1938). Substitution reactions and meso derivatives of BA. *J. Am. Chem. Soc.*, **60**, 1893–6.
117. Fieser, L. F. & Hershberg, E. B. (1939). Inter- and intra-molecular acylations with hydrogen fluoride. *J. Am. Chem. Soc.*, **61**, 1272–81.
118. Fieser, L. F. & Hershberg, E. B. (1940). Further observations on the use of hydrogen fluoride in acylations and cyclizations. *J. Am. Chem. Soc.*, **62**, 49–53.
119. Fieser, L. F., Hershberg, E. B., Long, L., Jr. & Newman, M. S. (1937). Hydroxy derivatives of benzo[a]pyrene and BA. *J. Am. Chem. Soc.*, **59**, 475–8.
120. Fieser, L. F. & Heymann, H. (1941). Synthesis of 11-hydroxybenzo[a]pyrene and 11-methylbenzo[a]pyrene. *J. Am. Chem. Soc.*, **63**, 2333–40.
121. Fieser, L. F. & Johnson, W. S. (1939a,b). (a) 11-MBA. *J. Am. Chem. Soc.*, **61**, 168–71. (b) Syntheses in the BA and chrysene series. *Ibid.*, **61**, 1647–54.
122. Fieser, L. F. & Johnson, W. S. (1940). Synthesis of 5-hydroxybenzo[a]pyrene and 8-i-PBA from 9,10-dihydrophenanthrene. *J. Am. Chem. Soc.*, **62**, 575–7.

123. Fieser, L. F. & Jones, R. N. (1938). Synthesis of 6,12- and 6,7-dimethyl-benz[a]anthracenes. *J. Am. Chem. Soc.*, **60**, 1940–5.
124. Fieser, L. F. & Newman, M. S. (1936). The synthesis of benz[a]anthracene derivatives related to cholanthrene. *J. Am. Chem. Soc.*, **58**, 2376–82.
125. Fieser, L. F. & Peters, M. A. (1932). Rearrangements in the condensation of methylated derivatives of 2-(α-naphthoyl)benzoic acid. *J. Am. Chem. Soc.*, **54**, 3742–51.
126. Fieser, L. F. & Seligman, A. M. (1936). An improved method for the synthetic preparation of 3-methylcholanthrene. *J. Am. Chem. Soc.*, **58**, 2482–7.
127. Fieser, L. F. & Seligman, A. M. (1938). 1-M- and 1,7-DMBAs. *J. Am. Chem. Soc.*, **60**, 170–176.
128. Fieser, L. F. & Seligman, A. M. (1939). Synthetic routes to meso substituted benz[a]anthracene derivatives. *J. Am. Chem. Soc.*, **61**, 136–42.
129. Flesher, J. W., Soedigdo, S. & Kelley, D. R. (1967). Syntheses of metabolites of 7,12-dimethylbenz[a]anthracene, 4-hydroxy-7,12-dimethyl-benz[a]anthracene, 7-hydroxymethyl-12-methylbenz[a]anthracene, their methyl ethers and acetoxy derivatives. *J. Med. Chem.*, **10**, 932–6.
130. Fu, P. P., Cortez, C., Sukumaran, K. B. & Harvey, R. G. (1979). Synthesis of the isomeric phenols of benz[a]anthracene from benz[a]anthracene. *J. Org. Chem.*, **44**, 4265–71.
131. Fu, P. P. & Harvey, R. G. (1977). [G-^{3}H]-7,12-DMBA-5,6-oxide. *J. Labelled Compd. Radiopharm.*, **13**, 619–21.
132. Fu, P. P., Lee, H. M. & Harvey, R. G. (1980). Regioselective catalytic hydrogenation of PAHs under mild conditions. *J. Org. Chem.*, **45**, 2797–803.
133. Fu, P. P. & Yang, S. K. (1979). A simple method for synthesis of specific deuterium and tritium labelled methylhydroxylated derivatives of 7,12-DMBA. *J. Labelled Compd. Radiopharm.*, **16**, 819–26.
134. Fuson, R. C. & Wassmundt, F. W. (1956). The reaction of phenyl 2-methoxy-1-naphthoate with Grignard reagents. A new route to fluorenones. *J. Am. Chem. Soc.*, **78**, 5409–13.
135. Gandhi, R. P., Chander, K., Vig, O. P. & Mukherji, S. M. (1957). PAH. Part IV. Synthesis of some 6-MBAs. *J. Indian Chem. Soc.*, **34**, 163–8.
136. Gaponenko, V. I., Kozlov, Y. P. & Skvarchenko, V. R. (1968). Preparation of a series of labelled polycyclic hydrocarbons. *Nauch. Dokl. Vyssh. Shk., Biol. Nauki*, 149–52. *Chem. Abst.*, **70**, 57521v.
137. Gates, M. (1982). Condensation of naphthoquinones with polar ethylenes. A reexamination. *J. Org. Chem.*, **47**, 578–82.
138. Gilman, H. & Leeper, R. W. (1951). Organometallic compounds of lead, tin and germanium. *J. Org. Chem.*, **16**, 466–75.
139. Giovanella, B. C., Abell, C. W. & Heidelberger, C. (1962). Preparation and purification of tritiated carcinogenic hydrocarbons. *Cancer Res.*, **22**, 925–30.
140. Girke, W. & Bergmann, E. D. (1976). Synthesis of 6-FBA derivatives. *Ber.*, **109**, 1038–45.
141. Goh, S. H. & Harvey, R. G. (1973). K-Region arene oxides of carcinogenic aromatic hydrocarbons. *J. Am. Chem. Soc.*, **95**, 242–3.
142. Gomes, L. M. (1974). Application of benzyl-3,4-dicarbomethoxyfurans to synthesis of BA derivatives. *C.R. Hebd. Séances Acad. Sci.*, **279**, 417–20.
143. Gribble, G. W., Allen, R. W., Anderson, P. S., Christy, M. E. & Colton, C. D. (1976). Oxidative deamination of aromatic 1,4-imines. A new synthesis of PAHs. *Tetrahedron Lett.*, 3673–6.
144. Groggins, P. H. & Newton, H. P. (1930). Studies in the Friedel–Crafts reactions. Naphthalene series I. Preparation of BAQ. *Industr. Engng Chem.*, **22**, 157–9.

145. Gschwend, H. W. & Hamden, A. (1975). Ortho-lithiation of aryloxazolines. *J. Org. Chem.*, **40**, 2008–9.
146. Gupta, S. C. S. & Chatterjee, D. N. (1954). Studies in catalytic dehydrogenation. *J. Indian Chem. Soc.*, **31**, 11–16.
147. Hadler, H. I. (1955). The synthesis of 7,12-DMBA-7,12-C^{14}. *J. Am. Chem. Soc.*, **77**, 1052–3.
148. Hadler, H. I. & Kryger, A. C. (1960). K-Region fission and addition products of 7,12-DMBA. *J. Org. Chem.*, **25**, 1896–901.
149. Hadler, H. I. & Raha, C. R. (1957). Synthesis of C^{14}-labelled anthracene, 9-methylanthracene and BA. *J. Org. Chem.*, **22**, 433–5.
150. Hallmark, R. K., Manning, W. B. & Muschik, G. M. (1981). The preparation of specifically deuterium-labelled BAs and 7,12-DMBAs. *J. Labelled Compd. Radiopharm.*, **18**, 331–45.
151. Harvey, R. G. (1985). Synthesis of the dihydrodiol and diol epoxide metabolites of carcinogenic polycyclic hydrocarbons. In *Polycyclic Hydrocarbons and Carcinogenesis. Am. Chem. Soc.* Symposium Series 283, American Chemical Society Monograph, pp. 35–62.
152. Harvey, R. G. & Arzadon, L. (1969). Metal ammonia reduction. V. The stereochemistry of reductive alkylation. *Tetrahedron*, **25**, 4887–94.
153. Harvey, R. G., Arzadon, L., Grant, J. & Urberg, K. (1969). Metal ammonia reduction. IV. Single stage reduction of polycyclic aromatic hydrocarbons. *J. Am. Chem. Soc.*, **91**, 4535–41.
154. Harvey, R. G., Cortez, C. & Jacobs, S. A. (1982). Synthesis of PAH via a novel annelation method. *J. Org. Chem.*, **47**, 2120–5.
155. Harvey, R. G., Goh, S. H. & Cortez, C. (1975). K-Region oxides and related oxidized metabolites of carcinogenic aromatic hydrocarbons. *J. Am. Chem. Soc.*, **97**, 3468–79.
156. Harvey, R. G. & Urberg, K. (1968). Metal–ammonia reduction. III. Stepwise transformation of PAH. *J. Org. Chem.*, **33**, 2206–11.
157. Hauptmann, S. & Hartig, S. (1963). Uber den Mechanismus der Reaktion von Oxalyl Bromide mit Aromaten in Abwesenheit von Katalysatoren. *J. Prakt. Chem.*, **20**, 197–201.
158. Haworth, R. D. & Mavin, C. R. (1933). A new route to chrysene and BA. *J. Chem. Soc.*, 1012–16.
159. Hayashi, M. (1927). A new isomerism of halogenohydroxybenzoyltoluic acids. *J. Chem. Soc.*, 2516–27.
160. Hayashi, M. (1930*a*,*b*,*c*). (*a*) A new isomerism of halogenohydroxybenzoyltoluic acids, Part II. 2-(5′-Chloro-2′-hydroxybenzoyl)-5(4?)-methylbenzoic acid. *J. Chem. Soc.*, 1513–19. (*b*) A new isomerism of halogenohydroxybenzoyltoluic acids. Part III. 2-(3′-Chloro-4′-hydroxybenzoyl)-3(or 6)-methylbenzoic acid. *Ibid.*, 1520–3. (*c*) A new isomerism of halogenohydroxybenzoyltoluic acids. Part IV. 2-(4′-Chloro-2′-hydroxybenzoyl)-3(or 6)-methylbenzoic acid. *Ibid.*, 1524–8.
161. Hayashi, M. & Turuoka, S. (1935). Derivatives of benzoylbenzoic acids. II. 3-Methyl-2-benzoylbenzoic acid and 6-methyl-2-benzoylbenzoic acid. *J. Chem. Soc. Japan*, **56**, 1084–92.
162. Hayashi, M., Turuoka, S., Morikawa, I. & Namikawa, H. (1936). Studies on the derivatives of benzoylbenzoic acids. *Bull. Soc. Chem. Japan*, **11**, 184–200.
163. Hewett, C. L. (1942). The condensation of some aromatic ketones with ethyl succinate. *J. Chem. Soc.*, 585–7.
164. Hulin, B. & Koreeda, M. (1984). A convenient mild method for the cyclization of 3- and 4-arylalkanoic acids via their trifluoromethanesulfonic anhydride derivatives. *J. Org. Chem.*, **49**, 207–9.

165. Inbasekaran, M. N., Witiak, D. T., Barone, K. & Loper, J. C. (1980). Synthesis and mutagenicity of A-ring reduced analogues of 7,12-DMBA. *J. Med. Chem.*, **23**, 278–81.
166. Inhoffen, H. H., Stoeck, G. & Lubcke, E. (1949). Total synthesis of 1,9-DMBA and 1,8,9-TMBA. *Annalen*, **563**, 177–85.
167. Ioffe, I. S. & Fedorova, N. M. (1941). The reaction of sulfonation. VII. Sulfonation of 7,12-benz[a]anthraquinone by sulfuric acid. *J. Gen. Chem. (U.S.S.R.)*, **11**, 619–25. *Chem. Abst.*, **35**, 6952[3].
168. Ioffe, I. S. & Fedorova, N. M. (1944). Sulfonation reaction. VIII. Sulfonation of 7,12-benz[a]anthraquinone with fuming sulfuric acid. *J. Gen. Chem. (U.S.S.R.)*, **14**, 88–95. *Chem. Abst.*, **39**, 927[6].
169. Ivanov, C. & Mladenova-Orlinova, L. (1964). A new synthesis of derivatives of benz[a]anthrone and dibenzo[a,h]anthrone. *Angew. Chem.*, **76**, 301–2.
170. Jacobs, S. A. & Harvey, R. G. (1981). Synthesis of 3-methylcholanthrene. *Tetrahedron Lett.*, **22**, 1093–6.
171. Jacquignon, P. & Croisy-Delcey, M. (1973). Formylation and oxidation of methylated homolog of benz[a]anthracene by lead tetraacetate. *C.R. Hebd. Séances Acad. Sci.*, **276**, 955–8.
172. Jerina, D. M. & Daly, J. W. (1976). Oxidation at carbon. In *Drug Metabolism – From Microbe to Man*, eds. D. V. Park & R. L. Smith, pp. 13–32. Taylor & Francis Ltd.: London.
173. Johnson, E. H., Weinmayr, V. & Adams, R. (1932). Substitution products of 2-(1-naphthoyl)benzoic acid. *J. Am. Chem. Soc.*, **54**, 3289–95.
174. Jones, R. N., Gogek, C. J. & Sharpe, R. W. (1948). The reaction of maleic anhydride with PAHs. *Can. J. Res.*, **26B**, 719–27.
175. Kelly, T. R., Magee, J. A. & Weibel, F. R. (1980). Synthesis of chartreusin aglycone. *J. Am. Chem. Soc.*, **102**, 798–9.
176. Kennaway, E. & Cook, J. W. (1932). Ring system of sterols and bile acids. *Chem. Ind. (London)*, 521.
177. Kloetzel, M. C., Broussalian, G. L., Warren, C. K. & Field, J. B. (1961). Polynuclear hydrocarbon derivatives. XI. Octadecanoylbenz[a]anthracenes and their derivatives. *J. Org. Chem.*, **26**, 1748–54.
178. Knapp, W. (1932). Action of o-phthaloyl chloride on 2-methoxynaphthalene and methyl-2-naphthyl sulfide. *Monatsh. Chem.*, **60**, 189–204.
179. Konieczny, M. & Harvey, R. G. (1979). Efficient reduction of polycyclic quinones, hydroquinones, and phenols to PAHs with hydriodic acid. *J. Org. Chem.*, **44**, 4813–16.
180. Krohn, K. & Baltus, W. (1982). Note on the synthesis of benz[a]anthraquinones. *Annalen*, 1579–81.
181. Larner, B. W. & Peters, A. T. (1952). New intermediates and dyes. III. *J. Chem. Soc.*, 1368–73.
182. Lee, H. M. & Harvey, R. G. (1979). Synthesis of biologically active metabolites of 7-MBA. *J. Org. Chem.*, **44**, 4948–53.
183. Letsinger, R. L., Jamison, J. D. & Hussey, A. S. (1961). Reactions of 2-benzhydrylphenylacetic acid; a new pyrone synthesis. *J. Org. Chem.*, **26**, 97–102.
184. Levy, L. A. & Kumar, S. V. P. (1983). Synthesis of methyl substituted BAs and BA derivatives. *Tetrahedron Lett.*, **24**, 1221–4.
185. Levy, L. A. & Pruitt, L. (1980). An expeditious synthesis of BA and some of its oxygenated derivatives. *J. Chem. Soc., Chem. Commun.*, 227–8.
186. Lijinsky, W. & Garcia, H. (1963). Preparation of carcinogenic polynuclear hydrocarbons labelled with tritium by Wilzbach's method. *Nature*, **197**, 688–90.

187. Lopp, A. & Gubergrits, M. (1981). Photochemical and thermal decomposition of 7,12-epidioxy-7,12-DMBA. *Zh. Obshch. Khim.*, **51**, 225–30. *Chem. Abst.*, **94**, 191271n.

188. Mackor, E. L., Dallinga, G., Kruizinga, J. H. & Hofstra, A. (1956). The basicities of the MBAs. *Rec. Trav. Chim.*, **75**, 836–44.

189. Manning, W. B. (1979). Regiochemical control in the Diels–Alder reactions of substituted naphthoquinones: orientation in the synthesis of BAQs. *Tetrahedron Lett.*, 1661–4.

190. Manning, W. B. (1981). Substituted styrene cycloaddition to juglone and derivatives – regiochemical control. *Tetrahedron Lett.*, **22**, 1571–4.

191. Manning, W. B. & Muschik, G. M. (1980). Synthetic precursors of BAs. 3,9- and 3,10-DimethoxyBAQs. *J. Chem. E ng Data.*, **25**, 289–90.

192. Manning, W. B., Muschik, G. M. & Tomaszewski, J. E. (1979). Preparation of derivatives of 8-, 9-, 10-, and 11-hydroxybenz[a]anthracene-7,12-diones, BAs and 7,12-DMBAs. *J. Org. Chem.*, **44**, 699–702.

193. Manning, W. B., Tomaszewski, J. E., Muschik, G. M. & Sato, R. I. (1977). A general synthesis of 1-, 2-, 3- and 4-substituted BAQs. *J. Org. Chem.*, **42**, 3465–8.

194. Manning, W. B. & Wilbur, D. J. (1980). Isolation and structure of the oxidized Diels–Alder adducts of certain styrenes and 1,4-naphthoquinone. *J. Org. Chem.*, **45**, 733–4.

195. Marschalk, C. & Dassigny, J. (1948). Structural problems in the BA series. *Bull. Soc. Chim. France*, 812–14.

196. Marschalk, C. & Dassigny, J. (1952). Problems of constitution in the BA series. *Bull. Soc. Chim. France*, 805–8.

197. Martin, R. H. (1943). Polymethylbenzoylnaphthoic acids. *J. Chem. Soc.*, 239–41.

198. Martin, R. H. & Stoffyn, P. (1950). Syntheses of carcinogenic hydrocarbons. *Bull. Soc. Chim. Belges*, **59**, 208–22. *Chem. Abst.*, **45**, 7095b.

199. Maruyama, K. & Otsuki, T. (1975). A photochemical reaction of 2-alkoxy-3-bromo-1,4-naphthoquinone with 1,1-diarylethylenes – a novel method of 5-aryl-7,12-BAQ synthesis. *Chem. Lett.*, 87–8.

200. Maruyama, K., Otsuki, T. & Mitsui, K. (1980a). Facile photochemical synthesis of polycyclic aromatic compounds. *J. Org. Chem.*, **45**, 1424–8.

201. Maruyama, K., Otsuki, T. & Mitsui, K. (1976). The photochemical synthesis of 5-aryl-7,12-BAQs from 1,4-naphthoquinones and 1,1-diarylethylenes. *Bull. Chem. Soc. Japan*, **49**, 3361–2.

202. Maruyama, K., Tai, S., Tojo, M. & Otsuki, T. (1981). Photochemical reaction of 2-bromo-3-methoxy-1,4-naphthoquinone with silylenol ether – one-pot synthesis of polycyclic aromatic compounds. *Heterocycles*, **16**, 1963–74.

203. Maruyama, K., Tojo, M., Iwamoto, H. & Otsuki, T. (1980b). Regioselective synthesis of D-ring substituted BAs by a one-pot photochemical reaction. *Chem. Lett.*, *Chem. Soc. Japan*, 827–30.

204. Marvel, C. S., Pearson, D. E. & Patterson, L. A. (1940). Cyclization of dienynes. VIII. Ring closures with alpha and beta cyclohexenylacetylene derivatives of octalin. *J. Am. Chem. Soc.*, **62**, 2659–65.

205. Matsuoka, M., Okamoto, T., Kitao, T. & Konishi, K. (1973). Synthesis of 8,11-disubstituted-7,12-BAQ dyes. *Nippon Kag. Kaishi*, 1328–32. *Chem. Abst.*, **79**, 106110g.

206. McCarthy, T. J., Connor, W. F. & Rosenfeld, S. M. (1978). Stereospecific addition of dimethylsulfonium methylide to 9,10-anthraquinone. *Synthetic Commun.*, **8**, 379–82.

207. Meyers, A. I., Temple, D. L., Haidukewych, D. & Mihelich, E. D. (1974).

Oxazolines. XI. Synthesis of functionalized aromatic and aliphatic acids. A useful protecting group for carboxylic acids against Grignard and hydride reagents. *J. Org. Chem.*, **39**, 2787–93.

208. Middleton, W. J. (1975). New fluorinating reagents. Dialkylaminosulfur fluorides. *J. Org. Chem.*, **40**, 574–8.

209. Mikhailov, B. M. (1946). Synthesis of polycyclic compounds. X. Mechanism of Wurtz reaction in the bimetallic derivatives of anthracene and benz[a]anthracene. *Izv. Akad. Nauk SSSR, Otdel Khim. Nauk*, 619–32. *Chem. Abst.*, **42**, 6350i.

210. Mikhailov, B. M. (1950). 7,12-DMBA. *Akad. Nauk SSSR, Inst. Org. Khim. Sintezy Org. Soedineii Sbornik I*, 56–7. *Chem. Abst.*, **47**, 8004i.

211. Mikhailov, B. M. & Blokhina, A. N. (1940). Synthesis of polycyclic compounds. IV. 12-Ethyl-7-methylbenz[a]anthracene and 12-ethyl-benz[a]anthracene, *J. Gen. Chem. (U.S.S.R.)*, **10**, 1793–7. *Chem. Abst.*, **35**, 4007[8].

212. Mikhailov, B. M. & Blokhina, A. N. (1949a,b). (a) Syntheses of polycyclic compounds. XIV. *Izv. Akad. Nauk SSSR, Otdel. Khim. Nauk*, 164–77. *Chem. Abst.*, **44**, 2962g. (b) Metalation of 9,10-dihydroanthracene and 7,12-DHBA. *Ibid*, 279–86. *Chem. Abst.*, **44**, 2963i.

213. Mikhailov, B. M. & Chernova, N. G. (1938). Synthesis of 7-alkyl derivatives of 12-methylbenz[a]anthracene. *C.R. Acad. Sci. URSS*, **20**, 579–81. *Chem. Abst.*, **33**, 5842[9].

214. Mikhailov, B. M. & Chernova, N. G. (1939). The Reformatsky reaction with 12-methyl-7-keto-7,12-dihydroBA. *J. Gen. Chem. (U.S.S.R.).*, **9**, 2171–2. *Chem. Abst.*, **34**, 4068[2].

215. Mikhailov, B. M. & Kozminskaya, T. K. (1947). Synthesis of polycyclic compounds. Methylation of anthracene and benz[a]anthracene. *Dokl. Akad. Nauk SSSR*, **58**, 811–13. *Chem. Abst.*, **45**, 9522f.

216. Mikhailov, B. M. & Kozminskaya, T. K. (1948). Synthesis of polycyclic compounds. New preparation of homologs of benz[a]anthracene. *Dokl. Akad. Nauk SSSR*, **59**, 509–11. *Chem. Abst.*, **42**, 6792[d].

217. Mikhailov, B. M. & Kozminskaya, T. K. (1951). Lithium compounds of BA and their reactions. *Zh. Obshch. Khim.*, **21**, 1276–83. *Chem. Abst.*, **46**, 2039g.

218. Mikhailov, B. M. & Kozminskaya, T. K. (1953). Syntheses in the series of BA with the aid of lithium reagents. *Zh. Obshch. Khim.*, **23**, 1220–4. *Chem. Abst.*, **47**, 12334f.

219. Mitra, A. K., Bannerjee, R. C. & Bhattacharya, R. (1971). A new synthesis of BA. *J. Indian Chem. Soc.*, **48**, 391–4.

220. Morreal, C. E. & Alks, V. (1975). BA derivatives via the Stobbe condensation. Synthesis of 3,9-dihydroxyBA. *J. Org. Chem.*, **40**, 3411–14.

221. Morreal, C. E. & Alks, V. (1977). Preparation of hydroxy derivatives of 7,12-DMBA. *J. Chem. Engng Data*, **22**, 118–21.

222. Morreal, C. E. & Bronstein, R. E. (1978). Synthesis of potentially estrogenic carcinogens: 3,9-dihydroxy-7,12-DMBA. *J. Chem. Engng Data*, **23**, 354–6.

223. Morreal, C. E., Sinha, D. K., Schneider, S. L., Bronstein, R. E. & Dawidzik, J. (1982). Antiestrogenic properties of substituted benz[a]anthracene-3,9-diols. *J. Med. Chem.*, **25**, 323–6.

224. Mosettig, E. & Kamp, V. D. J. (1930). Syntheses in the phenanthrene series. I. Acetylphenanthrenes. *J. Am. Chem. Soc.*, **52**, 3704–10.

225. Moszew, J. & Wachalewski, T. (1960). Synthetic plant growth regulators. VI. Benzyl derivatives of 1-naphthylacetic acid as plant growth regulators. *Roczniki Chem.*, **34**, 1387–96. *Chem. Abst.*, **55**, 22248i.

226. Mourev, H., Chovin, P. & Rivoal, G. (1946). Condensation of o-benzene-diacetonitrile with α-diketo compounds. Synthesis of aromatic and hydroaromatic polynuclear compounds. *Bull. Soc. Chim. France*, 106–9.

227. Mukherji, S. M. & Dabas, K. S. (1971a,b). (a) PAH. XVII. New syntheses of 4-M-, 1,6-DM- and 2,6-DMBAs. *Indian J. Chem.*, **9**, 1187–91. (b) PAH. XVIII. New approach to BAs. *Ibid.*, **9**, 1192–4.

228. Mukherji, S. M., Dhawan, S. N. & Handa, I. (1970c). PAH. XVI. Acid-catalyzed rearrangement of 2-oxo-4a-methyl-2,4a,5,6,8,9,10,11-octahydroBA. *Indian J. Chem.*, **8**, 864–7.

229. Mukherji, S. M., Handa, R. N. & Sharma, K. S. (1967). PAHs. X. Synthesis of BA by the Robinson–Mannich reaction. *Tetrahedron*, **23**, 3859–62.

230. Mukherji, S. M., Sawhney, S. N. & Sharma, K. S. (1965). PAHs. VI. A new synthesis of 6-MBA. *J. Indian Chem. Soc.*, **42**, 176–8.

231. Mukherji, S. M., Sharma, K. S. & Handa, R. N. (1966). BA derivatives by the Robinson–Mannich base synthesis. *Science Cult.*, **32**, 311.

232. Mukherji, S. M., Yadav, S. P. & Gandhi, R. P. (1970a,b). (a) PAH. XIV. New syntheses of 1-M- and 1,6-DMBAs. *Indian J. Chem.*, **8**, 679–82. (b) PAH. XV. Friedel–Crafts reaction of 9-methyl-1,2,3,4,4a,9,10,10a-octahydro-phenanthrene. *Ibid.*, **8**, 683–6.

233. Muller, A. & Hanke, F. G. (1949). Strukturanaloge Krebserzeugender Verbindungen. *Monatsh. Chem.*, **80**, 435–7. *Chem. Abst.*, **45**, 597i.

234. Muschik, G. M., Tomaszewski, J. E., Sato, R. I. & Manning, W. B. (1979). Synthesis of 1-, 2-, 3-, and 4-hydroxy isomers of BAQ, BA and 7,12-DMBA. *J. Org. Chem.*, **44**, 2150–3.

235. Nes, W. R. & Ford, D. L. (1962). The conversion of a steroid to 4,7-dimethyl-benz[a]anthracene by a model of a biochemical route. *Tetrahedron Lett.*, 209–12.

236. Nes, W. R. & Ford, D. L. (1963). The anthrasteroid rearrangement. XI. The conversion of anthrapregnatrien-20-one to 4,7-DMBA by a model of a biochemical route. *J. Am. Chem. Soc.*, **85**, 2137–41.

237. Newman, M. S. (1937). The synthesis of benz[a]anthracene derivatives related to benzo[a]pyrene. *J. Am. Chem. Soc.*, **59**, 1003–6.

238. Newman, M. S. (1938a,b). (a) The synthesis of 7,12-DMBA. *J. Am. Chem. Soc.*, **60**, 1141–2. (b) The synthesis of 8-chloro-7-methylbenz[a]anthracene and related compounds. *Ibid.*, **60**, 1368–70.

239. Newman, M. S. (1983). Synthesis of 7,11,12-TMBA. *J. Org. Chem.*, **48**, 3249–51.

240. Newman, M. S. & Addor, R. W. (1955). Synthesis and reactions of vinylene carbonate. *J. Am. Chem. Soc.*, **77**, 3789–93.

241. Newman, M. S. & Blum, S. (1964a,b,c,d). (a) Synthesis of fluorinated benz[a]anthracenes. *J. Org. Chem.*, **29**, 1414–16. (b) The synthesis of 6,8-dimethylbenz[a]anthracene and 6,7,8-trimethylbenz[a]anthracene. *J. Med. Chem.*, **7**, 466–8. (c) A new cyclization reaction leading to epoxides of aromatic hydrocarbons. *J. Am. Chem. Soc.*, **86**, 5598–600. (d) The behaviour of 3-fluorophthalic anhydride in Friedel–Crafts and Grignard reactions. *J. Org. Chem.*, **29**, 1416–18.

242. Newman, M. S., Cecil, J. H. & Hung, W. M. (1972). Synthesis of 5-fluoro-6,8-dimethylbenz[a]anthracene. *J. Med. Chem.*, **15**, 569–70.

243. Newman, M. S., Chatterji, R. & Seshadri (1961). The synthesis of 2-fluoro-7-methylbenz[a]anthracene. *J. Org. Chem.*, **26**, 2667–9.

244. Newman, M. S. & Cunico, R. F. (1972). The synthesis of 5-hydroxymethyl-, 5-acetoxymethyl-, and 5-mercapto-7,12-dimethylbenz[a]anthracenes and of 5,7,12-trimethylbenz[a]anthracene. *J. Med. Chem.*, **15**, 323–5.

245. Newman, M. S. & Davis, C. C. (1967). The syntheses of 5,6-dimethoxy-7,12-dimethylbenz[a]anthracene and 7,12-dimethyl-5,6-benz[a]anthraquinone. *J. Org. Chem.*, **32**, 66–8.
246. Newman, M. S., Dhawan, B. & Khanna, V. K. (1986). Synthesis of 10-hydroxymethyl-7,12-DMBA. *J. Org. Chem.*, **51**, 1631–2.
247. Newman, M. S. & Din, Z. U. (1971). A new synthesis of 7,12-dimethyl-benz[a]anthracene. *J. Org. Chem.*, **36**, 966–8.
248. Newman, M. S., Fikes, L. E., Hashem, M. M., Kannan, R. & Sankaran, V. (1978a). Synthesis and carcinogenic activity of 5-fluoro-7-(oxygenated methyl)-12-methylbenz[a]anthracenes. *J. Med. Chem.*, **21**, 1076–8.
249. Newman, M. S. & Galt, R. H. B. (1960). The syntheses of 3-fluoro- and 6-fluoro-7-methylbenz[a]anthracenes. *J. Org. Chem.*, **25**, 214–15.
250. Newman, M. S. & Gaertner, R. (1950). The synthesis of polynuclear aromatic hydrocarbons. Methylbenz[a]anthracenes. *J. Am. Chem. Soc.*, **72**, 264–73.
251. Newman, M. S. & George, M. V. (1961). The synthesis of 3,9-dimethyl-benz[a]anthracene. *J. Org. Chem.*, **26**, 4306–7.
252. Newman, M. S. & Hart, R. T. (1947). A new synthesis of benz[a]anthracene. *J. Am. Chem. Soc.*, **69**, 298–300.
253. Newman, M. S. & Hung, W. H. (1977). Structure–carcinogenic activity relationships in the benz[a]anthracene series. 1,7,12- and 2,7,12-trimethyl-benz[a]anthracenes. *J. Med. Chem..*, **20**, 179–81.
254. Newman, M. S. & Hussain, N. S. (1982). Synthesis of nuclear monobromo-benz[a]anthracenes. *J. Org. Chem.*, **47**, 2837–40.
255. Newman, M. S. & Ihrman, K. G. (1958). The behavior of o-aroylbenzoic acid types in acidic media. *J. Am. Chem. Soc.*, **80**, 3652–6.
256. Newman, M. S. & Kanakarajan, K. (1980). Synthesis of 8-hydroxy- and 11-hydroxy-7,12-dimethylbenz[a]anthracenes. *J. Org. Chem.*, **45**, 2301–4.
257. Newman, M. S. & Kannan, R. (1979). Syntheses of 8- and 9-fluoro-benzo[a]pyrenes and 9-fluoro- and 10-fluoro-7,12-dimethylbenz[a]anthracenes. *J. Org. Chem.*, **44**, 3388–90.
258. Newman, M. S. & Khanna, J. M. (1979). Synthesis of 12-fluoro-7-methyl-benz[a]anthracene and 7-fluoro-12-methylBA. *J. Org. Chem.*, **44**, 866–8.
259. Newman, M. S., Khanna, J. M., Kanakarajan, K. & Kumar, S. (1978b). Syntheses of 1-, 2-, 3-, 4-, 6-, 9-, and 10-hydroxy-7,12-dimethyl-benz[a]anthracenes. *J. Org. Chem.*, **43**, 2553–7.
260. Newman, M. S., Khanna, J. M., Khanna, V. K. & Kanakarajan, K. (1979a). Syntheses of 7,12-dimethylbenz[a]anthracene-3,4- and 1,4-diones. *J. Org. Chem.*, **44**, 4994–5.
261. Newman, M. S., Khanna, J. M. & Lilje, K. C. (1979b). Recommended syntheses for 7-methylbenz[a]anthracene, 12-methylbenz[a]anthracene, and 7,12-dimethylbenz[a]anthracene. *Org. Prep. Proc. Int.*, **11**, 271–4.
262. Newman, M. S. & Khanna, V. K. (1979). The synthesis of 10-fluoro-benzo[a]pyrene. *Bull. Soc. Chim. Belges*, **88**, 871–3.
263. Newman, M. S. & Khanna, V. K. (1980). Synthesis of 8-fluoro- and 10-fluoro-3-methylcholanthrenes. Observations on the Elbs reaction. *J. Org. Chem.*, **45**, 4507–8.
264. Newman, M. S., Kuivila, H. G. & Garrett, A. B. (1945). Normal and complex ionization of organic molecules in solvent sulfuric acid. *J. Am. Chem. Soc.*, **67**, 704–6.
265. Newman, M. S. & Kumar, S. (1978). A new 7,12-dimethylbenz[a]anthracene synthesis: 9-methoxy- and 10-methoxy-7,12-dimethylbenz[a]anthracenes. *J. Org. Chem.*, **43**, 370–1.

266. Newman, M. S. & Lilje, K. C. (1979). Synthesis of 7-fluorobenz[a]anthracene. *J. Org. Chem.*, **44**, 1347–8.

267. Newman, M. S., MacDowell, D. & Swaminathan, S. (1959). The synthesis of some monofluorobenz[a]anthracenes. *J. Org. Chem.*, **24**, 509–12.

268. Newman, M. S. & McCleary, C. D. (1941a,b). (a) Normal and pseudo esters of 2-benzoylbenzoic acid types. *J. Am. Chem. Soc.*, **63**, 1537–41. (b) The behavior of 3-methylphthalic anhydride in Friedel–Crafts and Grignard condensations. *Ibid.*, **63**, 1542–4.

269. Newman, M. S. & Naiki, K. (1962). The syntheses of 5-fluoro- and 4-fluoro-7,12-dimethylbenz[a]anthracenes. *J. Org. Chem.*, **27**, 863–5.

270. Newman, M. S. & Olson, D. R. (1974). A new hypothesis concerning the reactive species in carcinogenesis by 7,12-dimethylbenz[a]anthracene. The 5-hydroxy-7,12-dimethylbenz[a]anthracene–7,12-dimethylbenz[a]anthracen-5(6)one equilibrium. *J. Am. Chem. Soc.*, **96**, 6207–8.

271. Newman, M. S. & Orchin, M. (1938). The synthesis of 10-chloro-7-methyl-benz[a]anthracene and related compounds. *J. Am. Chem. Soc.*, **60**, 586–9.

272. Newman, M. S. & Orchin, M. (1939). The synthesis of 9-chloro-7-methyl-benz[a]anthracene and related compounds. *J. Am. Chem. Soc.*, **61**, 244–7.

273. Newman, M. S. & Otsuka, S. (1958). Syntheses of 1-M- and 4-MBAs. *J. Org. Chem.*, **23**, 797–9.

274. Newman, M. S., Prabhu, V. S. & Veeraraghavan, S. (1983). Synthesis of nuclear monobromobenz[a]anthracenes. *J. Org. Chem.*, **48**, 2926–8.

275. Newman, M. S., Sagar, W. C. & George, M. V. (1960). The synthesis of 1,12-dimethylbenz[a]anthracene. *J. Am. Chem. Soc.*, **82**, 2376–9.

276. Newman, M. S. & Sankaran, V. (1977). Improved synthesis of 7,12-dimethyl-benz[a]anthracene. *Tetrahedron Lett.*, 2067–8.

277. Newman, M. S., Sankaran, V. & Olson, D. R. (1976). Phenolic and ketonic tautomers in polycyclic aromatic hydrocarbons. *J. Am. Chem. Soc.*, **98**, 3237–42.

278. Newman, M. S. & Scheurer, P. R. (1956). The behavior of 3-chlorophthalic anhydride in Friedel–Crafts and Grignard condensations. *J. Am. Chem. Soc.*, **78**, 5004–7.

279. Newman, M. S. & Seshadri, S. (1962). The syntheses of 1-fluoro- and 1-fluoro-7-methylbenz[a]anthracenes. *J. Org. Chem.*, **27**, 76–8.

280. Newman, M. S., Swaminathan, S. & Chatterji, R. (1959). Synthesis of 9-fluoro-, 10-fluoro-, and 9-methoxy-7-methylbenz[a]anthracenes. *J. Org. Chem.*, **24**, 1961–4.

281. Newman, M. S. & Tuncay, A. (1980). Synthesis of 2-fluoro-7,12-dimethyl-benz[a]anthracene. *J. Org. Chem.*, **45**, 348–9.

282. Newman, M. S. & Veeraraghavan, S. (1983). Syntheses of 9-(trifluoromethyl)- and 10-(trifluoromethyl)-7,12-dimethylbenz[a]anthracenes. *J. Org. Chem.*, **48**, 3246–8.

283. Newman, M. S. & Venkateswaran, N. (1967). The syntheses of 4-bromo-7-methylbenz[a]anthracene and 4-chloro-7-methylbenz[a]anthracene. *J. Med. Chem.*, **10**, 728–9.

284. Newman, M. S., Venkateswaran, S. & Sankaran, V. (1975). Condensation of phthalaldehydic and o-acetylbenzoic acids with naphthalenes. *J. Org. Chem.*, **40**, 2996–7.

285. Newman, M. S. & Wise, P. H. (1941). The synthesis of 8-methoxy-7-methyl-benz[a]anthracene and related compounds. *J. Am. Chem. Soc.*, **63**, 2109–11.

286. Newman, M. S. & Wiseman, E. H. (1961). Synthesis of 11-fluoro-7-methyl-benz[a]anthracene. *J. Org. Chem.*, **26**, 3208–11.

287. Nicolaides, D. D. & Litinas, K. E. (1983). Bis–Wittig reaction of hexa-*p*-

phenyl-*o*-phenylenebismethylene-diphosphorane with *o*-quinones. Synthesis of polycyclic aromatic compounds. *J. Chem. Res.*, Synop., no. 3, 57.
288. O'Malley, R. F., Mariani, H. A., Buhler, D. R. & Jerina, D. M. (1981). Anodic fluorination of benz[a]anthracene. *J. Org. Chem.*, **46**, 2816–18.
289. Orchin, M. & Woolfolk, E. O. (1946). Molecular complexes with 2,4,7-trinitrofluorenone. *J. Am. Chem. Soc.*, **68**, 1727–9.
290. Pataki, J. & Balick, R. (1972). Relative carcinogenicity of some diethylbenz[a]anthracenes. *J. Med. Chem.*, **15**, 905–9.
291. Pataki, J. & Balick, J. (1974). Oxidation of 7,8,12-trimethylbenz[a]anthracene with lead tetraacetate. *Tetrahedron Lett.*, 3447–9.
292. Pataki, J. & Balick, R. F. (1977). Synthesis of potential metabolites of 7,12-dimethylbenz[a]anthracene. *J. Chem. Engng Data*, **22**, 114–15.
293. Pataki, J., Duguid, C., Rabideau, P. W., Huisman, H. & Harvey, R. G. (1971). Carcinogenic and adrenocorticolytic derivatives of benz[a]anthracene. *J. Med. Chem.*, **14**, 940–5.
294. Pataki, J., Wlos, R. & Cho, Y-J. (1968). Adrenocorticolytic derivatives of benz[a]anthracene. *J. Med. Chem.*, **11**, 1083–6.
295. Patrick, T. B., LeFaivre, M. H. & Koertge, T. E. (1976). Fluoroxytrifluoromethane reactions with polynuclear arenes. *J. Org. Chem.*, **41**, 3413–15.
296. Pearson, D. E., Cowan, D. & Beckler, J. D. (1959). A study of the entrainment method for making Grignard reagents. *J. Org. Chem.*, **24**, 504–9.
297. Peck, R. M. (1956). Functional derivatives of benz[a]anthracene. *J. Am. Chem. Soc.*, **78**, 997–1001.
298. Peck, R. M., O'Connell, A. P. & Creech, H. J. (1970). Relation of antitumor activity to structure in alkylating agents derived from PAH. *J. Med. Chem.*, **13**, 284–8.
299. Pepin, J. J., Andre-Louisfert, J. & Bisagni, E. (1970). Partially hydrogenated derivatives of 7,12-DMBA. III. Formation of octahydro-, decahydro- and dodecahydro-7,12-DMBAs. *Bull. Soc. Chim. France*, 3038–42.
300. Phillips, D. D. & Chatterjee, D. N. (1958*a*,*b*). (*a*) The Friedel–Crafts condensation of trans-2-hydroxycyclohexaneacetic acid lactone with aromatic hydrocarbons. II. *p*-Xylene, tetralin and 1-methylnaphthalene. *J. Am. Chem. Soc.*, **80**, 1911–15. (*b*) The Friedel–Crafts condensation of trans-2-hydroxycyclohexaneacetic acid lactone with aromatic hydrocarbons. I. Benzene and naphthalene. *J. Am. Chem. Soc.*, **80**, 1360–6.
301. Platt, K. L. & Oesch, F. (1981). Reductive cyclization of keto acids to polycyclic aromatic hydrocarbons by hydriodic acid–red phosphorus. *J. Org. Chem.*, **46**, 2601–3.
302. Poos, G. I., Arth, G. E., Beyler, R. E. & Sarett, L. H. (1953). Approaches to the total synthesis of adrenal steroids. *J. Am. Chem. Soc.*, **75**, 422–9.
303. Premasagar, V., Palaniswamy, V. A. & Eisenbraun, E. J. (1981). Methanesulfonic acid catalyzed cyclization of 3-arylpropanoic and 4-arylbutanoic acids to 1-indanones and 1-tetralones. *J. Org. Chem.*, **46**, 2974–6.
304. Priestly, G. M. & Warrener, R. N. (1972). A new route to isoindole and its derivatives. *Tetrahedron Lett.*, 4295–8.
305. Pullman, A. & Pullman, B. (1954). Sur les transformations métaboliques des hydrocarbures cancerogènes. *Bull. Soc. Chim. France*, **21**, 1097–104.
306. Rapson, W. S. & Shuttleworth, R. G. (1940). Production of polycyclic aromatic types through the cyclodehydration of unsaturated ketones. *J. Chem. Soc*, 636–41.
307. Reddy, M. P. & Rao, G. S. K. (1981). Applications of the Vilsmeier reaction. 13. Vilsmeier approach to PAHs. *J. Org. Chem.*, **46**, 5371–3.

308. Riegel, B. & Burr, J. G., Jr. (1948). Carcinogenic hydrocarbons. 9,11-DMBA and 8,9,11-TMBA. *J. Am. Chem. Soc.*, **70**, 1070–3.

309. Rigaudy, J., Barcelo, J. & Rabaud, M. (1969). Studies on 9-aminoanthracenes. V. Oxidation of 9-aminoanthracene. Diazotization by nitrogen oxides. *Bull. Soc. Chim. France*, 3538–49.

310. Rivett, D. E. A., Swain, G. & Todd, A. R. (1949). Some synthetic experiments leading to formation of MBAQs. *J. Chem. Soc.*, 37–42.

311. Rosen, B. I. & Weber, W. P. (1977). Synthesis of 7,12-benz[a]anthraquinones via Diels–Alder reaction of 1,4-phenanthraquinones. *J. Org. Chem.*, **42**, 3463–5.

312. Sammes, P. G. & Dodsworth, D. J. (1979). Simple one-step route to substituted anthraquinones. *J. Chem. Soc., Chem. Commun.*, 33–4.

313. Sandin, R. B. & Fieser, L. F. (1940). Synthesis of 7,12-dimethyl-benz[a]anthracene and of a thiophene isolog. *J. Am. Chem. Soc.*, **62**, 3098–105.

314. Sangaiah, R., Gold, A. & Toney, G. E. (1983). Synthesis of a series of novel polycyclic aromatic systems: isomers of BA containing a cyclopenta-fused ring. *J. Org. Chem.*, **48**, 1632–8.

315. Schoental, R. (1952). Friedel–Crafts succinoylation of anthracene. Synthesis of 1- and 4-hydroxyBAs. *J. Chem. Soc.*, 4403–6.

316. Scholl, R. & Neuberger, W. (1912). MBAQ Series. *Monatsh. Chem.*, **33**, 507–33. *Chem. Abst.*, **7**, 1494[8].

317. Scholl, R., Seer, C. & Zinke, A. (1921). MBAQ Series. *Monatsh. Chem.*, **41**, 583–602. *Chem. Abst.*, **15**, 3836[6].

318. Scholl, R. & Tritsch, W. (1911). MBAQ Series. *Monatsh. Chem.*, **32**, 997–1018. *Chem. Abst.*, **6**, 631[5].

319. Sempronj, A. (1939). Some derivatives of benz[a]anthracene-7,12-dione-7-sulfonic acid. *Gazz. Chim. Ital.*, **69**, 448–53. *Chem. Abst.*, **34**, 416[9].

320. Sharma, K. S. & Mukherji, S. M. (1966). PAH. VII. Synthesis of 3,6-DMBA. *J. Indian Chem. Soc.*, **43**, 197–203.

321. Sheikh, Y. M., Cazer, F. D., Hart, R. W. & Witiak, D. T. (1979). Facile preparation of 2- and 3-fluoro-7,12-dimethylbenz[a]anthracenes. *J. Org. Chem.*, **44**, 3715–17.

322. Sheikh, Y. M., Ekwuribe, N., Dhawan, B. & Witiak, D. T. (1982). Synthesis of 5-fluoro-7,12-dimethyl-benz[a]anthracene-3,4-dione: nucleophilic displacement of fluorine in polyaromatic hydrocarbons. *J. Org. Chem.*, **47**, 4341–4.

323. Smith, D. C. C. (1962). Synthesis of 3-methoxyBA and of 2-methoxynaphthacene. *J. Chem. Soc.*, 673–4.

324. Smith, J. G., Welankiwar, S. S., Chu, N. G., Lai, E. H. & Sondheimer, S. J. (1981). Synthetic routes to BAs via transient 1-benzylisobenzofuran derivatives. *J. Org. Chem.*, **46**, 4658–62.

325. Smith, W. M., Jr., Pratt, E. F. & Creech, H. J. (1951). Isocyanates of 12-methyl- and 7,12-dimethylbenz[a]anthracenes. *J. Am. Chem. Soc.*, **73**, 319–22.

326. Snyder, H. R. & Werber, F. X. (1950). Polyphosphoric acid as a dehydrating agent. II. Intramolecular acylation. *J. Am. Chem. Soc.*, **72**, 2965–7.

327. Sukumaran, K. B. & Harvey, R. G. (1980). Synthesis of *o*-quinones and dihydro diols of polycyclic aromatic hydrocarbons from the corresponding phenols. *J. Org. Chem.*, **45**, 4407–13.

328. Susan, A. B., Rohrig, T. P. & Wiley, J. C., Jr. (1981). Stability upon storage, analysis and purification of [14]C- and ^{3}H-labeled PAHs and their metabolites. *J. Labelled Compd. Radiopharm.*, **18**, 1449–55.

329. Susan, A. B. & Wiley, J. C., Jr. (1982). Uniform tritium labeling of PAHs. In *PAHs: Formation, Metabolism and Measurement*, eds. M. Cooke & A. J. Dennis, pp. 1153–9. Battelle Press (Pub. 1983): Columbus.

330. Szmuszkovicz, J. & Modest, E. J. (1950). Condensation of phenylcycloalkenes with maleic anhydride. II. Synthesis of substituted benzo[c]phenanthrenes. *J. Am. Chem. Soc.*, **72**, 566–70.

331. Tada, K. & Takitani, R. (1961). Benz[a]anthracene derivatives. *Kyoritsu Yakka Daigaku Kenkyu Nempo*, **5**, 18–20. *Chem. Abst.*, **55**, 15443f.

332. Tada, K., Takitani, R., Nakagome, H. & Iwasaki, K. (1968). Benz[a]anthracene derivatives. IV. Synthesis of meso-substituted benz[a]anthracene-5,6-diones and their related compounds. *Kyoritsu Yakka Daigaku Kenkyu Nempo*, **13**, 19–25. *Chem. Abst.*, **71**, 3177q.

333. Tanaka, M. (1935). A new hypothesis on amino and carbonyl radicals of aminoanthraquinone and its derivatives. *J. Chem. Soc., Japan*, **56**, 353–6. *Chem. Abst.*, **29**, 4760[6].

334. Tanaka, M. & Morikawa, K. (1930). A new hypothesis of hydroxyl and carbonyl radicals. IV. Synthesis of dihydroxybenzanthraquinone. *J. Chem. Soc., Japan*, **51**, 361–3. *Chem. Abst.*, **25**, 3647[9].

335. Tochtermann, W., Malchow, A. & Timm, H. (1978). Polycyclic compounds. X. Partially hydrogenated BAs. *Ber.*, **111**, 1233–8. *Chem. Abst.*, **89**, 24029e.

336. Tomaszewski, J. E., Manning, W. B. & Muschik, G. M. (1977). A facile synthesis of BAQs. *Tetrahedron Lett.*, 971–4.

337. Tsunoda, T. (1951a,b). (a) Condensation between phthalic anhydride and various aromatic compounds by Friedel–Crafts reaction. *J. Soc. Org. Syn. Chem., Japan*, **9**, 127–132. *Chem. Abst.*, **47**, 10516e. (b) Condensation products from 2-acetylaminonaphthalene. *Ibid.*, **9**, 195–7. *Chem. Abst.*, **47**, 10516e.

338. Tsunoda, T. (1952). Condensation products from 1-naphthol with phthalic anhydride. *J. Soc. Org. Syn. Chem.*, Japan, **10**, 292–4. *Chem. Abst.*, **47**, 10516ef.

339. Tsunoda, T. (1953). Condensation between phthalic anhydride and various aromatic compounds by the Friedel–Crafts reaction. VII. o-(Monochloro-1-naphthoyl)-2-benzoic acids and 4-chloro-1,8-phthaloylnaphthalene. *J. Soc. Org. Syn. Chem., Japan*, **11**, 108–10. *Chem. Abst.*, **48**, 3328e.

340. Tsunoda, T. (1954). Condensation between phthalic anhydride and various aromatic compounds by Friedel–Crafts reaction. IX. The halogen derivatives of o-(2-naphthoyl)benzoic acid. *J. Soc. Org. Syn. Chem., Japan*, **12**, 412–14. *Chem. Abst.*, **51**, 14663i.

341. Tsunoda, T. (1956). Naphthoylbenzoic acid derivatives. *Chiba Daigaku Kogakubu Kenkyu Hokoku*, **7**, 19–82. *Chem. Abst.*, **54**, 9861d.

342. Turner, D. L. (1954). Oxidation of aromatic alcohols with manganese dioxide. *J. Am. Chem. Soc.*, **76**, 5175–6.

343. Uemura, M., Take, K. & Hayashi, Y. (1983). Regioselective synthesis of anthraquinones via (Arene)chromium tricarbonyl complexes. *J. Chem. Soc., Chem. Commun.*, 858–9.

344. Velluz, L. (1939). Photooxidizability of 1,2-cyclosubstituted diphenylanthracenes. *Bull. Soc. Chim. France*, **6**, 1541–8.

345. Vig, O. P., Kessar, S. V., Kubba, V. P. & Mukherji, S. M. (1955). Polynuclear aromatic hydrocarbons. Part I. A new route to anthracene and BA derivatives. *J. Indian Chem. Soc.*, **32**, 697–701.

346. Vig, O. P., Kessar, S. V. & Mukherji, S. M. (1954). A novel synthesis of 6-MBA. *Nature*, **174**, 834.

347. Vingiello, F. A. & Borkovec, A. (1955a,b). (a) The synthesis of six isomeric 7-(dimethylphenyl)benz[a]anthracenes. *J. Am. Chem. Soc.*, **77**, 3413–15.

80   *Chemistry*

(*b*) The synthesis of 12-phenylBA and the three isomeric 12-(monomethyl-phenyl)BAs. *Ibid.*, **77**, 4823–4.

348. Vingiello, F. A. & Borkovec, A. (1956*a*,*b*). (*a*) The synthesis of the six isomeric 12-(dimethylphenyl)benz[a]anthracenes. *J. Am. Chem. Soc.*, **78**, 1240–2. (*b*) The use of alumina in aromatic cyclodehydration. *Ibid.*, **78**, 3205–7.

349. Vingiello, F. A., Borkovec, A. & Shulman, J. (1955). The synthesis of 7-phenylbenz[a]anthracene and three isomeric 7-(monomethyl-phenyl)benz[a]anthracenes. *J. Am. Chem. Soc.*, **77**, 2320–2.

350. Vingiello, F. A., Borkovec, A. & Zajac, W., Jr. (1958). An unusual Elbs-type reaction observed during a study of the cyclization of ketones. *J. Am. Chem. Soc.*, **80**, 1714–16.

351. Vingiello, F. A. & Delia, T. J. (1961). Cleavage of 7-substituted benz[a]anthracenes. *J. Org. Chem.*, **26**, 1005–8.

352. Vingiello, F. A. & Lewis, C. I. (1968). Synthesis of substituted 7-(1-naphthyl)-benz[a]anthracene. *J. Chem. Engng Data*, **13**, 439–40.

353. Vingiello, F. A. & Menon, C. S. (1974). 1,2-Aryl shifts in BAs. *J. Math. Sci.*, **1**, 15–17.

354. Vingiello, F. A., Ojakaar, L. & Kelsey, R. (1965). 7- and 12-(*o*-halophenyl)BAs. *J. Med. Chem.*, **8**, 144.

355. Vingiello, F. A. & Thornton, J. R. (1966). A study of electronic and steric effects on the course of an aromatic cyclodehydration reaction versus an Elbs reaction. *J. Org. Chem.*, **31**, 659–63.

356. Vingiello, F. A., Yanez, J. & Campbell, J. A. (1971). A new approach to the synthesis of dibenzo[a,l]pyrenes. *J. Org. Chem.*, **36**, 2053–6.

357. Waldmann, H. (1931). Concerning BAQ. *J. Prakt. Chem.*, **131**, 71–81.

358. Waldmann, H. & Steskal, G. (1930). Several derivatives of benz[a]anthracene-7,12-dione. *J. Prakt. Chem.*, **127**, 201–9.

359. Watanabe, M. & Snieckus, V. (1980). Tandem directed metalation reactions. Short syntheses of PAHs and ellipticine alkaloids. *J. Am. Chem. Soc.*, **102**, 1457–60.

360. Weitzberg, M., Aizenshtat, A., Jerushalmy, P. & Blum, J. (1980). An improved synthesis of carbocyclic and heterocyclic arene imines. *J. Org. Chem.*, **45**, 4252–4.

361. Weizmann, C. & Bergmann, E. (1936). Methoxylated *o*-benzoylbenzoic acids. *J. Chem. Soc.*, 567–9.

362. Wildeman, J., Borgen, P. C., Pluim, H., Rouwette, P. H. F. M. & van Leusen, A. M. (1978). Synthesis of naphthalenes from *o*-substituted benzyl sulfones and Michael acceptors. *Tetrahedron Lett.*, 2213–16.

363. Wiley, J. C., Jr., Menon, C. S., Fischer, D. L. & Engel, J. F. (1975). Metabolites of polycyclic aromatic hydrocarbons. II. Isomeric K-region phenols and methyl ethers of benz[a]anthracene. *Tetrahedron Lett.*, 2811–14.

364. Winternitz, F., Mousseron, M. & Vinas, J. (1952). The cyclization of some arylcycloalkaneacetic acids. *Bull. Soc. Chim. France*, 1035–42.

365. Wood, J. L., Barker, C. L. & Grubbs, C. J. (1979). Photooxidation products of 7-12-DMBA. *Chem. Biol. Interact.*, **26**, 339–47.

366. Wood, J. L. & Fieser, L. F. (1940). Sulfhydryl and cysteine derivatives of benz-[a]anthracene, 7-methylbenz[a]anthracene and benzo[a]pyrene. *J. Am. Chem. Soc.*, **62**, 2674–81.

367. Wood, J. L. & Fieser, L. F. (1941). Thiocyanation of carcinogenic hydrocarbons. *J. Am. Chem. Soc.*, **63**, 2323–31.

368. Wood, J. L. & Fieser, L. F. (1951). Derivatives of 7,12-DMBA. *J. Am. Chem. Soc.*, **73**, 4494–5.

369. Wunderly, S. W. & Weber, W. P. (1978). Synthesis of 8-methoxy- and 11-

methoxyBAQs via Diels–Alder reaction of 1,4-phenanthraquinone. *J. Org. Chem.*, **43**, 2277–9.

370. Yagi, H., Vyas, K. P., Tada, M., Thakker, D. R. & Jerina, D. M. (1982). Synthesis of enantiomeric bay-region diol epoxides of benz[a]anthracene and chrysene. *J. Org. Chem.*, **47**, 1110–17.
371. Zajac, W. W., Jr. & Denk, R. H. (1962). Reaction of nitriles with hydrazine hydrate and Raney nickel. Synthesis of PAH. *J. Org. Chem.*, **27**, 3716–17.
372. Zaugg, H. E. (1946). A synthesis of 5,6-dihydro-7-hydroxyBA. *J. Am. Chem. Soc.*, **68**, 2492–4.

PART 2: BIOLOGY

B. TIERNEY

Historical aspects

With the onset of research into the carcinogenicity of pure chemicals, the benz[a]anthracene (BA) nucleus was regarded, in these early studies, as a basic requirement for the demonstration of carcinogenicity. Kennaway (1930) had observed that the application of a pure polycyclic aromatic hydrocarbon (PAH) to mice produces tumours. At the same time Hieger (1930) was investigating the fluorescence characteristics of particular fractions obtained from coal tar which possessed carcinogenic activity. The fluorescence spectra of these fractions were similar to the fluorescence spectrum of BA. These observations led investigators to propose that the ring system of BA, a compound which is only weakly carcinogenic in itself, provides the basis for a potentially carcinogenic molecule and that cancer-producing properties are developed by substitution at suitable positions (Barry *et al.*, 1935).

Initially, because of the strong carcinogenic activity of 3-methylcholanthrene (3-MC) and dibenz[a,h]anthracene, substituents at positions 8 and 9 on the BA nucleus were regarded as particularly favourable for carcinogenicity (see figure). The chemical synthesis of a large number of compounds based on BA, which varied in the position, number and type of substituents, was undertaken in England by Cook and his associates at the Royal Free Hospital, London, and in the USA by Fieser and co-workers in Harvard and Newman at Ohio State University. The biological activities of these compounds were examined under the supervision of Kennaway in London and Shear in the USA. In a fascinating series of experiments, the structural features superfluous to the cancer-producing properties of substituted BAs were revealed. By 1935, the London group had examined 69 compounds based on BA, of which 25 gave a positive carcinogenic response (437 tumours in 1220 mice); in contrast, of 71 compounds not related to BA which were tested for carcinogenic activity, only six were positive (Barry *et al.*, 1935). With the synthesis and biological testing of all 12 possible monomethyl BA isomers Shear (1938) demonstrated that a methyl group at the C-7 position resulted in a most carcinogenic compound, being as potent as 3-MC, cholanthrene or 7,8-dimethylbenz[a]anthracene (see figure). These types of experiments culminated in the synthesis and testing of 7,12-dimethyl-benz[a]anthracene (7,12-DMBA), one of the most potent chemical carcinogens ever examined (Bachmann *et al.*, 1938). This chemical is now widely used in animal model tumour systems. The remarkable enhancement in carcinogenicity of the weak carcinogen BA by the introduction of a simple methyl group at the C-7 position, and the further enhancement (the effect being not merely additive) by the introduction of two methyl groups at the C-7 and C-12 positions, is still not completely understood. Observations made by Fieser (1938) 'that the angular benzene ring of the BA derivatives is an important feature of the structure' and that 'substitution of alkyl groups in the angular ring of the molecule

Structures of some chemicals examined for carcinogenic activity prior to 1940.

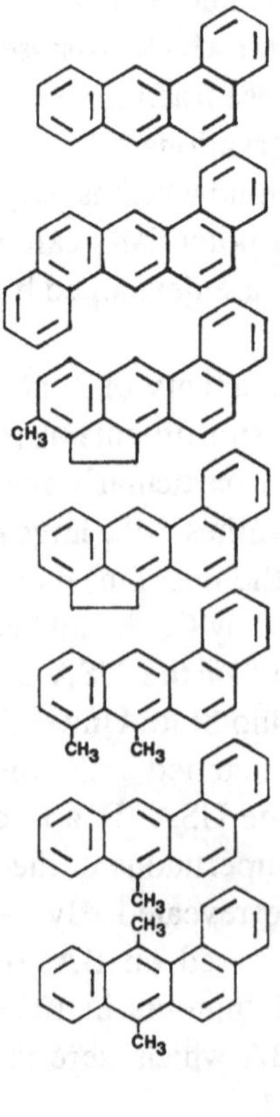

Benz[a]anthracene (BA)

Dibenz[a,h]anthracene

3-Methylcholanthrene (3-MC)

Cholanthrene

7,8-Dimethylbenz[a]anthracene

7-Methylbenz[a]anthracene (7-MBA)

7,12-Dimethylbenz[a]-anthracene (7,12-DMBA)

seems unfavourable for the development of cancer-producing properties' may well have relevance today. The extensive literature of this period has been reviewed by Fieser (1938) and by Cook and Kennaway (1940).

In addition to variations in the structure of the cancer-producing chemical it was also clear that carcinogenic activity was dependent on a number of other factors such as the species of animal employed and the mode of administration. In these early studies chemicals were being examined as complete carcinogens. It was not until the nineteen-forties that it was recognized that there are stages in the progression of cancer in which noncarcinogenic, promoting, substances exert critical control (Mottram, 1944; Berenblum and Shubik, 1947). Also at this time the possible significance of metabolism in the activation of chemicals was realized. PAHs are chemically relatively inert and researchers suggested that rather than acting directly on a cell the PAH may be converted metabolically into an active species which may then react with cellular macromolecules to cause cell transformation. The initial indication that metabolism of PAHs was occurring came from the extracts of urine and faeces of animals which had been treated with a particular PAH; they showed that in many cases elimination was preceded by hydroxylation. Thus the 4-phenol was formed from BA as a metabolite in mice and rats (Berenblum and Schoental, 1943) as it was also from 7,12-DMBA (Dickens, 1945). That these types of hydroxylated metabolites may result from the metabolic formation of an epoxide was suggested by Boyland (1950) and recent findings have strongly suggested that a diol epoxide and in particular that which occurs in a bay-region (Jerina and Lehr, 1978) is the ultimate carcinogenic form of a PAH.

There have been a number of excellent reviews on PAHs as chemical carcinogens to which the interested reader is referred (Badger, 1954; Bun-Hoi, 1964; Arcos and Argus, 1968; Dipple *et al.*, 1984a).

8

Metabolism

8.1 Introduction

Polycyclic aromatic hydrocarbons are metabolized by the mixed function oxidase system to forms more readily excretable by the cell; usually by making the PAH more polar and therefore more water soluble. The principal enzymes involved in this process are those consisting of the haem-containing cytochrome P-450 (which requires both NADPH and molecular oxygen) and epoxide hydrolase. These enzymes are located mainly as membrane-bound proteins in the endoplasmic reticulum or nuclei of cells although some cytosolic forms are known. They exist in 'multiple forms' some of which have been isolated and purified. These isoenzymes, which are present in a variety of tissues, can be selectively induced by treatment of the animal with various chemicals (commonly used cytochrome P-450 inducers are 3-MC and phenobarbital), and these various induced states can result in different metabolic pathways for the compounds under study.

Cytochrome P-450 introduces a hydroxyl group into an alkyl group, or an epoxide group across the double bond of an aromatic system. Epoxide hydrolase can then metabolize the epoxide further to a *trans*-dihydrodiol. If this *trans*-dihydrodiol contains an adjacent double bond then cytochrome P-450 may act for a second time to form a diol epoxide. Although these events are designed as detoxification routes current evidence suggests that the formation of a diol epoxide, particularly a bay-region diol epoxide, are in fact steps of metabolic activation. The formation of a bay-region diol epoxide or epoxide (that is, a compound in which the epoxide is generated in the angular portion of a PAH, see Fig. 8.1; for benz[a]anthracene an epoxide formed across the 1,2 bond is the bay-region epoxide) represents a species with an enhanced mutagenic and sometimes carcinogenic activity compared with that of the parent hydrocarbon and is regarded, in many cases, as the ultimate carcinogenic form of a PAH (for a more extensive discussion see Chapter 11).

The hydroxyl, epoxide or diol epoxide metabolites formed by the mixed function oxidase system may be subject to a variety of further modifications both nonenzymatic and enzymatic. Nonenzymatically the epoxide group can be hydrated to form a dihydrodiol, it may rearrange to form a phenol, or a phenol may be produced from an unstable dihydriol. The epoxide may react with electrophilic centres on DNA, RNA or proteins to form covalent adducts. Enzymatically the diol epoxide can be converted to a tetrol by epoxide hydrolase; it may be significant that the bay-region diol epoxide is often a poor substrate for epoxide hydrolase. The epoxide may be conjugated to glutathione via one of the glutathione-S-transferases, and these glutathione conjugates further converted into the related mercapturic acids which are found in the urine. The presence of hydroxyl groups on the PAH allows enzymic glucuronide and sulphate conjugation and also enzymic dehydrogenation of vicinal dihydrodiols to yield catechols (via dihydrodiol dehydrogenase). Alkyl alcohols may be oxidized further to aldehydes and then to carboxylic acids.

An interesting recent development has been the observation that methyl groups may be introduced metabolically into an aromatic nucleus; thus benz[a]anthracene may be converted into the moderate carcinogen 7-methylbenz[a]anthracene which may be further metabolized to the strong carcinogen 7,12-dimethylbenz[a]anthracene. There are thus a wide variety of metabolites formed from PAH, and metabolic studies have been carried out in a number of different species, tissues and cell types, each with its own preferred metabolic pathway. Although liver is a tissue often used in metabolism experiments, this is not a target tissue for a number of PAH. More relevant are metabolic studies in whole animals or which involve target tissues, such as skin, as the metabolizing enzyme source. Also marked differences have been observed when results from experiments using whole cells were compared with those

Fig. 8.1. Benz[a]anthracene; numbering and regions with specific names.

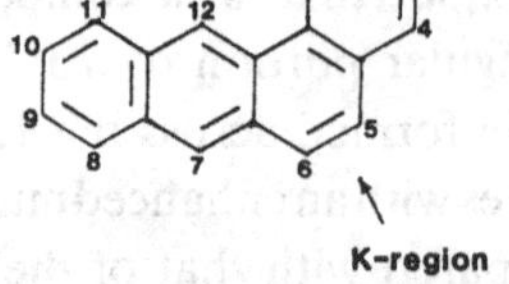

using broken cells. Therefore caution has to be applied when extrapolating metabolism data to account for the observed carcinogenicity of a compound, although studies on the types of metabolites formed, the metabolic pathways followed, and the mutagenicity and carcinogenicity of various metabolites, have considerably aided our current understanding of the metabolic activation of carcinogens.

Certain metabolites of PAHs exist as stereoisomers and the metabolic pathway followed by a particular PAH can be extremely selective as to which stereoisomer is formed, and which stereoisomer is a favoured substrate for a particular enzyme. Each *trans*-dihydrodiol can exist in either a diaxial or diequatorial conformation; the latter is usually energetically favoured, but in the case of steric hinderance or other factors, a diaxial conformation may be adopted (Fig. 8.2). Each *trans*-dihydrodiol is optically active and contains asymmetric carbon atoms. Thus it can exist in two enantiomeric forms, (+) and (−), each with its own absolute stereochemistry. The further oxidation of the dihydrodiol to a diol epoxide is possible, the epoxide group can be *syn* or *anti* to the benzylic hydroxyl group [i.e. may be on the same side, (*syn*), or below (*anti*) the plane of the ring, relative to the benzylic hydroxyl group, see Fig. 8.2]. These two geometric isomers can exist in two enantiomeric forms making a total of four optically active diol epoxide isomers possible

Fig. 8.2. A, different conformations adopted by a *trans*-dihydrodiol of a PAH; B, different diol epoxide geometric isomers.

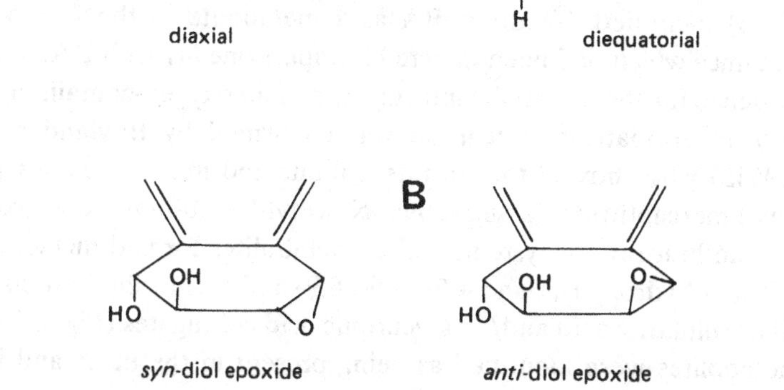

diaxial   diequatorial

syn-diol epoxide   anti-diol epoxide

[(+)-*syn*, (−)-*syn*, (+)-*anti* and (−)-*anti*], each with its own absolute configuration.

The configuration of the metabolites formed *in vitro*, determined mainly from studies employing rat liver, have shown a marked stereoselective preference for forming dihydrodiols with an [R,R] absolute stereochemistry, the enantiomeric ratio being little affected by the state of induction of the animals used. However, subtle alterations in the structure of the chemical being metabolized can cause marked stereochemical changes i.e. the metabolically formed K-region *trans*-dihydrodiol undergoes a progressive alteration from [R,R] to [S,S] absolute stereochemistry as the chemical structure is changed from BA to 7-MBA to 12-MBA and finally to 7,12-DMBA. The [R,R]-dihydrodiol stereoisomer is usually a better substrate for cytochrome P-450 than the enantiomeric [S,S] isomer, forming predominantly the *anti*-diol epoxide, although this may depend upon the state of induction of the liver. The effect of the preferred conformation adopted by a dihydrodiol (diaxial or diequatorial), on the subsequent ratio of *syn*- to *anti*-diol epoxide has not been conclusively established. Certainly the adoption of a diaxial conformation, as with the 1,2-dihydrodiol of BA, does not necessarily result in the directing of metabolic oxidation away from the adjacent double bond, as is found with certain diaxial dihydrodiols of B[a]P and B[e]P. In the identification of metabolites there are essentially two approaches: either sufficient quantities of the metabolites are made to allow adequate chemical characterization, or the metabolites formed are compared with reference chemical compounds of known structure. Obviously it is necessary in the former case that a sufficiently rigorous examination be carried out, otherwise only a tentative structural identification can be made.

8.2   Metabolism of benz[a]anthracene

In experiments with whole animals Berenblum and Schoental (1943) identified 4-hydroxy-BA as a metabolite in the faeces of rats and mice which had been injected intraperitoneally with BA. This early evidence for the metabolic introduction of an oxygen-containing species into an aromatic hydrocarbon was confirmed by Boyland and Sims (1964*b*) who showed that in rats, rabbits and mice the major product was a mercapturic acid derivative, N-acetyl-S-(5,6-dihydro-6-hydroxy-5-benzanthracenyl)-L-cysteine; other metabolites formed included 3-, 4-, 8- and 9-hydroxy BA and 4,5-, 5,6-, 8,9- and 10,11-dihydrodiols of BA, all as sulphuric acid and/or glucuronic acid conjugates (Fig. 8.3). These metabolites were identified as being present in the urine and in some

cases the bile and faeces of the animals under study. The K-region mercapturic acid metabolite represented about 1% of the dose of hydrocarbon administered to the rats; the related K-region dihydrodiol was
present only as a minor product, and no K-region phenols were detected.
The comparative metabolism of BA in rats, rabbits and mice revealed
no qualitative differences between the species.

In experiments employing rat liver microsomes (Boyland *et al.*, 1964*a*),
the metabolism of BA yielded as a major product the 8,9-dihydrodiol;
minor products which were detected included the 1,2- and 5,6-dihydro-
diol and the 3- and 4-hydroxy BA phenols. The hypothesis that dihydrodiols and phenols might arise from an intermediate epoxide group
(formed metabolically by the introduction of oxygen across an aromatic
double bond) was examined experimentally by Boyland and Sims
(1965*a*). The metabolic pathway followed by BA 5,6-epoxide in rat liver
homogenate does produce dihydrodiols and a phenol as well as glucuronide conjugates. Calculation of the electron density of the various double
bonds present in BA shows that the K-region double bond has the highest
electron density, with the 8,9- and 10,11-bonds being next highest (Pullman and Pullman, 1952). Therefore it was proposed that these positions
on the BA molecule would be most susceptible to attack by the metabolizing enzymes involved in the insertion of an epoxide group across the
double bond. The isolation of a metabolically formed K-region epoxide
of BA from rat liver incubations has been reported (Grover *et al.*, 1971)
and the enantiomeric composition of the K-region epoxide formed from

Fig. 8.3. Probable pathways in benz[a]anthracene metabolism. Formulae in
parentheses are those of compounds whose presence as metabolites is
uncertain. From Boyland and Sims (1964*b*).

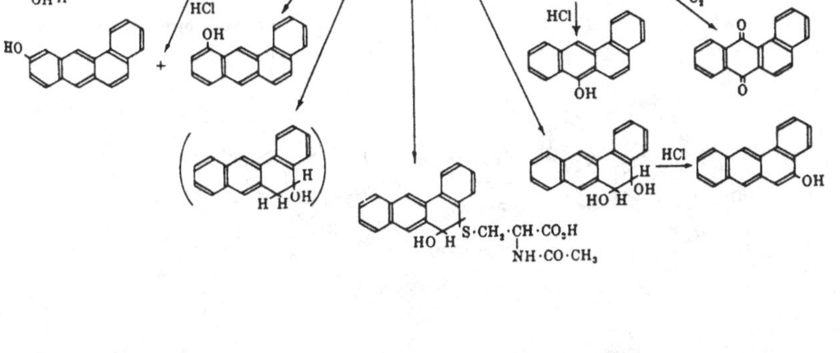

BA in the presence of rat liver microsomes has been shown to be markedly affected by whether the animal is untreated, phenobarbital treated or 3-MC treated (Yang and Chiu, 1985).

The involvement of non-K-region positions, such as the 8,9-bond, in the metabolic formation of epoxides and dihydrodiols of BA has also been demonstrated (Sims, 1971). Such dihydrodiols have an adjacent isolated double bond. The proposal that the active metabolic species obtained from PAHs is the result of further oxidation of non-K-region dihydrodiols to give a diol epoxide developed from the studies described above, as well as evidence from mutagenicity and carcinogenicity experiments which showed that the K-region epoxide was not involved in the metabolic activation of benzanthracene (see Chapters 10 and 11). Booth and Sims (1974) described, for the first time, the metabolic formation of a diol epoxide, 8,9-dihydro-8,9-dihydroxy-BA 10,11-oxide from the 8,9-dihydrodiol using rat liver microsomes (Fig. 8.4). The formation of a dihydrodiol was, therefore, not necessarily a metabolic end point; further metabolism to form an epoxide at the vicinal double bond does occur.

The relevance of oxidation at non-K-region positions, and in particular at the bay-region bond, has been emphasized by Jerina who formulated the bay-region hypothesis in an attempt to explain and predict the carcinogenicity of polycyclic aromatic hydrocarbons. This theory, based on quantum mechanical calculations, postulates that a diol epoxide on a saturated, angular benzene ring in which the epoxide forms part of a bay-region of the polycyclic hydrocarbon should be a highly reactive

Fig. 8.4. Metabolic pathway for the formation of 8,9-dihydro-8,9-dihydroxy-BA 10,11-epoxide. From Booth and Sims (1974).

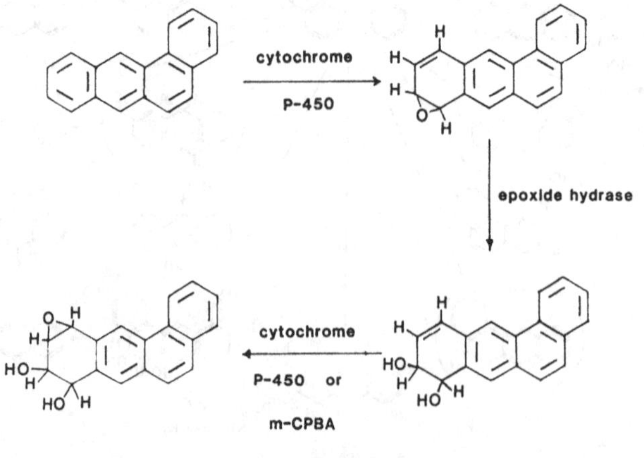

metabolite which may also be the ultimate carcinogenic form of the polycyclic hydrocarbon (Jerina and Lehr, 1978).

These theoretical proposals prompted a re-examination of the metabolism of BA using fully characterized synthetic non-K-region *trans*-dihydrodiols as standards and more efficient systems (HPLC) for resolving those metabolites formed. All five possible *trans*-dihydrodiols were detected on metabolism of BA with rat liver microsomes (Tierney *et al.*, 1978*b*), the 8,9- and 5,6-dihydrodiols of BA predominating. Similar results were obtained by Thakker *et al.* (1979*a*) using liver microsomes from induced and uninduced rats as well as a purified and reconstituted cytochrome P-448/epoxide hydrolase system. Only trace amounts of phenols were produced indicating that the arene oxides of BA must be good substrates for epoxide hydrolase. When epoxide hydrolase was omitted from the system only phenols and the K-region epoxide were detected, and the extent of metabolism of BA was substantially reduced suggesting that certain of these metabolites are potent inhibitors of the cytochrome P-450 dependent monooxygenase system.

The absolute stereochemistry of the dihydrodiols formed by liver enzymes has been determined (Thakker *et al.*, 1979*b*,*c*); the major metabolically formed enantiomer for each dihydrodiol has the [R,R] configuration. For the 3,4-dihydrodiol of BA this is also the most tumourigenic enantiomer (see Chapter 11). These findings on the marked stereospecificity of the mixed function oxidase system and epoxide hydrolase are similar to those described for other polycyclic hydrocarbons, such as benzo[a]pyrene.

Each *trans*-dihydrodiol can exist in two enantiomeric forms, and each *trans*-dihydrodiol can be further metabolized to a diol epoxide in which the epoxide group is either *syn* or *anti* to the benzylic hydroxyl group. The further metabolism of BA *trans*-1,2-dihydrodiol to both *syn* and *anti* vicinal diol epoxides (Yang and Chou, 1980*a*) provides an example of the vicinal metabolism of a double bond adjacent to a dihydrodiol whose hydroxyl groups exist in a quasi-diaxial conformation due to steric hinderance. Previously, from studies carried out on B[a]P and B[e]P dihydrodiols, it was speculated that a quasi-diaxial conformation of a dihydrodiol would result in metabolism occurring at positions distal to the dihydrodiol (Thakker *et al.*, 1978; Wood *et al.*, 1979).

The metabolism of optically pure BA (−)-[1R,2R]- and (+)-[1S,2S]-dihydrodiols showed there to be varying degrees of stereoselectivity depending on the constitutive forms of cytochrome P-450 in the rat liver microsomal preparation. Thus the (−)-dihydrodiol enantiomer formed predominantly the *anti*-diol epoxide with 3-MC microsomes, and the *syn*-diol epoxide with control and PB-microsomes, whilst the (+) enantiomer formed the *syn*-diol epoxide with control, 3-MC and PB-microsomes (Chou *et al.*, 1983). However, in addition to these findings, Vyas *et al.* (1983) observed that substantial amounts of bis-dihydrodiols were also formed suggesting that quasi-diaxial hydroxyl groups may indeed direct some metabolism away from the vicinal double bond.

Further metabolism of precursors to the bay-region diol epoxide i.e. the (−)-[3R,4R]-dihydrodiol, to the *anti*-diol epoxide can occur (Fig. 8.5); in contrast the (+)-[3S,4S]-enantiomer appears to be very poorly, if at all, metabolized by rat liver microsomes to a diol epoxide (Thakker *et al.*, 1979*b*, 1982). The overall conversion of the (−)-[3R,4R]-dihydrodiol to the highly tumourigenic bay-region diol epoxide was very small (<16% of the total metabolites). This may be contrasted with the metabolic conversion of similar stereochemical dihydrodiols derived from B[a]P, phenanthrene and chrysene where >65% are converted to the bay-region diol epoxide. For both enantiomers of BA 3,4-dihydrodiol the major metabolites formed were bis-dihydrodiols and a novel microsomal metabolite identified as BA 3,4-quinone (Thakker *et al.*, 1982).

Quantum mechanical calculations on the ease of carbonium ion formation at the bay-region suggest that BA should be a strong carcinogen. The observed weak carcinogenicity of BA may be due to the low conversion of the hydrocarbon to the 3,4-dihydrodiol (2–4% of the total meta-

Fig. 8.5. Stereochemical course of the metabolic conversion of BA to the bay-region diol epoxide by phenobarbital induced rat liver microsomes. Data from Thakker *et al.* (1979, 1982).

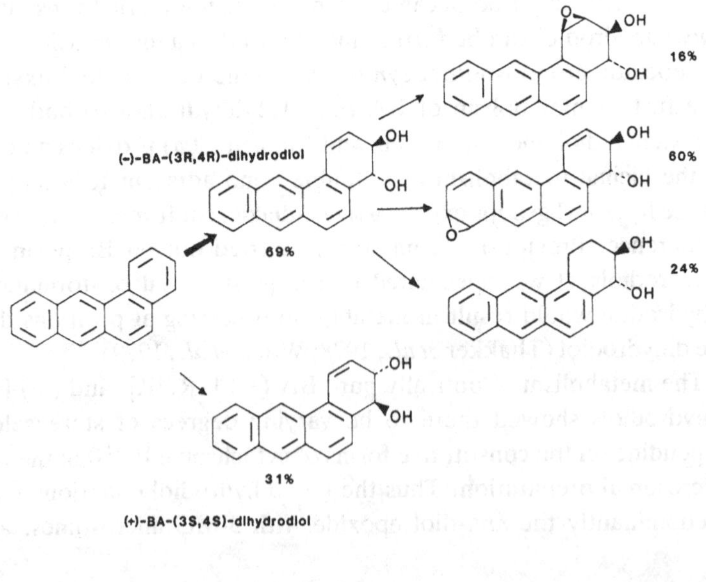

bolites with rat liver preparations) and the subsequent poor conversion of the *trans*-3,4-dihydrodiol to a bay-region diol epoxide; however, in each case the most active stereochemical isomer is preferentially formed. In intact cells (MacNicoll *et al.*, 1981) and in a target tissue such as mouse skin (MacNicoll *et al.*, 1980*b*, 1981) the 3,4-dihydrodiol represents a major metabolite of those free dihydrodiol products formed; also being formed are water-soluble metabolites probably in the form of sulphate esters, glucuronides and glutathione conjugates. Therefore there is no simple answer to the observed weak carcinogenicity of BA: factors such as the type of metabolite formed, the amount of metabolite formed, the substrate specificity of the cytochrome P-450 and epoxide hydrolase enzyme system, the stereochemistry of the metabolites, and the rate of conversion into water-soluble conjugates all probably contribute to the formation (or lack of formation) of the ultimate carcinogenic form of BA.

The alternative sites on BA for the formation of a diol epoxide are at the 8-, 9-, 10- and 11-positions. The conversion of the *trans*-8,9-dihydrodiol to a diol epoxide has been described (Booth and Sims, 1974). Also Cooper *et al.* (1980*a*) has reported the conversion of the 10,11-dihydrodiol to a diol epoxide with liver microsomes. Although both these non-bay-region diol epoxides may thus be formed metabolically, and although both the *trans*-8,9- and 10,11-dihydrodiols are major metabolites from rat liver microsomes (Tierney *et al.*, 1978*b*; Jacob *et al.*, 1981), hamster embryo cells (MacNicoll *et al.*, 1981) and mouse skin (MacNicoll *et al.*, 1980*b*) they do not possess significant carcinogenic activity (see Chapter 11). The 10,11-diol 8,9-epoxide does not form an adduct with DNA using a rat liver microsomal system (Cooper *et al.*, 1980*a*) to DNA in hamster embryo cells, or in mouse skin *in vivo* (Cooper *et al.*, 1980*c*,*f*). In contrast the 8,9-diol 10,11-epoxide does bind to DNA of mouse skin *in vivo* (Cooper *et al.*, 1980*f*), to hamster embryo cells in culture (Cooper *et al.*, 1980*c*) and in rat liver microsomal systems (MacNicoll *et al.*, 1979*b*). No stereochemical studies have yet been carried out on the metabolic route of these non-bay-region diol epoxides; such studies may provide insight into the *in vivo* activity of such metabolites.

It has recently been demonstrated (Flesher *et al.*, 1984) that rat liver cytosol preparations fortified with 5-adenosyl-L-methionine will introduce methyl groups into BA at the C-7 and C-12 positions. The introduction of such methyl groups at these positions show that it is possible that the weak carcinogen BA may be enzymatically altered *in vivo* to give the moderate carcinogen 7-MBA, or even the strong carcinogen 7,12-DMBA. Such observations may be important in the assessment of risk when considering the exposure of populations to supposed weak carcinogens such as BA.

8.3   Metabolism of monosubstituted benz[a]anthracenes
8.3.1   *1-Methylbenz[a]anthracene*
Approximately equal amounts of the two enantiomeric forms of the K-region epoxide are formed when 1-MBA is metabolized by liver microsomes prepared from phenobarbital-treated rats (Weems *et al.*, 1985).

8.3.2   *4-Methylbenz[a]anthracene*
Cerniglia *et al.* (1983) have reported that the metabolism of 4-MBA by the fungus *Cunninghamella elegans* formed 4-OHMBA and the *trans*-8,9- and 10,11-dihydrodiol related to the hydroxymethyl metabolite; each dihydrodiol had an [S,S] absolute configuration. This indicates there may be differences in the stereoselectivity of the fungal cytochrome P-450 monooxygenase-epoxide hydrolase systems when compared with the rat liver enzyme system where the predominant enantiomer of the dihydrodiols formed usually has an [R,R] configuration. The presence of a methyl group in the 4-position appears to direct metabolism away from the K-region and the 3,4-bond.

8.3.3   *6-Fluorobenz[a]anthracene*
The major metabolites formed from 6-fluoro-BA by a rat liver S-10 fraction are the *trans*-8,9-dihydrodiol and various phenols. No K-region dihydrodiols were detected in this study (Sheikh *et al.*, 1981).

8.3.4   *6-Methylbenz[a]anthracene*
The rat liver microsomal metabolism of the carcinogen 6-MBA formed the 3-OH, 4-OH and 5-OH 6-MBA phenols, the *trans*-3,4-, 5,6-, 8,9- and 10,11-dihydrodiols and the 4-OH-6-MBA-*trans*-10,11-dihydrodiol as identifiable metabolites. 6-OHMBA and its phenolic and dihydrodiol metabolites are also formed (Yang *et al.*, 1980*b*; Mushtaq *et al.*, 1985). It is interesting that the presence of a methyl group at the C-6 position does not prevent cytochrome P-450 catalysed epoxidation at that position, nor the action of epoxide hydrolase. Similar oxidative metabolism at methyl-substituted aromatic double bonds has been shown to occur with 8-MBA (Yang *et al.*, 1979*a*) and 11-MBA (Yang, 1982*a*). Another interesting aspect in the metabolism of 6-MBA is that the 10,11-

dihydrodiol is preferentially metabolized to give the 4-phenol, rather than oxidative metabolism occurring at the isolated 8,9-double bond to produce the diol epoxide. The behaviour of this dihydrodiol is similar in this respect to the 3,4-dihydrodiol of BA (Thakker *et al.*, 1982). There are significant changes in the quantitative pattern of metabolites formed from 6-MBA when control rats or rats treated with 3-MC or pheno-barbital were used as the source of liver (Yang *et al.*, 1980*b*; Mushtaq *et al.*, 1985).

8.3.5 *7-Methylbenz[a]anthracene*

This compound is the most carcinogenic of the monomethylated BAs (Shear, 1938). There have been no reports on the metabolism of 7-MBA in whole animals. Incubation of 7-MBA with rat liver homoge-nates has indicated that metabolism occurs on the aliphatic side chain to form 7-OHMBA and on the aromatic ring to form the *trans*-8,9-dihydrodiol as the major metabolites. The 5,6-dihydrodiol can also be detected. A combination of ring and alkyl oxidation also results in the 7-OHMBA-8,9-dihydrodiol as a metabolite (Sims, 1967*a*, 1970*a*). In these studies evidence was also presented for the presence of a glutath-ione conjugate in the aqueous phase, S-5,6-dihydro-(6-hydroxy-7-methyl-5-benz[a]anthracenyl) glutathione. Using HPLC rather than tlc, the separation of 7-MBA metabolites can be more effectively accomplished, and all five possible *trans*-dihydrodiols formed as metabo-lites from rat liver have now been identified (Tierney *et al.*, 1977). NMR data indicated that both the *trans*-1,2- and -8,9-dihydrodiols exist predo-minantly in a quasi-diaxial conformation, presumably due to steric inter-actions in the bay-region for the 1,2-dihydrodiol and with the adjacent 7-methyl group for the 8,9-dihydrodiol. These conformational effects are reflected in the relative retention times of the dihydrodiols on HPLC (Fig. 8.6), which can then be used in predicting the preferred conforma-tion of the dihydrodiols of unsubstituted and substituted PAH (Tierney *et al.*, 1979; Chiu *et al.*, 1982). The formation of *trans*-dihydrodiols, including the 3,4-dihydrodiol, has been reported in target tissues such as mouse skin (Tierney *et al.*, 1977) and rat lung (Grover *et al.*, 1973) and metabolites of this kind also occur as the result of fungal metabolism (Cerniglia *et al.*, 1982).

The presence of a methyl group at the 7-position of BA does not alter the stereoselective properties of the rat liver microsomal mono-oxygenase system with respect to the preferential formation of [R,R] dihydrodiol enantiomers. Thus the predominant enantiomer formed by the four non-K-region *trans*-dihydrodiols of 7-MBA has an [R,R] configuration (Yang and Fu, 1984*a*), as has also been shown for BA dihydrodiols. The metabolic formation by rat liver microsomes of the K-region epoxide of 7-MBA has been reported (Keysell *et al.*, 1973), and the major enantiomer has the [R,R] absolute configuration (Weems *et al.*, 1985). There has been no direct evidence for the metabolic formation of diol epoxides.

Two interesting observations on the hepatic metabolism of 7-MBA have been made in the laboratory of Flesher. The bio-alkylation of 7-MBA can occur using rat liver cytosol fortified with S-adenosyl-L-methionine, to give the strong carcinogen 7,12-DMBA. This introduction of a methyl group into the 12-position of 7-MBA may represent an important metabolic step in the carcinogenic activity of 7-MBA (Flesher *et al.*, 1984). The second observation, by Flesher and Myers (1985), concerns the oxidative metabolism of the methyl group of 7-MBA. Incubation of 7-MBA with hepatic cytosol results in the formation of hydroxymethyl derivatives with no apparent ring oxidation occurring. The novel enzyme involved in this alkyl hydroxylation did not appear to involve the microsomal system and did not require an NADP- or NADPH-generating system (Flesher and Myers, 1985).

Fig. 8.6. Relative retention times on normal phase HPLC of *trans*-dihydrodiols of BA, 7-MBA and 7,12-DMBA and their relationship to the preferred conformation adopted.

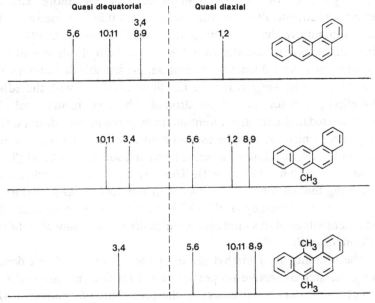

8.3.6   *Other 7-substituted benz[a]anthracene derivatives*
The hepatic microsomal metabolism of 7-fluoro-BA (Chiu *et al.*, 1982, 1984) and 7-bromo-BA (Fu and Yang, 1983*a*) is qualitatively similar to that reported for BA: *trans*-3,4-, -5,6-, -8,9- and -10,11-dihydrodiols being formed, the predominant enantiomer in each case having an [R,R] configuration. The presence of a fluorine or bromine atom at the 7-position causes the 5,6- and 8,9-dihydrodiols to adopt a quasidiaxial conformation (as with 7-MBA), due to electronic repulsion and steric effects between the halogen atom and the *peri* hydroxyl oxygen (Chiu *et al.*, 1982; Fu and Yang, 1983*a*). The metabolic oxidation at various positions on the BA nucleus differs significantly between BA and 7-FBA. Thus using untreated liver microsomes as the metabolizing system, the 5,6-dihydrodiol represented 45% of all the metabolites formed from BA whereas it represented only 10% of the total metabolites formed from 7-FBA. The 10,11-dihydrodiol was the most abundant metabolite formed from 7-FBA but it was a relatively minor metabolite of BA (Chiu *et al.*, 1984). With no direct comparison between the metabolism of BA, 7-MBA and 7-FBA in a target tissue being reported in the literature, it is difficult to reconcile the observed differences in the hepatic metabolic pathways for these PAH with the three-fold enhancement in carcinogenicity of 7-FBA, and 20-fold enhancement in carcinogenicity of 7-MBA, when compared with the carcinogenicity exhibited by BA (Wood *et al.*, 1982).

7-NitroBA is reported to be noncarcinogenic (Shear *et al.*, 1940); however, metabolic studies using rat liver microsomes (Fu and Yang, 1983*b*) have demonstrated both the *trans*-3,4- and -8,9-dihydrodiols to be major metabolites. Each has an [R,R] configuration, the *trans*-3,4-dihydrodiol existing in a quasi-diequatorial conformation, the *trans*-8,9-dihydrodiol in a mixture of quasi-diaxial and diequatorial conformations. The nitro substituted PAHs are a recently identified group of environmental pollutants which possess very high mutagenic activity (Rosenkranz and Mermelstein, 1983). The findings of Fu and Yang (1983*b*), indicating that high levels of the 3,4-dihydrodiol are formed from 7-nitroBA, suggest that a marked alteration has occurred in the sites preferentially available for metabolism on the BA nucleus, when substituted by the deactivating NO_2 group at the 7-position.

8.3.7   *8-Methylbenz[a]anthracene*
The rat liver microsomal metabolism of 8-MBA gives all five possible *trans*-dihydrodiols, 8-OHMBA and the *trans*-3,4-, -5,6- and -10,11-dihydrodiols derived from 8-OHMBA, together with the 1-, 2-,

3- and 4-phenol derivatives of 8-MBA (Yang *et al.*, 1980*b*). The metabolism of this compound is of interest because it shows that the methyl group on a substituted PAH does not necessarily block the action of the microsomal enzymes; that the metabolic formation of methyl-substituted arene oxides can occur and that this methyl-substituted arene oxide can be acted on further by epoxide hydrolase to form a *trans*-dihydrodiol (Yang *et al.*, 1979*a*). The type of enantiomer formed is dependent on the cytochrome P-450 isoenzyme composition in the rat liver enzyme preparations (Yang *et al.*, 1982*b*).

8.3.8   *11-Methylbenz[a]anthracene*

Liver microsomes from PB-treated rats formed *trans*-3,4-, -5,6-, -8,9- and -10,11-dihydrodiols as metabolites. The predominant enantiomer in each case had the [R,R] configuration (Yang *et al.*, 1982*a*).

8.3.9   *12-Methylbenz[a]anthracene*

The metabolism of 12-methylbenz[a]anthracene by rat liver homogenates was reported by Sims (1967*a*) to give 12-OHMBA, the *trans*-5,6- and -8,9-dihydrodiols, the 12-OHMBA *trans*-8,9-dihydrodiol and 12-MBA 3- and 4-phenols. The use of HPLC has allowed identification of many other metabolites, including the *trans*-3,4- and -10,11-dihydrodiols (though in this study hydroxylation of the 12-methyl group was a minor metabolic pathway) (Yang *et al.*, 1980*b*). In examining the absolute stereochemistry of the *trans*-dihydrodiols formed from 12-MBA, Fu *et al.* (1982) reported that the stereochemistry of the major enantiomer of the *trans*-K-region dihydrodiol formed by hepatic microsomes from 3-MC induced rats was [5S,6S]. By comparison, when BA is incubated under similar conditions the [5R,6R] K-region dihydrodiol is the major enantiomer. These contrasting results exemplify the observation that a methyl group on a PAH may alter the stereoselective preference of the rat liver microsomal drug-metabolizing enzyme system toward the substrate molecule in the formation of a dihydrodiol metabolite. Indeed the position of a methyl substituent on the BA nucleus can alter the enantiomeric ratio of those optically active metabolites formed. The major 5,6-epoxide stereoisomer formed from the metabolism of 12-MBA with hepatic microsomes of PB-treated rats again had the opposite stereochemistry [5R,6R] to those formed in the metabolism of either 1-MBA or 7-MBA (Weems *et al.*, 1985).

The moderately active carcinogen, 12-MBA, may be converted to the strong carcinogen 7,12-DMBA by a bioalkylation substitution reaction. Thus Flesher *et al.* (1984) reported that rat liver cytosol preparations, fortified by the addition of S-adenosyl-L-methionine, add on a methyl group in the 7-position of 12-MBA to form 7,12-DMBA. It has also been reported by the same group (Flesher and Myers, 1985) that selective oxidation of the methyl group of 12-MBA may be accomplished by hepatic cytosol preparations without any apparent oxidation of the ring positions. Whether this cytosolic enzyme is quantitatively responsible for all the hydroxymethyl derivatives found metabolically is not known.

8.4   Metabolism of disubstituted benz[a]anthracenes

8.4.1   *3- and 5-Fluoro-7-methylbenz[a]anthracene*
The major hepatic metabolic pathway involved in the metabolism of 3- and 5-fluoro-7-MBA is the formation of the *trans*-8,9-dihydrodiol together with hydroxylation of the methyl group. With 3-fluoro-7-MBA significant amounts of the *trans*-10,11-dihydrodiol were also formed. Neither compound produced K-region dihydrodiols to any great extent (Sheikh *et al.*, 1981).

8.4.2   *6-Fluoro-12-methylbenz[a]anthracene*
The major hepatic metabolite formed from 6-fluoro-12-MBA *in vitro* by an S-10 fraction is the 12-hydroxymethyl derivative. Other predominant metabolites are the *trans*-8,9- and -10,11-dihydrodiols; no K-region dihydrodiol was detected (Sheikh *et al.*, 1981).

8.4.3   *7,12-Dimethylbenz[a]anthracene*
In experiments on the metabolism of 7,12-DMBA in whole animals Dickens (1945) reported the presence of the 4-phenol in the faeces of rats after intraperitoneal injection of 7,12-DMBA. The elimination of PAH metabolites in the faeces rather than the urine would appear to be a common feature of their metabolic distribution. Treatment of mice with 7,12-DMBA either on the dorsal skin of the nose or the skin on the back, or by intravenous injection resulted in the majority of the metabolites being excreted in the faeces (Sanders *et al.*, 1984). Absorption of 7,12-DMBA from the skin was rapid, only 18% of the applied dose remaining at the application site after 24 h; neither 7,12-DMBA nor its metabolites accumulated significantly in other body tissues, but were excreted rapidly (Sanders *et al.*, 1984).

Using *in vitro* techniques to examine the metabolism of 7,12-DMBA in mouse skin, a target tissue for 7,12-DMBA, it has been shown that all five possible *trans*-dihydrodiols are formed (DiGiovanni *et al.*, 1977; MacNicoll *et al.*, 1980b; Weston *et al.*, 1983), together with dihydrodiols related to 7-OHM-12-MBA (MacNicoll *et al.*, 1979a). A comparison of the metabolites formed from 7,12-DMBA by mouse, rat and human skin showed very little 3,4-dihydrodiol (the precursor to the bay-region diol epoxide) being formed by human skin, the major metabolite being the 1,2-dihydrodiol (Weston *et al.*, 1983), illustrating that there can be marked metabolic differences from the same type of tissue obtained from different species. The metabolism of 7,12-DMBA in mouse epidermal cells (DiGiovanni *et al.*, 1980*b*) similarly results in the formation of *trans*-dihydrodiols and hydroxymethyl derivatives, although phenolic metabolites predominated both within the cell (unconjugated) and in the medium (conjugated with glucuronic acid). Interestingly, although the 8,9-dihydrodiol was excreted rapidly from the cell, the 3,4-dihydrodiol was retained within the cell over the time period of the experiment. The metabolism of 7,12-DMBA in hamster epidermal cells (the hamster is a species in which the two-stage skin tumour model has yet to be conclusively demonstrated) also shows extensive conversion of 7,12-DMBA to water-soluble phenolic derivatives conjugated with glucuronic acid (DiGiovanni *et al.*, 1983*c*) and results suggest that lack of metabolism cannot account for the relative resistance of hamsters to epidermal carcinogenesis.

The metabolism of 7,12-DMBA by early passage cultures of mouse and hamster embryo cells, which are often used as a source of metabolizing enzyme in mutagenicity assays, results in extensive conversion of 7,12-DMBA to organic and particularly water-soluble metabolites (Sims, 1970*b*; Diamond, 1971; Gentil *et al.*, 1977; Baird *et al.*, 1978*b*). The major organic-soluble metabolites have been identified as the *trans*-8,9-dihydrodiol, *trans*-3,4-dihydrodiol and 7-OHM-12-MBA (Sims, 1970*b*; Gentil *et al.*, 1977; Huberman *et al.*, 1979*a*); and the water-soluble metabolites as phenol derivatives conjugated with glucuronic acid (Baird *et al.*, 1978*b*). Most of the 7,12-DMBA metabolites are from oxidation of the aromatic ring rather than of the methyl groups. In view of the large amounts of 8,9-dihydrodiol found in the medium it does not seem that this metabolite forms a glucuronic acid conjugate readily. The glucuronides of 7,12-DMBA phenols would be expected to detoxify, and make more readily excretable, those phenolic derivatives cytotoxic to the cells.

Hamster embryo cells have been used as a source of metabolizing enzyme when 7,12-DMBA and its weakly carcinogenic analogues such as 2-fluoro-7,12-DMBA (Oravec *et al.*, 1983) and 5-fluoro-7,12-DMBA (Daniel *et al.*, 1979) have been compared. Each readily forms a *trans*-8,9-dihydrodiol. The presence of a fluorine atom at C-2 greatly reduced metabolism at positions -1, -2, -3 and -4, whilst the presence of a fluorine atom at C-5 reduced metabolism at the K-region; the effect of metabolism at the bay-region was not reported for this latter compound. The metabolizing capability of hamster embryo cells has been compared with that of a human hepatoma cell line (DiGiovanni *et al.*, 1984); the two were quantitatively similar, although the hepatoma cell line produced primarily water-soluble conjugates which were neither sulphates nor glucuronides; this difference in metabolic pathway may account in part for the higher levels of binding to DNA and higher cell-mediated mutagenicity found with hamster embryo cells compared with human hepatoma cells. A marked alteration in metabolic pattern is observed in the metabolism of 7,12-DMBA by hamster embryo cells when benzo[e]pyrene is present. Benzo[e]pyrene, which is an inhibitor of the carcinogenic effect of 7,12-dimethylbenz[a]anthracene in mouse skin initiation-promotion assays, inhibits the secondary oxidation of 7,12-DMBA dihydrodiols (Baird *et al.*, 1984), in particular the *trans*-3,4-dihydrodiol (which was, in fact, formed in greater amounts in the presence of benzo[e] pyrene).

The lung represents a target tissue for polycyclic aromatic hydrocarbons, but the metabolism of 7,12-DMBA has not been studied extensively in this organ. One report (Palmer *et al.*, 1978) does describe the metabolism of 7,12-DMBA by mouse lung and tracheal tissue, and by cultured mouse macrophages to predominantly the *trans*-8,9-dihydrodiol. These important observations suggest that macrophages within the lung may contribute not only in the phagocytosis of insoluble particles which may have polycyclic aromatic hydrocarbons absorbed on them, but also the macrophages may metabolize the hydrocarbon to active metabolic forms which can be taken up by the surrounding tissue.

Because of its ready availability and richness in the cytochrome P-450 mixed function oxidase system, liver (a non-target organ), is the tissue in which the metabolism of 7,12-DMBA has been studied most extensively. Probably the most comprehensive examination of the metabolites formed has been carried out by Chou and Yang (1979*b*) where a total of 28 metabolites were identified from the incubation of phenobarbital-induced rat liver microsomes with 7,12-DMBA; 14 metabolites were obtained as products from incubations containing 12-OHM-7-MBA, 12 metabolites as products from incubations containing 7-OHM-12-MBA, and 9 metabolites as products from incubations containing 7,12-DiOH-MBA (Fig. 8.7). Both the aliphatic side chain and the aromatic nucleus of 7,12-DMBA underwent oxidation, the side chains to hydroxymethyl, aldehyde and carboxylic acid derivatives, the aromatic ring to *trans*-dihydrodiols (the 5,6-dihydrodiol predominating) and phenols. The

104   *Biology*

dihydrodiols formed from 7,12-DMBA included *trans*-3,4-, -5,6-, -8,9-
and -10,11-dihydrodiols; the phenols included 2-, 3- and 4-phenol derivatives, and in addition dihydrodiols and phenols of hydroxymethyl metabolites were also detected (Chou and Yang, 1979b). The exact sequence
of events involving hydroxylation of the methyl group and dihydrodiol

Fig. 8.7. Reversed-phase HPLC separation of the *in vitro* rat liver microsomal
metabolites of (a) 7,12-DMBA, (b) 12-OHM-7-MBA, (c) 7-OHM-12-MBA and
(d) 7,12-diOH-DMBA. From Chou and Yang (1979b).

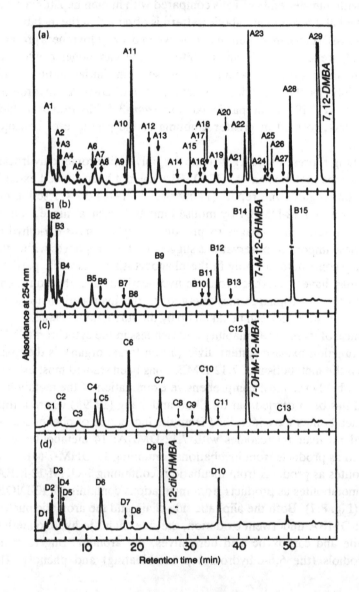

formation *in vivo* is not known although it has been demonstrated, using rat liver microsomes, that 7-OHM-12-MBA and 12-OHM-7-MBA can be metabolized further to form hydroxymethyl dihydrodiols and phenols (Chou and Yang, 1979*b*; Christou *et al.*, 1984).

Previously it had been shown that 7,12-DMBA metabolites such as dihydrodiols, phenols and hydroxymethyl derivatives were formed in rat liver homogenates containing 7,12-DMBA (Boyland and Sims, 1965*b*, 1967*b*; Flesher *et al.*, 1967; Sims, 1970*a*). There was no evidence of metabolic attack at the K-region of 7,12-DMBA, nor of the formation of glutathione conjugates, using rat liver homogenates. In contrast, with rat liver microsomes (Sims and Grover, 1967*b*) or hamster liver preparations (Gentil *et al.*, 1974), K-region dihydrodiol formation was apparent. Comparisons have also been made between hepatic nuclei and microsomes in the quantitative and qualitative metabolism of 7,12-DMBA (Chou *et al.*, 1981). The major difference between the two cell fractions was in the rate of metabolism, higher levels being observed with microsomes; quantitatively a similar metabolic profile was obtained using either of the two cell fractions. Hepatic cytosol is reported to be involved in the selective hydroxylation of the methyl groups of 7,12-DMBA to hydroxymethyl derivatives without any apparent oxidation of the ring positions (Flesher and Myers, 1985).

Pretreatment of rats with cytochrome P-450 enzyme inducers stimulates the metabolism of 7,12-DMBA (Levin and Conney, 1967; Jellinck and Gondy, 1966; Boyland and Sims, 1967*b*; Yang and Dower, 1975). Pretreatment with 3-MC caused a decrease in the amount of hydroxymethyl derivatives and an increase in the ring hydroxylation productions, whereas pretreatment with PB caused a small increase in metabolism mainly involving the methyl and hydroxymethyl groups. Observations of these variations led to suggestions of possible multiple forms of the cytochrome P-450 enzyme system (Boyland and Sims, 1967*b*; Levin and Conney, 1967). More recently (Yang *et al.*, 1980*c*; Wilson *et al.*, 1984), using more precise analytical techniques such as HPLC, it has been demonstrated with hepatic microsomes from animals in various states of induction i.e. treated with chemicals such as 3-MC or PB, or by using various reconstituted enzyme systems each containing a highly purified form of cytochrome P-450, that the metabolic profile of 7,12-DMBA can be substantially altered (Table 8.1).

Variations in age and diet (Sims and Grover, 1967*b*, 1968) and species (Sims and Grover, 1968; Gentil *et al.*, 1974) can also have a marked effect on the hepatic metabolism of 7,12-DMBA. Very young rats between the ages of 15 and 50 days possess an enhanced ability to metabo-

Table 8.1 *Regioselectivity of 7,12-DMBA metabolism by purified P-450 cytochromes*

| P-450 | Percent distribution of metabolites | | | | | | |
| | Dihydrodiols | | | Hydroxymethyl metabolites | | HMMBA Metabolites[a] | Phenols[b] |
	5,6-	8,9-	3,4-	7-	12-		
Uninduced							
microsomes	16 ±6.0[c]	16 ±0.6	7.5±0.6	32±8.0	16 ±0.3	6.0±1.3	7.0±1.8
PB-induced							
microsomes	24 ±3.0	13 ±2.0	7.5±2.3	10±2.0	23 ±5.7	22 ±4.0	2.0±0.4
P-450a	7.0±0.9	8.0±0.3	2.3±0.3	71±7.0	8.5±2.1	3.5±0.6	<0.2
P-450b	32 ±8.0	8.5±2.0	0.1±0.04	33±4.0	20 ±3.4	6.0±1.5	1.4±0.2
P-450e	18 ±7.0	4.0±1.6	0.1±0.04	22±4.0	46 ±2.0	9.9±2.0	<0.1
P-450h	29 ±9.0	7.0±0.4	<0.5	33±1.4	31 ±2.7	<0.5	<0.3
P-450 PCN	17 ±2.0	<0.5	<0.5	50±5.0	33 ±4.0	<0.5	<0.5
MC-induced							
microsomes	21 ±3.0	49 ±4.0	0.6±0.1	15±1.2	<0.1	6.4±0.3	7.5±1.2
P-450c	22 ±3.0	28 ±6.0	0.5±0.1	30±7.0	<0.1	12 ±1.0	7.0±2.0
P-450d	31 ±7.0	24 ±1.0	<0.2	26±3.0	1.5±0.3	7.5±0.4	10 ±1.0

[a] Includes 7,12-dihydroxymethylbenz[a]anthracene as well as aldehydes and phenols formed by further metabolism of 7-hydroxymethyl-12-methyl- or 12-hydroxymethyl-7-methylbenz[a]anthracene.
[b] Includes 2-, 3- and 4-phenols of 7,12-DMBA.
[c] All assays were performed in triplicate.
From Wilson *et al.* (1984).

lize 7,12-DMBA, these effects possibly being due to stimulation of enzyme activity by diet. Hamsters and mice are resistant to the induction of adrenal necrosis by 7,12-DMBA, (believed to be caused in the rat by a metabolite of 7,12-DMBA (see Chapter 8, p. 109). Such effects are not reflected in lower metabolizing capability of hepatic microsomes and homogenates prepared from these species, indeed a higher metabolic capability is reported in liver preparations from hamster compared with rat (Gentil *et al.*, 1974).

The instability of metabolic derivatives of 7,12-DMBA, particularly the *trans*-dihydrodiols and related epoxides and diol epoxides, has made the chemical synthesis of reference compounds difficult. Nevertheless the chemical preparation of the K-region epoxide has been reported (Sims, 1973) and its conversion enzymatically by rat liver microsomal fractions and homogenates (presumably by epoxide hydrolase) into the related *trans*-dihydrodiol, its conjugation with glutathione, and its conversion into phenols under acid conditions, have been described (Sims, 1973; Keysell *et al.*, 1973). There have been no reports on the isolation of non-K-region epoxides. The identification of non-K-region dihydrodiols, and in particular the *trans*-3,4-dihydrodiol (the precursor to the bay-region diol epoxide) was aided by the use of HPLC and the availability of authentic reference compounds. Thus the metabolic formation of 7,12-DMBA 3,4-dihydrodiol (Tierney *et al.*, 1978*b*; Chou and Yang, 1978; Yang *et al.*, 1979*b*) as well as the 3,4-dihydrodiols of 7-OHM-12-MBA, 12-OHM-7-MBA and 7,12-DiOH-DMBA (Chou and Yang, 1978) has been reported from rat liver preparations. Although *trans*-3,4-dihydrodiols are readily formed from the hydroxymethyl derivatives of 7,12-DMBA and indeed hydroxylation of the 7-methyl group may direct metabolism towards the 3,4-bond (Christou *et al.*, 1984), current evidence on the carcinogenicity of hydroxymethyl compounds suggests that they are not significantly involved in the metabolic activation of 7,12-DMBA (see Chapter 11). The metabolic formation of the *trans*-1,2-dihydrodiol has not been demonstrated in rat liver preparations. Although it may be postulated that the bay-region double bond (between C-1 and C-2) is adjacent to the 12-methyl group and thus steric effects may hinder the formation of the 1,2-dihydrodiol, this is in contrast to the observed formation of the 1,2-dihydrodiol from 7,12-DMBA using human skin as a source of metabolizing enzyme (Weston *et al.*, 1983). Thus enzymatic oxidation at the bay-region double bond of 7,12-DMBA is possible. The metabolic formation of the 2-phenol has been reported from rat liver microsomal incubations (Chou *et al.*, 1979*a*). Whether this formation is due to nonenzymatic rearrangement of the 1,2-epoxide

Table 8.2 *Comparison of the enantiomeric composition of the trans-5,6-dihydrodiol metabolite formed in the metabolism of various substituted BAs by liver microsomes from 3-MC-treated rats*

PAH	Enantiomer (%)		Optical purity (%)[a]
	R,R.	*S,S.*	
BA	81	19	62
8-MBA	90	10	80
11-MBA	75	25	46
7-Bromo-BA	98	2	96
7-Fluoro-BA	81	19	62
7-MBA	53	47	6
12-MBA	5	95	90
7,12-DMBA	6	94	88

[a] The optical purity is defined as the difference between the percentage of the two enantiomers.
From Yang and Fu (1984*b*).

(Jerina and Daly, 1974) or, possibly, hydroxylation of the aromatic nucleus by a direct insertion mechanism is not known. An unusual metabolite is reported to be formed from 7,12-DMBA by rat liver microsomes, involving peroxide formation between C-7 and C-12. The product from the transannular peroxidation of 7,12-DMBA is reduced further to give *cis*-7,12-dihydroxy-7,12-dimethylbenz[a]anthracene (Chen and Tu, 1976).

The absolute configurations of the various metabolically formed non-K-region *trans*-dihydrodiols of 7,12-DMBA have not been described. Interesting observations have been made on the absolute configuration of the metabolically formed K-region dihydrodiol of 7,12-DMBA. The predominant enantiomer formed by liver microsomes, whether from control, phenobarbital or 3-MC induced rats, has an [5S,6S] absolute configuration. When these findings are compared with the absolute configuration of the 5,6-dihydrodiol of BA [5R,6R], 7-MBA (approximately 1:1; [5R,6R]:[5S,6S]) and 12-MBA (approximately 5:95; [5R,6R]:[5S,6S]) it is clear that the introduction of a methyl group at the 7-position, and more particularly at the 12-position plays a crucial role in the stereoselective metabolism (Table 8.2) which occurs at the K-region 5,6-double bond (Yang and Fu, 1984*b*).

The absolute configuration of the K-region epoxide of 7,12-DMBA has been the subject of controversy. The initial assignment by Mushtaq *et al.* (1984) of the 7,12-DMBA 5,6-epoxide enantiomer predominantly formed by liver microsomes from 3-MC treated rats was [5R,6S]. This has recently been challenged by Balani *et al.* (1985); metabolism of 7,12-

DMBA by microsomes from 3-MC induced rats, as well as by homo-genous cytochrome P-450c, produces the 5,6-epoxide highly enriched (75%) in the [5S,6R]-enantiomer. This is in accordance with theoretical predictions on the proposed steric model for the catalytic binding site of cytochrome P-450c (Van Bladeren *et al.*, 1985).

The further hepatic metabolism of dihydrodiols, epoxides, phenols and hydroxymethyl derivatives of 7,12-DMBA to water-soluble conju-gates has not been extensively studied, in relation to the characterization of such products. An exception to this is the 7-hydroxymethylsulphate ester formed as a hepatic metabolite of 7,12-DMBA (Watabe *et al.*, 1982, 1985), after hydroxylation of the methyl groups. This sulphate ester conjugation of the hydroxymethyl groups by a rat liver cytosolic sulphotransferase results in a species which is a potent, intrinsic, mutagen toward *Salmonella typhimurium* and can bind to DNA and protein. This water-soluble conjugate represents therefore an interesting example of a metabolite, other than an epoxide, which possesses significant biologi-cal activity.

Metabolism of 7,12-dimethylbenz[a]anthracene in the adrenal gland
7,12-DMBA differs from other PAHs in its ability to cause necrosis in the two inner zones of the adrenal cortex; the zona fasciculato and the zona reticularis, of the adult rat, resulting in the induction of adrenal apoplexy (Huggins and Morii, 1961). It is possible to suppress the necro-sis by pretreatment of the animal with certain PAHs and amines (Huggins and Fukunishi, 1964a; Dao, 1964; Wheatley *et al.*, 1966b). Adrenal nec-rosis is a very specific effect both in terms of the hydrocarbons which elicit the response and the animal in which the response occurs: mice, hamster and immature rats do not exhibit adrenal necrosis whereas the mature rat does. Other hormone-dependent tissues, such as the testes and ovaries, are also affected by 7,12-DMBA; the cytochrome P-450 enzymes located in these tissues are regulated by pituitary peptide hor-mones (Guenthner *et al.*, 1979; Lee *et al.*, 1980). The cytochrome P-450 located in the adrenal gland may be different from that in the liver as it is not inducible by PAHs (Sims, 1970c; Guenthner *et al.*, 1979). These specific parameters have led investigators to examine the role that metabolism plays in the effect of 7,12-DMBA on the adrenal gland.

It was quickly recognized that a major hepatic metabolite of 7,12-DMBA, 7-OHM-12-MBA, has an enhanced capability to induce adreno-corticolysis compared with 7,12-DMBA itself (Boyland *et al.*, 1965c). In contrast hydroxylation of the 12-methyl group of 7,12-DMBA results in the complete loss of activity toward the adrenal gland. The 12-methyl group is necessary for 7,12-DMBA induced necrosis as 7-OHMBA also has no effect on adrenal glands of the mature rat (Boyland *et al.*, 1965c). Adrenal glands from adult rats can metabolize 7,12-DMBA, those from mice and infant rats do not (Jellinck *et al.*, 1967). Unlike the hepatic metabolism of 7,12-DMBA, adrenal metabolism *in vitro* results primarily in ring oxidation products (8,9-dihydrodiol) rather than hydroxylation of the methyl groups (Sims, 1970c). More recent studies have identified other dihydrodiols of 7,12-DMBA and 7-OHM-12-MBA, (including the 3,4-dihydrodiol) as metabolites from rat adrenal homogenates and rat adrenocortical cells (Montelius *et al.*, 1982; Swallow *et al.*, 1983). Both studies showed that there is a high and selective binding of 7,12-DMBA metabolites to soluble and microsomal proteins suggesting that the cytotoxic effects of these hydrocarbons on adrenocortical cells *in vivo* could result from reactions with proteins (Swallow *et al.*, 1983). It is still not clear how 7,12-DMBA exerts its effect on the adrenal gland, whether the bay-region dihydrodiol is important, whether the metabolites generated in the liver (such as 7-OHM-12-MBA) are transported to the adrenal gland, or whether the metabolism that occurs *in situ* within the adrenal gland itself is the important factor.

Metabolism of 7,12-dimethylbenz[a]anthracene in mammary tissue and cells
Mammary cancer can be induced rapidly in female rats by oral administration, intravenous injection or by the direct application to the mammary gland of 7,12-MBA (see Chapter 11). Because of the potency and reproducibility of the induction of mammary cancer by 7,12-DMBA, this system is widely used as a model to study carcinogenic events in mammary tissue (Huggins, 1979).

The particular susceptibility of mammary tissue to 7,12-DMBA induced carcinogenesis has been examined in relation to the metabolic products that are formed from 7,12-DMBA. In common with other organs, mammary tissue metabolizes 7,12-DMBA to hydroxymethyl derivatives (Tamulski *et al.*, 1973). Rat epithelial cell aggregates and fibroblasts prepared from mammary tissue form *trans*-dihydrodiols, the *trans*-8,9-dihydrodiol predominating (Shepherd and Bryan, 1977; Cooper *et al.*, 1982) and similar results have been observed using mammary cells prepared from human tissue (Grover *et al.*, 1980; MacNicoll *et al.*, 1980a). The majority of the metabolites formed from rat or human mammary cell preparations are water-soluble products (Grover *et al.*, 1980; MacNicoll *et al.*, 1980a; Cooper *et al.*, 1982) presumably in the form of glucuronides, sulphate esters and glutathione conjugates. Factors which can affect the susceptibility of rats to 7,12-DMBA induced mammary carcinoma include genetic background and physiological state. Metabolic comparisons which have been made between mammary cells isolated from rat strains which differ in their susceptibility to mammary cancer have not revealed any significant differences in their ability to metabolize 7,12-DMBA. The authors concluded that the specific susceptibility of certain rat strains to mammary cancer does not reside in differences in the ability of the mammary cells to activate these carcinogens metabolically (Moore *et al.*, 1983). In contrast when comparisons were made between the metabolizing ability of mammary cells obtained from rats whose susceptibility to mammary cancer results from differences in their physiological states (pregnant and virgin rats), a significantly altered ability to activate 7,12-DMBA in the mammary glands was found (Moore and Gould, 1984). This difference was of a quantitative rather than qualitative nature, mammary epithelial cells derived from pregnant rats (resistant to mammary cancer) showing a consistently lower capability to metabolize 7,12-DMBA than those derived from virgin rats. Thus the difference in the susceptibility to mammary cancer due to physiological states may be caused, at least in part, by differences in the amount of metabolically activated carcinogen formed.

The rat mammary gland is composed of two major cell populations, the parenchymal population containing ductal and myoepithelial cells, and the stromal population composed of fibroblasts, endothelial cells and various lymphatic cells types. It is small lesions, which appear to be located in the epithelial cells of the inner lining of the mammary duct, which are thought to proliferate to produce mammary cancer (Sinha and Dao, 1975). Metabolic comparisons using fibroblasts and epithelial cell aggregates from rat mammary tissue did not show any significant differences (Cooper *et al.*, 1982); four *trans*-dihydrodiols were identified (the 1,2-dihydrodiol was not detected). Similar results were found by Gould (1982*a*) who also compared the metabolism of 7,12-DMBA with B[a]P (a weak mammary carcinogen) and aflatoxin B_1 (a non-mammary carcinogen) in rat mammary parenchymal and stromal enriched cell populations. Whilst aflatoxin B_1 was not activated by either cell types, and 7,12-DMBA was activated by both cell types, B[a]P was activated by the stromal but not the parenchymal cell types (it is in the latter in which mammary carcinomas are believed to arise). This suggested that the organ specificity shown by 7,12-DMBA in the mammary gland may, in part, be explained by the intra-organ relationship between cell types that activate a carcinogen, and cell types that undergo neoplastic transformation.

8.5   Metabolism of trisubstituted benz[a]anthracenes

8.5.1   *Fluorine-substituted 7,12-dimethylbenz[a]anthracenes*

The comparative metabolism of 2-, 3-, 4-, 5- and 6-fluoro-7,12-dimethylbenz[a]anthracene in phenobarbital, naphthoflavone and 3-MC treated rat liver S-10 fractions has been examined (Sheikh *et al.*, 1981). Hydroxylation of the methyl groups was a major route of metabolism although only with phenobarbital-induced rat liver preparations were there significant amounts of hydroxylation at the 12-methyl group. Also only 7,12-DMBA and 6-fluoro-7,12-DMBA (a known carcinogen) yielded 3,4-dihydrodiols, precursors to the appropriate bay-region diol epoxide. The K-region dihydrodiol formation was inhibited by substitution of a fluorine atom at C-4 on 7,12-DMBA, whereas formation of the 8,9-dihydrodiol was stimulated by substitution of a fluorine at C-4 and C-5. The authors concluded that their results provided evidence for both electronic and steric influences on BA analogue metabolism. Steric effects seem to be important in the production of 5,6-dihydrodiols, whilst electronic effects, in conjunction with a consideration of the various resonance structures, may explain the modulating influence of fluorine substitution on the biofunctionalization of specific double bonds relative to those of the parent PAH (Sheikh *et al.*, 1981).

9

DNA, RNA and protein interactions

9.1 Introduction

The transformation of a normal cell into a malignant cell, after exposure to a chemical carcinogen, is the result of a complex series of biochemical events. It is generally believed that the initial step involves the reaction of an electrophile (formed from the carcinogen either directly or by metabolism) with cellular macromolecules such as DNA, RNA and protein. Which of these cellular macromolecules represents the critical target for the chemical carcinogen in the initiation of the carcinogenic process has been the subject of much theoretical discussion. The somatic mutation theory proposes that some permanent inheritable change in the nucleotide sequence occurs as the result of an alteration, deletion or rearrangement of the primary structure of DNA. Alternatively, epigenetic changes in cellular transcription and translation may bring about malignant cell transformation; such epigenetic changes also occur in normal development and differentiation (see Rubin, 1980; Marquardt, 1979a; and Barrett and Ts'o, 1978, for a fuller discussion of these hypotheses). The weight of evidence currently favours the somatic mutation theory, and underlies the widespread acceptance of the use of short-term mutation assays, such as the Ames Test, to indicate compounds with potential carcinogenic activity (many chemical carcinogens are mutagens). The DNA adducts formed *in vivo* and *in vitro* after attack by PAHs have been, in general, well characterized in terms of their chemical structure: it is often known which bases are involved, whereabouts on the base the PAH has bound and what type of functional group on the PAH is responsible for such binding.

Although the structures of the adducts are well known, and the amounts of such adducts present in the DNA can be determined, in certain instances there is only a poor correlation between the extent of DNA binding and the carcinogenic potency of a PAH. It seems there-fore that other factors must also play a part. One area which is of great current interest is whether there are any specific sequences of DNA to which a carcinogen may be preferentially bound, and whether such specific interactions may involve activation of oncogenes present in DNA. Such switching on of the oncogene could be due to binding of the carcinogen to the promoter region 'upstream' of the oncogene or result from alterations to the gene itself. Techniques are now becoming available which will allow such experiments to be carried out. Thus each of the Ha-*ras*-1 oncogenes present in MNU-induced mammary car-cinomas become activated by $G \rightarrow A$ mutations in the second nucleotide of codon 12 (Zarbl *et al.*, 1985). The considerable interest, therefore, in car-cinogen–DNA interactions is reflected in the space devoted to the topic in this chapter. Nevertheless there are certain carcinogenic substances for which it is difficult to reconcile their biological activity with DNA binding; for example, asbestos is a potent lung carcinogen and certain implants of chemically inert plastic film can cause tumours. The adducts formed with RNA by PAHs have not been as extensively investigated as those formed with DNA, although similar levels of binding occur.

The majority of the information available on carcinogen–protein and –peptide interactions is related to their metabolism by enzymes such as cytochrome P-450 and the subsequent conjugation of the metabolites with cellular entities such as glutathione and sulphate moities. Much less attention has been devoted to the possible transforming effects carcin-ogen-protein binding may have on a cell. In general, carcinogen-protein binding is of the same magnitude as carcinogen–DNA binding. Selective binding to specific proteins does occur, both in the cytosol and the nucleus of cells. The functional role of such interactions remains to be explored.

Finally it should be noted that experiments using PAHs, in particular when 7,12-DMBA has been used, have required that precautions should be taken to exclude light (due to the extreme photosensitivity of certain PAHs and their metabolites) and extremes of pH. Several publications, for example, Baird and Dipple (1977), Baird (1978*a*), have drawn atten-tion to these problems in relation to light-sensitive DNA-bound 7,12-DMBA adducts (where exposure to light over 24 h results in a complete loss of such adducts) and the sensitivity of certain 7,12-DMBA adducts to acid (Dipple *et al.*, 1985).

9.2   Binding of benz[a]anthracene to DNA and RNA

The covalent binding of the weak carcinogen BA to nucleic acids has been studied primarily in biological systems such as mouse skin, mouse or hamster embryo cells, and using rat liver preparations. Much of the work has been performed in the laboratory of Grover and Sims, and concerns the identification and characterization of the BA adducts formed in these biological systems.

Initial experiments examined the binding of BA to the DNA of hamster embryo cells; the major hydrocarbon adduct was derived from the 8,9-diol 10,11-epoxide (Swaisland *et al.*, 1974). It was also shown that rat liver microsomal preparations can activate BA 8,9-dihydrodiol to bind to DNA (Swaisland *et al.*, 1974). These findings implicating the 8,9-diol 10,11-epoxide as a metabolite involved in the metabolic activation of BA to DNA have been confirmed and extended using more powerful analytical techniques, such as HPLC, to describe the nucleic acid adducts formed by BA in rat liver preparations (MacNicoll *et al.*, 1979*b*), hamster embryo cells (Cooper *et al.*, 1980*c,d,f*) and by mouse skin (Cooper *et al.*, 1980*f*). Fluorescence spectral data on the BA adducts present in DNA isolated from mouse skin and hamster embryo cells which have been treated with BA, suggest the presence of a phenanthrene-like chromophore consistent with metabolic activation occurring in the 8,9,10,11-ring (Vigny *et al.*, 1980).

The adducts formed by the reaction of BA 8,9-diol 10,11-epoxide with DNA and RNA have characteristics of N^2-guanine derivatives (Hemminki *et al.*, 1980); NMR spectroscopy of the RNA adducts shows that the linkage is through the 11-position of the diol epoxide (Fig. 9.1) (Cary *et al.*, 1980). The NMR spectra of two of the adducts are almost identical, they also have similar pK values and stability in either acid or alkali, suggesting these adducts may be the result of the reaction of the (+) and (−) enantiomeric forms of the diol epoxide with guanine; only one of these adducts was found in RNA isolated from hamster embryo cells that had been treated with BA, possibly indicating stereospecific metabolism of the parent hydrocarbon (Cary *et al.*, 1980). The BA

Fig. 9.1. Proposed structure of the guanosine-*anti*-BA 8,9-diol 10,11-epoxide adduct, in which a carbonium ion, formed at the 11-position by the opening of the epoxide ring in the *anti*-BA 8,9-diol 10,11-epoxide has reacted with the exocyclic amino group of guanosine. From Cary *et al.* (1980).

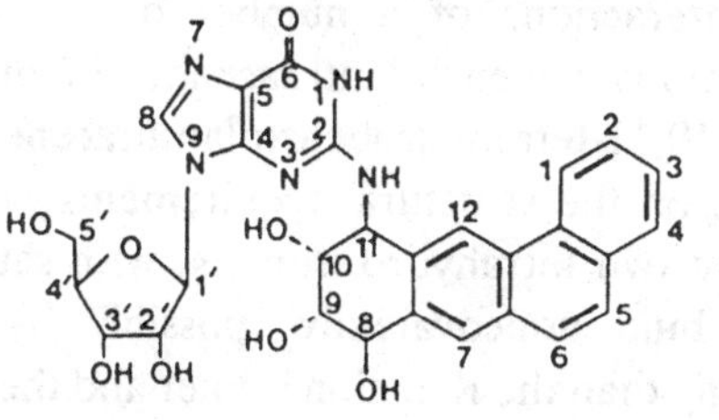

adducts present in RNA isolated from hamster embryo cells treated with BA were products of the reaction of BA 8,9-diol 10,11-epoxide with guanosine and adenosine (Cooper *et al.*, 1980*d*), similar results were obtained after reaction of BA with RNA *in vitro* (Phillips *et al.*, 1978).

Nucleic acid adducts have also been found resulting from the reaction of the bay-region 3,4-diol 1,2-epoxide in mouse skin and hamster embryo cells which had been treated with BA (Cooper *et al.*, 1980*d,f*). The principal base attacked is deoxyguanosine (Cooper *et al.*, 1980*d*), though the structural characterization of this adduct has not, so far, been reported. The exceptional biological activity (both in terms of muta-genicity and carcinogenicity) shown by the 3,4-dihydrodiol and the 3,4-diol 1,2-epoxide, when compared with that exhibited by BA itself or other, non-bay-region, dihydrodiols and diol epoxides of BA (Wood *et al.*, 1977*a,b*; Wislocki *et al.*, 1978) strongly implicates the bay-region diol epoxide as the ultimate carcinogenic form of BA. Only weak skin tumour-initiat-ing activity is associated with the 8,9-dihydrodiol and 8,9-diol 10,11-epoxide though it should be noted that relative to the parent hydrocarbon this activity is similar to that of the B[a]P 7,8-dihydrodiol and 7,8-diol 9,10-epoxide relative to B[a]P (Slaga *et al.*, 1978). Single strand breaks may be caused in DNA by BA 8,9-diol 10,11-epoxide (Cooper *et al.*, 1983) usually at the guanine sites. The relative contributions which the DNA adducts described above derived from BA 3,4-diol 1,2-epoxide and BA 8,9-diol 10,11-epoxide make to the observed weak biological activity of BA are still, at present, the subject of considerable discussion.

As well as the 3,4- and 8,9-dihydrodiols a third non-K-region dihydro-diol, the 10,11-dihydrodiol is produced during the metabolism of BA by mouse skin or rat liver microsomes (MacNicoll *et al.*, 1980*b*). How-ever, although the 10,11-dihydrodiol can form the 10,11-diol 8,9-epoxide surprisingly this entity does not contribute to the binding of BA to DNA in a rat liver microsomal system (Cooper *et al.*, 1980*a*), in hamster embryo cells, or in mouse skin *in vivo* (Cooper *et al.*, 1980*c,f*). The metabolic formation of a dihydrodiol or its diol epoxide therefore does not necessarily result in binding to DNA.

The noncovalent DNA interactions of a number of 'metabolite models', such as 1,2,3,4-tetrahydrobenz[a]anthracene, 5,6-dihydro-benz[a]anthracene and 8,9,10,11-tetrahydrobenz[a]anthracene (Fig. 9.2), have provided evidence on the structural requirements of meta-bolites for DNA binding. The two tetrahydro isomers, with saturated 1,2,3,4- or 8,9,10,11-rings, bind noncovalently (possibly by inter-calation) to DNA more strongly than the K-region isomer and the PAHs phenanthrene or anthracene (Shahbaz *et al.*, 1983). Other studies have compared the rates of covalent binding of various actual and potential metabolites of BA and B[a]P to electron-rich entities such as nucleic acids. The reactivities to DNA decreased in the order *anti*-BP-7,8-diol 9,10-epoxide > *anti*-BA-3,4-diol 1,2-epoxide > *anti*-BA-8,9-diol 10,11-epoxide (Phillips *et al.*, 1978; Hemminki *et al.*, 1980), and are in accordance with the predicted greater reactivity of epoxides formed in the bay-region of a hydrocarbon relative to epoxides formed in other positions.

Although the formation of phenols of PAHs is generally thought to be a process of detoxification, recently the further metabolism and subsequent binding to DNA of phenols of BA has been described (Hewer *et al.*, 1984). These DNA adducts have chromatographic properties similar to diol epoxide–deoxyribonucleoside adducts, though the precise role of such phenols in the carcinogenicity of BA has yet to be determined.

The type of tissue in which the reaction of BA with DNA occurs can result in large differences in the adduct profile; thus higher levels of the DNA adduct from the bay-region diol epoxide of BA were found in DNA isolated from BA-treated mouse skin or hamster embryo cells (Table 9.1) than in that obtained from a rat liver microsomal incubation (MacNicoll *et al.*, 1981). The extent of BA–DNA adduct formation can also be significantly affected by the location of the DNA within the cell. When nuclear and mitochondrial DNA are isolated from mouse embryo cells which have been treated with BA, much higher levels of adduct formation are present in the mitochondrial DNA (Allen and Coombs, 1980). The same effect is observed for more potent carcinogens such as B[a]P and 7,12-DMBA, there being a good correlation between the carcinogen–mitochondrial DNA binding and carcinogenic potential (Allen and Coombs, 1980).

Generally the work carried out on the interaction of BA metabolites with DNA has involved racemic mixtures; in view of the interesting

Fig. 9.2. Structures of some benz[a]anthracene analogues.

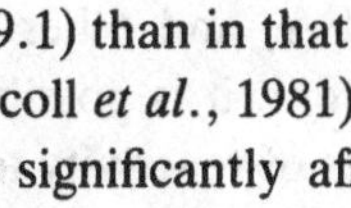

1,2,3,4-tetrahydroBA

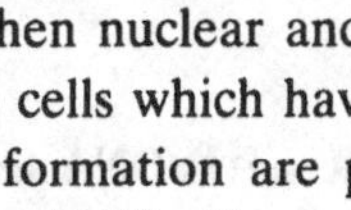

5,6-dihydroBA

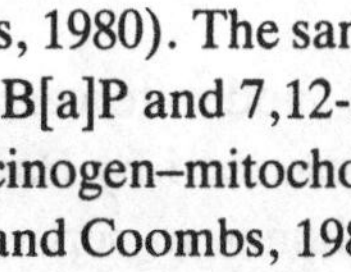

8,9,10,11-tetrahydroBA

Table 9.1 *Benz[a]anthracene–deoxyribonucleoside adducts formed in incubations of the hydrocarbon with rat-liver microsomal fractions, mouse skin or with hamster embryo cells*

	Benz[a]anthracene–nucleoside adducts[a] derived from	
Metabolic system	*anti*-BA-3,4-diol 1,2-oxide (%)	*anti*-BA-8,9-diol 10,11-oxide (%)
Rat-liver microsomal fraction	19.0	81.0
Mouse skin	45.8	54.2
Hamster embryo cells	33.4	66.6

[a] The amounts of hydrocarbon–DNA adducts derived from the 2 diol-epoxides are expressed as percentages of the total amounts of hydrocarbon–DNA adducts that co-eluted after HPLC, with authentic benz[a]anthracene–DNA adducts derived from either the *anti*-BA-3,4-diol 1,2-oxide or *anti*-BA-8,9-diol 10,11-oxide. From MacNicoll *et al.* (1981).

studies from several laboratories on the high degree of stereoselectivity required by dihydrodiols and diol epoxides of BA, and other hydrocarbons, for the initiation of the carcinogenic event, it is possible that such enantiomers may also show different degrees of reactivity towards a chiral substrate such as DNA.

9.3   Binding of monosubstituted benz[a]anthracenes to DNA and RNA
9.3.1   *7-Methylbenz[a]anthracene*
The formation of DNA adducts by the moderate carcinogen 7-methylbenz[a]anthracene (7-MBA) was first described by Baird and Brookes (1973*a*) who used Sephadex LH-20 columns to separate the 7-MBA-deoxyribonucleoside adducts from other products. The application of this chromatographic technique to the examination of carcinogen adducts has since been widely used and allows comparisons to be made between adducts from different sources, such as radioactive *in vivo* adducts with synthetically prepared marker adducts. It also allows separation of radiolabelled carcinogen adducts from extraneous radioactivity, and thus the actual amount of hydrocarbon bound to DNA can be determined. Baird and Brookes (1973*a*) found that the [³H]7-MBA–deoxyribo nucleoside adducts were present as two peaks after separation by Sephadex LH-20 chromatography (Fig. 9.3), and that similar chromatographic profiles were obtained from enzymic digests of DNA isolated from mouse embryo cells, mouse skin and human embryo cells, suggesting similar pathways of metabolic activation. The [³H]7-MBA–deoxyribonucleoside

adduct profile from mouse embryo cells which had been treated with [³H]7-MBA was different from that obtained from the enzymic digest of DNA treated with 7-MBA 5,6-epoxide or 7-BrMBA (Baird *et al.*, 1973*b*). These data do not support mechanisms of binding of 7-MBA to DNA in cells that require metabolic activation of the methyl group or the formation of a K-region epoxide. Similar results were found with 7-MBA–ribonucleoside adducts isolated from the RNA of mouse embryo cells treated with 7-MBA (Baird *et al.*, 1976).

Fluorescence spectral data on DNA isolated from either hamster embryo cells or mouse skin which had been treated with 7-MBA (Fig. 9.4) showed spectra similar to 9-methylanthracene indicating that the 1,2,3,4-ring

Fig. 9.3. Sephadex LH-20 elution profiles of enzymic digests of (a) mouse skin DNA isolated from mice treated topically with [³H]7-MBA for 24 h; (b) mouse skin DNA isolated from mice treated topically with [³H]7-MBA for 48 h; and (c) DNA isolated from mouse embryo cells treated for 72 h with [³H]7-MBA. From Baird and Brookes (1973*a*). - - -, A_{254}; ——, radioactivity.

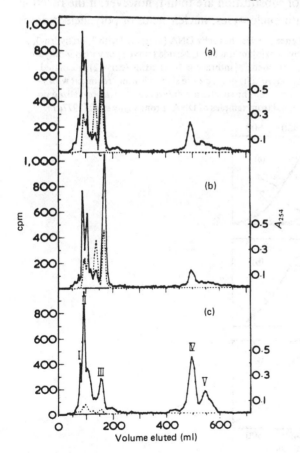

of 7-MBA is saturated when bound to DNA (Vigny *et al.*, 1977*a*; Moschel *et al.*, 1979). Sephadex LH-20 chromatography of DNA nucleoside adducts from mouse skin treated with 7-MBA *in vivo* showed similarities with the chromatographic profile of BA 3,4-diol 1,2-epoxide reacted with DNA (Tierney *et al.*, 1977) consistent with the above fluorescent data.

9.3.2   *7-Bromomethylbenz[a]anthracene*

7-Bromomethylbenz[a]anthracene (7-BrMBA) is a carcinogen which, unlike most PAHs, has a direct acting capability and does not necessarily require metabolic activation. The direct reaction of 7-BrMBA with nucleosides has been studied in dimethylacetamide, where nucleophilic substitution of the bromine atom in the 7-bromomethyl group by the N-7 of guanine, N-1 of adenine and N-3 of cytosine occurs (Dipple *et al.*, 1971*a*). Similar adducts have been detected after the reaction of DNA with other direct acting alkylating agents (Lawley, 1966). Different sites of substitution are found, however, if the reaction between 7-BrMBA with nucleosides, nucleic acids or polynucleotides is

Fig. 9.4. Fluorescence spectra shown by DNA (a) treated with 3,4-dihydro-3,4-dihydroxy-7-methylbenz[a]anthracene 1,2-oxide (curve 1) or with 8,9-dihydro-8,9-dihydroxy-7-methylbenz[a]anthracene 10,11-oxide (curve 2) or isolated (b) from hamster embryo cells or (c) mouse skin following treatment with 7-methylbenz[a]anthracene. The spectra are difference spectra normalized on their maxima obtained from samples of DNA. From Vigny *et al.* (1977*a*).

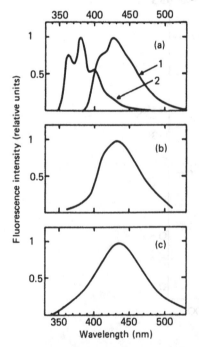

in aqueous solution. Under this condition reaction mainly occurs on the exocyclic amino group of guanine, adenine and possibly cytosine (Dipple *et al.*, 1971*a*). Adducts of this latter type have been identified as being present in the DNA of mouse skin after topical application of 7-BrMBA (Rayman and Dipple, 1973*a*). There was a poor correlation when comparisons were made between the carcinogenicity of 7-BrMBA and of 7-bromomethyl-12-methylbenz[a]anthracene (Dipple and Slade, 1971*b*) with the binding of these compounds to the DNA of mouse skin, both in terms of the total extent of reaction and the extent of attack on any specific nucleoside residue in DNA (Rayman and Dipple, 1973*b*).

There has been widespread use of 7-BrMBA in studies investigating the repair of carcinogen-DNA adducts. The 7-BrMBA adducts present in DNA have been well characterized and are chemically stable; these facts, coupled with the ease of use of a direct acting carcinogen such as 7-BrMBA have provided a model system for studying DNA repair in both mammalian (Lieberman and Dipple, 1972) and bacterial (Vennit and Tarmy, 1972) cells. The early studies in mammalian cells demonstrated that 7-BrMBA induced unscheduled DNA synthesis in nondividing human lymphocytes and that there was a time-dependent removal of 7-BrMBA adducts; the adenine adducts were removed more extensively than the guanine adducts (Lieberman and Dipple, 1972). These findings have been confirmed and extended in other cell lines such as a human cell line (HeLa S-3) and a Chinese hamster cell line (V-79379A) where again the carcinogen-modified adenine residues were excised more readily than the carcinogen-modified guanine residues (Dipple and Roberts, 1977). The data strongly support an excision repair mechanism though complete excision of all the damaged DNA is not necessary for DNA replication and subsequent cell survival (Dipple and Roberts, 1977). When the repair of 7-BrMBA was studied in normal human cells and in those defective in their repair of ultraviolet damage, the results suggested that different cellular mechanisms are involved in the repair of DNA damage resulting from ultraviolet irradiation and that resulting from 7-BrMBA treatment (McCaw *et al.*, 1978). The interaction of 7-BrMBA with DNA caused distortion in the DNA structure, and this distortion is recognized by a possible repair enzyme from *E. coli*, endonuclease V (Demple and Linn, 1982), the cleavage at the methylbenz[a]anthracene adducts being usually 5' to the lesion.

9.3.3   *7-Hydroxymethylbenz[a]anthracene*
The binding of the weak carcinogen 7-hydroxymethylbenz[a]an-

thracene to DNA *in vitro* requires metabolic activation, ATP, and is time-dependent (Wettstein *et al.*, 1979). There is only a single peak in the hydrocarbon-deoxyribonucleoside region on Sephadex LH-20 chromatography (Moschel *et al.*, 1979); the characteristics of this presumed adduct have not yet been described.

9.3.4   *12-Methylbenz[a]anthracene*

The binding of 12-methylbenz[a]anthracene (12-MBA) to DNA isolated from mouse embryo cells is similar to that of 7-MBA, as judged by the profiles of enzymic digests of adducted DNA after Sephadex LH-20 chromatography (Moschel *et al.*, 1979). However, the fluorescence spectra of the 12-MBA–DNA adducts are quite different from those of 7-MBA adducts and more closely resemble those of 7,12-DMBA–DNA adducts. The 12-MBA adduct emission spectra are broad and lack resolution, and they occur at longer wavelengths than model compounds such as those with an anthracene nucleus. The effects, both for 12-MBA and 7,12-DMBA may be related to the presence of a methyl group in the bay-region and the intermolecular interaction of the hydrocarbon chromophore and the attached nucleoside, suggesting that binding may occur through the intermediacy of a 3,4-diol 1,2-epoxide (Moschel *et al.*, 1979).

9.4   Binding of disubstituted benz[a]anthracenes to DNA and RNA
9.4.1   *7,12-Dimethylbenz[a]anthracene*
Mouse skin

When 7,12-DMBA has been compared with B[a]P in its ability to initiate tumours in mouse skin, B[a]P is a much weaker skin tumour initiator; 10 nmol of 7,12-DMBA compared with 200 nmol of B[a]P per mouse being required for 100% tumour incidence in mice (DiGiovanni *et al.*, 1980*a*). This difference in oncogenic potential is not quantitatively reflected in the binding of the two hydrocarbons to DNA; 7,12-DMBA does bind to mouse skin DNA to a greater extent than B[a]P, but only at a 2- to 4-fold higher level (Brookes and Lawley, 1964; Phillips *et al.*, 1979*a*; Bigger *et al.*, 1983). Therefore there has been an extensive examination of the types of individual hydrocarbon adducts formed in mouse skin DNA to see whether these may account for the strong carcinogenicity of 7,12-DMBA.

Fluorescence spectral measurements provide the most direct method of analysis of the binding of 7,12-DMBA to mouse skin DNA. The treatment of mouse skin *in vivo* with 7,12-DMBA and the subsequent isolation of the mouse skin DNA and its examination by fluorescence spectroscopy shows such DNA has characteristics consistent with hydro-carbon-adduct formation, with the retention of a substituted anthracene-like nucleus as would be expected after oxidation at C-1, -2, -3 and -4 in 7,12-DMBA (Vigny *et al.*, 1977*b*). When DNA, isolated from mouse skin which has been treated with 7,12-DMBA, is hydrolysed enzymatically to nucleosides the carcinogen nucleoside adducts can be separated into three major peaks by Sephadex LH-20 chromatography and HPLC. The fluorescence spectra of these nucleoside adduct peaks are all anthracene-like, again supporting the concept of metabolic activation occurring in the 1,2,3,4-ring. Conversely, the fluorescence evidence does not support activation through the K-region or at the 8-, 9-, 10-, and 11-positions, nor does it support binding through the methyl groups which would leave the benz[a]anthracene nucleus intact (Vigny *et al.*, 1981). Similar findings have been made in mouse (Moschel *et al.*, 1977) and hamster embryo cells (Ivanovic *et al.*, 1978).

The direct analysis between 7,12-DMBA mouse skin DNA adducts formed *in vivo* and those DNA adducts formed by the reaction of non-K-region diol epoxides with DNA has been limited by the difficulties encountered (mainly due to stability) in the chemical synthesis of such diol epoxides. Nevertheless current evidence (Cooper *et al.*, 1980*e*) suggests that the bay-region diol epoxide is responsible, in part, for the 7,12-DMBA–DNA adducts isolated from mouse skin treated with 7,12-DMBA. By comparison with adducts tentatively characterized in the mouse embryo cells system as bay-region *anti*-diol epoxide deoxyguanosine and deoxyadenosine adducts and a bay-region *syn*-diol epoxide deoxyadenosine adduct (Dipple *et al.*, 1983; Sawicki *et al.*, 1983), it has been shown that qualitatively the same adducts are present, as three major peaks on HPLC (Fig. 9.5) in mouse skin DNA from animals treated topically with 7,12-DMBA (Bigger *et al.*, 1983). Interestingly, at higher doses of 7,12-DMBA the *syn*-diol epoxide deoxyadenosine adduct (peak C, Fig. 9.5) increases significantly until it represents as much as 40% of the total DNA binding; this may be compared with the much lower levels of adenosine binding by the weaker carcinogen B[a]P (Bigger *et al.*, 1983). A correlation between binding to deoxyadenosine and tumourigenic potential for a series of PAH has previously been pointed out by DiGiovanni *et al.* (1979*b*). Using mouse epidermal homogenates they showed that although poly(G) had the highest capacity to bind hydrocarbons, there was no correlation between binding to poly(G) and mouse skin carcinogenicity whereas there was good agreement between binding of various PAHs to poly(A) and mouse skin tumourigenicity. At present one can only speculate as to how such

124   *Biology*

binding to adenosine may be involved in initiating carcinogenesis; deoxy-adenosine-rich sequences are present in DNA, and such sequences are involved in the regulation of gene expression in eukaryotic cells (Breathnach and Chambron, 1981; Moreau *et al.*, 1981). The preferential binding of 7,12-DMBA is to reiterated rather than unique regions of DNA isolated from murine skin at low doses of the carcinogen (Shoyab, 1978). Equal levels of binding of 7,12-DMBA to main band and satellite DNA have been reported (Zieger *et al.*, 1972). The significance of these types of observations on the position of carcinogen binding within the genome remains to be established.

Recently, advances have been made in the analysis of carcinogen-DNA adducts allowing very low levels of modification, possibly as low as one adduct per 10^{10} nucleotides, may be measured. The method does not require the carcinogen to be radiolabelled and utilizes the incorporation of ^{32}P into DNA constituents by polynucleotide kinase-catalysed ^{32}P-phosphate transfer from γ-^{32}P ATP after exposure of the DNA, either *in vitro* or *in vivo*, to a carcinogen (Randerath *et al.*, 1983; Gupta, 1985). The application of this technique to 7,12-DMBA–DNA adducts

Fig. 9.5. HPLC elution profiles of 7,12 DMBA-deoxyribonucleoside adducts isolated from the skin of male mice treated topically with (a) 0.14 μmol [^{3}H]7,12-DMBA (2.4 Ci/mmol) and (b) 0.003 μmol [^{3}H]7,12-DMBA (45.7 Ci/mmol). Mice were killed 24 h after 7,12-DMBA treatment. For further description see text. From Bigger *et al.* (1983).

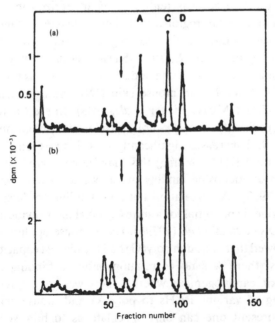

formed in the dermis and epidermis of mouse skin has allowed some interesting observations to be made. While initial binding to DNA was higher in the epidermis, the adducts were ten times more persistent in the dermal DNA. This study was carried out over a period of 42 weeks, much longer than previous studies. It was found that there is a pool of persistent adducts which are present in subpopulations of dormant cells, and it was proposed that such cells, in the absence of promoting stimulus, are incapable of division because of the adductation and/or mutation of genes critical for growth (proto-oncogenes) and may thus correspond to the 'latent tumour cells', as defined by Berenblum and Shubik (1947, 1949*b*) in their classical analysis of the attributes of tumour initiation and promotion (Randerath *et al.*, 1985*b*). The treatment of such quiescent initiated cells *in vivo* with TPA results in a rapid loss of the persistent adducts, possibly reflecting a stimulation of cell division (Randerath *et al.*, 1985*a*). Since the initiated cells contain altered genes which may include oncogenes, the expression of such genes may occur; the activation of oncogenes in 7,12-DMBA-induced skin tumours has been described previously (Balmain *et al.*, 1984).

Considerable progress has been made in determining the genetic events which may underlie the initiation of carcinogenesis. A single base pair substitution may alter a non-transforming proto-oncogene to an activated oncogene capable of causing cellular transformation. (For a review see Land *et al.*, 1983.) The transformation of NIH 3T3 fibroblasts by DNA isolated from 7,12-DMBA-induced mouse skin carcinomas has been shown to be related to the transfer of an activated cellular homologue of the Harvey-*ras* oncogene (Balmain and Pragnell, 1983). This is consistent with the findings that oncogenes related to the *ras* genes of Harvey or Kirsten sarcoma viruses are activated preferentially in tumours arising in epithelial tissues (Pulciani *et al.*, 1982; Cooper, 1982). The treatment *in vitro* of the c-Ha-*ras*-1 proto-oncogene with a PAH (B[a]P) results in a transforming oncogene when such modified DNAs are introduced into NIH 3T3 cells (Marshall *et al.*, 1984), supporting the concept that chemical modification of DNA is a necessary step in the multistage process of tumour induction. The activation of Ha-*ras*-1 oncogenes in 7,12-DMBA induced tumours probably involves mutations in codon 61 (Yuasa *et al.*, 1983; Taparowsky *et al.*, 1983). The transformation observed in NIH 3T3 cells is often not seen in primary cultures or senescent cells, suggesting possibly that the NIH 3T3 cells are already partially transformed and that some biological event, such as the acquisition of immortality, is required before the transforming gene can be phenotypically expressed. Evidence to support this comes from Newbold and Overall (1983) who showed that EJC-Ha-*ras*-1 lacks complete trans-forming activity when transfected into normal fibroblasts (which have a limited lifespan) but can fully transform fibroblasts that have been newly 'immortalized' by carcinogens.

Minor alterations in the structure of a chemical may have a marked effect on its carcinogenicity, and this type of structure–activity relation-ship has been examined at the level of DNA binding. The substitution of fluorine at C-10 of 7,12-DMBA results in a compound with increased tumour initiating activity (DiGiovanni *et al.*, 1983*a*). This is also reflected in the levels of DNA binding found in mouse epidermal cells treated either *in vivo* or in culture with 7,12-DMBA or the 10-fluoro derivative, higher levels of binding being found with the latter compound, though the HPLC profiles were qualitatively the same (DiGiovanni *et al.*, 1985). The adducts which were present at a lower level in DNA isolated from mouse skin treated with 10-fluoro-7,12-DMBA were those correspond-ing to the formation of adducts from *syn-* and *anti*-diol epoxides with deoxyadenosine. Only the adduct resulting from the binding of the *anti*-diol epoxide with deoxyguanosine was enhanced; these findings therefore suggest the importance of deoxyguanosine adducts and the *anti*-diol epoxide isomer during 7,12-DMBA-induced mouse skin car-cinogenesis.

Although the major carcinogen adducts present in mouse skin DNA, after treatment with 7,12-DMBA, have been tentatively identified, other minor adducts remain which cannot be accounted for directly by a bay-region diol epoxide metabolite (Cooper *et al.*, 1980*e*), nor do they seem to arise from hydroxylation of the methyl group (MacNicoll *et al.*, 1979*a*; Dipple *et al.*, 1979*a*), although adducts of this type, containing a hydroxy-lated methyl group, have now been reported (DiGiovanni *et al.*, 1983*b*) to be present in the DNA of 7,12-DMBA-treated mouse skin.

It has been known for a number of years that a wide variety of chemi-cals, including PAHs (Slaga and Boutwell, 1977*a*; Slaga *et al.*, 1979*c*; DiGiovanni *et al.*, 1982*b*), benzoflavones (Slaga and Bracken, 1977*b*; Lesca, 1981) and antioxidants such as butylated hydroxytoluene (Slaga and Bracken, 1977*b*) are capable of inhibiting the carcinogenic activity of 7,12-DMBA in mouse skin. Where the effects of these chemicals on the total binding of 7,12-DMBA to DNA have been examined there has, in general, been an inhibition of DNA–carcinogen binding correlat-ing with the inhibition of the initiating activity of 7,12-DMBA (Kinoshita and Gelboin, 1972; Cohen *et al.*, 1979; Lesca, 1981; DiGiovanni *et al.*, 1982*b*). More recently (Dipple *et al.*, 1984*b*) experiments have demon-strated the effects of these types of inhibitors on the individual

Table 9.2 *Effect of benzoflavones on the binding of 7,12-DMBA to DNA in the skin of female NIH Swiss mice*

| | | Adducts in μmol/mol DNA-P | | | |
Benzoflavone	Time (h)	Total	*anti-*dGuo	*syn-*dAdo	*anti-*dAdo
None	6	1.9	0.56	0.46	0.41
	24	1.8	0.54	0.44	0.39
	48	1.2	0.40	0.27	0.24
5,6- (1000 μg)	6	1.3	0.34	0.38	0.23
	24	1.3	0.37	0.35	0.23
	48	1.1			
7,8- (25 μg)	6	0.3	0.09	0.07	0.07
	24	0.4	0.14	0.09	0.09
	48	0.4			
7,8- (100 μg)	6	0.2	0.06	0.06	0.04
	24	0.3	0.10	0.07	0.07
	48	0.2	0.07	0.04	0.05

From Dipple *et al.* (1984*b*).

carcinogen adducts present after separation on HPLC. The potent inhibitor 7,8-benzoflavone caused a reduction in the amount of 7,12-DMBA binding to DNA, there being no specific variation in the levels of individual adducts, suggesting that 7,8-benzoflavone inhibits the formation of both the *syn-* and *anti-*diol epoxides (Table 9.2). In contrast, antioxidants such as butylated hydroxytoluene had very little effect on the overall total DNA binding or on individual adduct levels, suggesting that oncogenesis induced by 7,12-DMBA may require changes in the target tissue, other than changes to its DNA, to complete the process of tumour initiation and it is at this step that butylated hydroxytoluene acts (Dipple *et al.*, 1984*b*). Strains of mice which differ markedly in their susceptibility to 7,12-DMBA induced carcinogenesis also showed no difference in total DNA binding or in the HPLC profile of individual adducts, suggesting differences in their susceptibilities do not arise at the level of metabolic activation and consequent binding to DNA (Dipple *et al.*, 1984*b*).

Mammary tissue
Mammary cancer can be induced rapidly in female rats by 7,12-DMBA. The induction of mammary cancer is dependent on a number of factors such as the age, strain, sex and hormonal status of the animal; inhibition of mammary cancer can occur if the animal is pregnant or lactating (see Huggins, 1979, for a review). These modulating factors have proved

of great interest to researchers attempting to understand how 7,12-DMBA causes mammary cancer.

Within 24 h of a single dose of 7,12-DMBA, covalent binding of the hydrocarbon to the DNA, RNA and proteins present in breast tissue of rats can be detected (Prodi *et al.*, 1970; Janss and Ben, 1978). The binding of 7,12-DMBA to mammary gland DNA has been well correlated with the age-related incidence of mammary tumours in Sprague–Dawley rats (Janss *et al.*, 1972; Janss and Ben, 1978); thus the binding of 7,12-DMBA is highest in 50- to 60-day virgin rats, which also have the highest mammary tumour incidence, and lower levels of 7,12-DMBA DNA binding are found in younger and older animals. The type of DNA adducts present in mammary tissue exposed to 7,12-DMBA appear to be similar to those described and characterized in mouse skin and mouse embryo cell DNA. The adducts in mammary tissue DNA probably result from attack by the bay-region diol epoxide of 7,12-DMBA and possibly 7-hydroxymethyl-12-MBA on guanine and adenine (Tay and Russo, 1981; Cooper *et al.*, 1982; Daniel and Joyce, 1983, 1984; Vigny *et al.*, 1985). Adducts of this type have also been detected after treatment of human mammary cells with 7,12-DMBA (Grover *et al.*, 1980).

The way in which the presence of 7,12-DMBA DNA adducts may alter the expression of such modified DNA is not fully understood yet. The activation of a specific oncogenic locus, that involving the Ha-*ras*-1 oncogene, has been reported to occur in 7,12-DMBA-induced tumours (Yuasa *et al.*, 1983; Taparowsky *et al.*, 1983). There appear to be significant differences in the way such an oncogene becomes mutagenic in mammary tumours initiated by different chemicals. Each of the Ha-*ras*-1 oncogenes present in mammary tumours induced by N-nitroso-N-methylurea become activated by the same G→A transitions in the second nucleotide of codon 12; in contrast, the activation of the Ha-*ras*-1 oncogene in 7,12-DMBA-induced mammary tumours does not involve such a transition and may involve mutations in codon 61, specifically at the two deoxyadenosine residues (Zarbl *et al.*, 1985).

Although evidence has been presented for the resistance of 7,12-DMBA adducts to DNA repair processes in mouse embryo cells (Dipple and Hayes, 1979*a*), relatively high levels of DNA repair of 7,12-DMBA adducts exist in mammary cells derived from parous rats, which are resistant to 7,12-DMBA induced mammary cancer, when compared with repair levels in mammary cells obtained from young and old virgin rats (Tay and Russo, 1981). In the same study the qualitative examination of individual 7,12-DMBA adducts revealed similar patterns in the three types of rat. This suggested that the observed complete refractoriness of the parous rat mammary gland to 7,12-DMBA-induced carcinogenesis may be due not to different metabolic activation pathways or to the formation of different adducts, but to the lower binding capacity and to the more efficient DNA repair processes present in lactating mammary tissue (Tay and Russo, 1981). The possible importance of DNA repair processes has also been noted in a study carried out on 7,12-DMBA induced mammary cancer in Long–Evans versus Sprague–Dawley rats (the former strain is more resistant to mammary cancer). Higher levels of 7,12-DMBA adduct removal were observed in the Long–Evans strain, both in the liver and mammary gland (Daniel and Joyce, 1984), which may reflect the greater activity of repair enzymes in the Long–Evans strain rat.

Pretreatment of rats with N^6,O^2-dibutyl cyclic adenosine $3',5'$-monophosphate (DBcAMP) prevents the induction of mammary carcinoma (Cho-Chung *et al.*, 1983). The mechanism by which this effect occurs has been studied by Huang *et al.* (1984) in relation to the level of 7,12-DMBA binding to DNA, and alterations in gene expression. Lower levels of 7,12-DMBA binding to DNA are found in susceptible rats which have been treated with DBcAMP. In addition examination of the gene transcription products from young virgin rats which had been treated with DBcAMP showed the products now resembled those of the old virgin gland (which are resistant to the effects of 7,12-DMBA). It has also been shown that DBcAMP transforms the cAMP system of an undifferentiated young virgin gland into that of a highly differentiated older virgin gland (Cho-Chung *et al.*, 1983). Thus specific patterns of transcription may be imposed on the young virgin gland by DBcAMP; these may lead to a loss of growth potential and promote differentiation resulting in a cellular mechanism which is similar to that of the old virgin gland (Huang *et al.*, 1984). How these alterations at the genetic level may relate to the lowering of 7,12-DMBA binding to DNA and cause suppression of mammary tumour incidence is not known.

Structural alterations in the 7,12-DMBA molecule can also cause inhibition of 7,12-DMBA-induced mammary cancer. Substitution of a fluorine atom at the 2-position of 7,12-DMBA results in a compound which is essentially non-carcinogenic and non-mutagenic (Slaga *et al.*, 1979*a*; Harvey and Dunne, 1978). The levels of DNA binding of 7,12-DMBA and its 2-fluorine substituted analogue have been examined in target (mammary) and non-target (liver) tissue from rats treated with these hydrocarbons (Daniel and Joyce, 1983). Although considerably lower levels of binding to DNA were found in animals treated with the noncarcinogenic 2-fluoro-7,12-DMBA (when compared with 7,12-DMBA-treated animals), this was not the case when the level of 7,12-DMBA binding to DNA isolated from target and non-target tissue was examined. Approximately equal levels of binding of 7,12-DMBA to DNA were found between liver and mammary tissue, suggesting that adduct formation alone was not sufficient to account for the observed difference in susceptibility to tumour initiation by 7,12-DMBA (Daniel and Joyce, 1983, 1984). These findings on the similarity of 7,12-DMBA adduct levels in target and non-target tissues are in contrast with an earlier report by Janss and Ben (1978), where a higher level of 7,12-DMBA binding to DNA isolated from mammary glands was observed, when compared with binding to liver. Differences in the route of administration and DNA isolation and analysis may account for these discrepancies.

There is a good correlation between the age-dependent induction of mammary cancer (reaching a maximum at the age of 50–60 days for the female rat) and the rate of DNA synthesis (Nagasawa and Yanai, 1974; Nagasawa *et al.*, 1976). This enhanced level of DNA synthesis may be related to the increased density of terminal end-buds and terminal ducts present in the mammary glands of young virgin rats (55 days old), fewer terminal end-buds and terminal ducts being present in older, non-susceptible rats (180 days old) which also had lower levels of DNA synthesis (Russo and Russo, 1978). That 7,12-DMBA-induced mammary tumours arise in the ductal structures has been described previously (Sinha and Dao, 1975). They appear to originate from the epithelial cells of the inner lining of the mammary duct. However fibroblasts and epithelial cell aggregates derived from mammary tissue were similar in their ability to metabolize and metabolically activate 7,12-DMBA, there being little difference either quantitatively or qualitatively, in the binding of 7,12-DMBA to DNA and protein isolated from the two cell types (Cooper *et al.*, 1982).

There appear, therefore, to be a number of factors which may contribute towards 7,12-DMBA-induced mammary cancer susceptibility including the initiation level, the role of DNA synthesis, the type of cell structure present in the mammary gland, the DNA repair potential of the different cell types and sensitivity to agents which may have promotional effects, such as hormones and dietary fat.

Liver
Although liver is resistant to the carcinogenic action of 7,12-DMBA (except when the compound is administered during liver regeneration: Marquardt *et al.*, 1970) experiments using this tissue have led to two

important observations: (a) that the metabolite 7-OHM-12-MBA can contribute to the observed binding to DNA of 7,12-DMBA; and (b) that variations in the products of metabolic activation are observed with tissues from different sources.

The formation of hydroxymethyl metabolites of 7,12-DMBA has been well documented (Palmer *et al.*, 1978; Chou and Yang, 1979*b*) and such metabolites are able to bind to DNA (Chou and Yang, 1978; Dipple *et al.*, 1979*b*; MacNicoll *et al.*, 1979*a*), and exhibit a distinctive fluorescence spectrum consistent with activation in the bay-region to form a diol epoxide (Ivanovic *et al.*, 1978). However, until recently 7-OHM-12-MBA was not considered to contribute significantly to the binding of 7,12-DMBA to DNA in mouse embryo cells (Dipple *et al.*, 1979*b*) or in mouse skin (MacNicoll *et al.*, 1979*a*). The formation of such 7-OHM-12-MBA–DNA adducts has now been reported *in vivo* in the liver of rats treated intraperitoneally with 7,12-DMBA (Joyce and Daniel, 1982) and similar observations have also been made regarding 7,12-DMBA adducts isolated from mouse skin (DiGiovanni *et al.*, 1983*b*).

Rat liver microsomal or homogenate preparations are frequently used for the examination of the metabolic activation and the mutagenicity of carcinogens. However, large differences exist in the DNA–carcinogen adduct profiles found after HPLC, when such substituted DNA from hepatic preparations are compared with that obtained from intact cultured cells (Bigger *et al.*, 1978, 1980*a*) or with substituted DNA obtained from tissues susceptible to the carcinogen, such as mouse skin (Bigger *et al.*, 1978). HPLC of 7,12-DMBA adducts generated by hepatic preparations show strong similarities with those adducts formed by the reaction of the K-region epoxide with DNA, whereas those formed in mouse embryo cells or mouse skin do not (Bigger *et al.*, 1978). The formation of DNA adducts derived from the K-region epoxide of 7,12-DMBA by hepatic preparations are dependent on the concentration of the hydrocarbon (Fig. 9.6); such concentration effects are not observed in intact mouse embryo cells (Bigger *et al.*, 1980*a,b*). Whilst at certain concentrations adducts which are derived from diol epoxides were also observed, in no case was an exactly similar HPLC adduct profile obtained from DNA which had been incubated with 7,12-DMBA in the presence of hepatic preparations when compared with that from a target tissue such as mouse skin (Bigger *et al.*, 1980*b*), showing the need for caution in the use and interpretation of short-term mutagenicity tests which employ liver as the activating system.

Although the formation of K-region oxidation products is favoured by the hepatic metabolism of 7,12-DMBA, when the *trans*-3,4-dihydrodiol of 7,12-DMBA is further metabolized by hepatic microsomes in the presence of DNA, covalent binding to DNA of the 7,12-DMBA metabolite is observed, indicative of the formation of a bay-region epoxide (Chou and Yang, 1978). Whereas lower levels of binding to DNA were found when the 3,4-dihydrodiol of 12-OHM-7-MBA was employed (Table 9.3) (suggesting possible steric interference in the bay-region) higher levels of binding to DNA occur with 7-OHM-12-MBA and its 3,4-dihydrodiol, compared with the analogous 7,12-DMBA compound (Chou and Yang (1978)).

Mouse embryo cells in culture
Experiments which have been carried out, mainly in the laboratory of Dipple, on the binding of 7,12-DMBA to the DNA of mouse embryo cells have allowed substantial advances to be made in our understanding of the type of 7,12-DMBA metabolites and DNA bases involved in such binding. These studies are particularly relevant because the carcinogen adducts present in this cell line are also present in a target tissue such as mouse skin (Bigger *et al.*, 1978, 1983).

Initial information on the type of 7,12-DMBA adducts present in DNA isolated from mouse embryo cells which had been treated with 7,12-DMBA, was obtained from their fluorescence spectra and suggested oxidation was occurring at C-1, -2, -3 and -4 of the 7,12-DMBA molecule, consistent with the metabolic formation of a bay-region diol epoxide (Moschel *et al.*, 1977). The fluorescence spectral characteristics of 7,12-DMBA adducts showed a lack of resolution and shifts to longer wavelengths when compared with the 7-MBA adduct fluorescence spectra;

Fig. 9.6. Sephadex LH-20 column chromatography of 7,12-DMBA-deoxyribonucleoside adducts formed by enzymic digestion of calf thymus DNA treated with (a) 320 nmol [^{3}H]7,12-DMBA, or (b) 24 nmol [^{3}H]7,12-DMBA in the presence of hepatic microsomes. The single-headed arrows denote the position of elution of 4-(*p*-nitrobenzyl)pyridine, the double-headed arrows denote the position of added 7,12-DMBA 5,6-epoxide-deoxyribonucleoside UV-absorbing markers. From Bigger *et al.* (1980*b*).

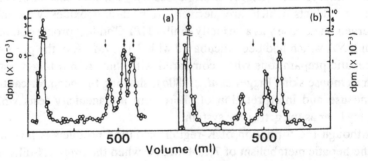

Volume (ml)

Table 9.3 In vitro DNA-binding activities of 7,12-DMBA and its metabolites upon further metabolism with liver microsomes

[³H]-7,12-DMBA and its metabolites[a]	Specific activity (mCi/mmol)	DNA-binding activity[b] (pmol/mg DNA)	
		− Microsomes	+ Microsomes
7,12-DMBA	190	5	53
7-OHM-12-MBA	96	6	97
12-OHM-7-MBA	130	8	68
7,12-(OH)₂DMBA	130	4	21
7,12-DMBA-trans-3,4-diol	130	16	137
12-OHM-7-MBA-trans-3,4-diol	130	16	69
7-OHM-12-MBA-trans-3,4-diol	130	32	178
7,12-DMBA-trans-8,9-diol[c]	130	8	43
7-OHM-12-MBA-trans-8,9-diol[d]	130	4	17

[a] The hydrocarbons were used at 80 nmol per ml reaction of mixture. The amount of 7,12-(OH)₂DMBA-trans-3,4-diol obtained was not sufficient for this experiment. We have observed that the trans-3,4-diols are considerably less stable than the other trans-diols under identical storage conditions (dried under nitrogen and stored at −20°C). Hence the experimental data reported herein were obtained by using the metabolites within 24 h of purification.
[b] Average values of duplicate samples which agree within 10% of the values shown. To convert to the unit of μmol of polycyclic aromatic hydrocarbon bound per mol of DNA phosphate, multiply the values by 3.23.
[c] The ultraviolet–visible absorption and fluorescence spectra, retention times in both HPLC systems, and mass spectra were identical those of the synthetic standard.
[d] The ultraviolet–visible absorption and fluorescence spectra were the same as those of 7,12-Me₂BA-trans-8,9-diol. The identity was confirmed by mass spectral analysis (M⁺ at m/c 306) and by its inability to form vicinal cis-acetonide.
From Chou and Yang (1978).

these spectral properties may reflect the presence of the methyl group at the 12-position interacting with the attached nucleoside, thus providing evidence for reaction through a bay-region diol epoxide (Moschel et al., 1979).

The binding of 7,12-DMBA to the DNA of mouse embryo cells is inhibited by the addition of 1,1,1-trichloropropene-2,3-oxide. This compound blocks the action of epoxide hydrolase thus suggesting that epoxides, or the product of enzymic action on an epoxide, a trans-dihydrodiol, are necessary intermediates in the binding of 7,12-DMBA to DNA (Dipple and Nebzydoski, 1978). The introduction of matrices containing phenylboronic acid (which interacts specifically with molecules containing cis-diol groups) has considerably aided the determination of the relative contributions which the syn- and anti-bay-region diol epoxide make in the binding to DNA by 7,12-DMBA. As can be seen in Fig. 9.7 only the anti-diol epoxide will generate an adduct which contains a *cis*-diol group which would be expected to interact with the boronic acid group. Using this system, Sawicki *et al.* (1983) have shown that both the *syn*- and *anti*-diol epoxide make a substantial contribution to the observed DNA adducts present in mouse embryo cells treated with 7,12-DMBA. Fluorescence spectra of these individual 7,12-DMBA adducts, after separation on HPLC, also support the structural identification of these adducts as being derived from *syn*- and *anti*-bay-region diol epoxides (Moschel *et al.*, 1983; Sawicki *et al.*, 1983). Of the three major adducts present on HPLC (labelled A, C and D on Fig. 9.8) two are derived from the *anti*-diol epoxide (A and D) and one from the *syn*- isomer(C). The *syn*- isomer also makes a contribution to the minor adducts present. The ^{14}C pre-labelling of purine bases in the DNA of mouse embryo cells has allowed the further characterization of the 7,12-DMBA–deoxyribonucleoside adducts by determining which bases are associated with which peak on HPLC; thus of the three major adducts present in Fig. 9.8, A is a bay-region *anti*-diol epoxide–deoxyguanosine adduct, C is a bay-region *syn*-diol epoxide–deoxyadenosine adduct and D is an *anti*-diol epoxide–deoxyadenosine adduct (Dipple *et al.*, 1983).

These findings on the structure of the 7,12-DMBA adducts differ substantially in two respects from that described for the less potent carcinogen B[a]P, which is probably the most intensely studied PAH. Firstly there is a large contribution to DNA binding made by the *syn*-diol epoxide of 7,12-DMBA and secondly there is extensive binding of metabolized 7,12-DMBA to deoxyadenosine, which is the only detected target for the *syn*-diol epoxide. Because the *syn*-diol epoxide of B[a]P has been

Fig. 9.7. Relative stereochemistry of 7,12-DMBA *anti*- and *syn*-bay-region diol epoxides and their expected reaction products with nucleoside residues (R) in DNA. From Sawicki *et al.* (1983).

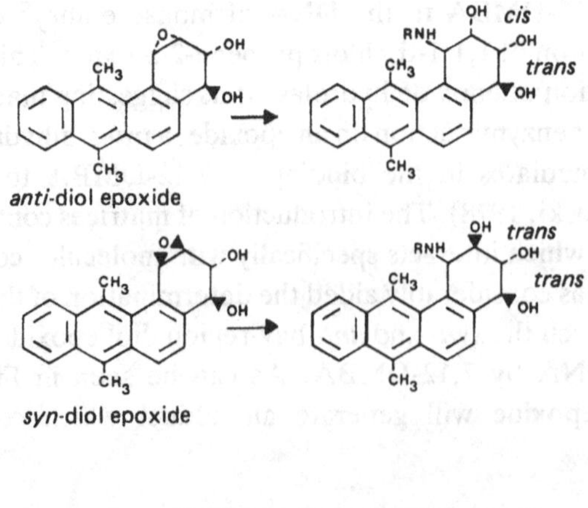

found to be less carcinogenic than the *anti*-isomer, interest has largely centred on the *anti*-isomer. However, 7,12-DMBA has a methyl group in its bay-region and this may alter the stability and reactivity of such isomers. In addition a correlation between binding to adenine and tumourigenesis in mouse skin has been commented on previously (DiGiovanni *et al.*, 1979*b*). Given the greater carcinogenic potency of 7,12-DMBA compared with B[a]P, the above observations suggest that reactions on deoxyadenosine residues may be important in the initiation of the carcinogenic process (Dipple *et al.*, 1983).

The moderate carcinogen 7-OHM-12-MBA is also activated by the

Fig. 9.8. HPLC separations of deoxyribonucleoside adducts from mouse embryo cells treated with [^{3}H]7,12-DMBA for (a) 24 h and (b) 6 h. The arrow denotes the position of an added UV-absorbing marker of toluene. For further description see text. From Sawicki *et al.* (1983).

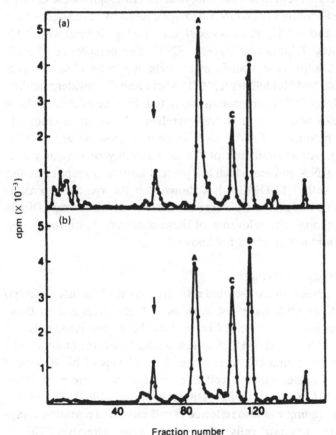

formation of a diol epoxide, which can then bind to DNA in mouse embryo cells; however, adducts of this type are not present in adduct hydrolysates of 7,12-DMBA bound to mouse embryo DNA, suggesting that the activation of 7,12-DMBA does not involve a preliminary conversion to the hydroxymethyl derivative (Dipple *et al.*, 1979*b*).

The 7,12-DMBA adducts in DNA which has been isolated from mouse embryo cells treated with 7,12-DMBA show marked differences to those adducts isolated from DNA incubations containing rat liver microsomes and 7,12-DMBA. These differences stem principally from the fact that the type of adduct being formed is concentration dependent in the microsomal system, whereas no such concentration effect is found in intact mammalian cells (Bigger *et al.*, 1980*b*). Findings such as these suggest limitations in the use of microsomal systems as models for target tissue activation.

The role of DNA repair seems very limited in the removal of 7,12-DMBA adducts present in mouse embryo cells. Although mouse embryo cell cultures efficiently excise DNA damage caused by carcinogens such as 7-BrMBA and 3-MC, no such excision of damage is seen with 7,12-DMBA adducts (Dipple and Hayes, 1979*a*). The persistence of 7,12-DMBA–DNA adducts in transformable cells has been observed previously (Kuroki and Heidelberger, 1971) where also the covalent binding of 7,12-DMBA to RNA and protein was noted. In none of these cellular macromolecules was there a strong correlation between carcinogenic potency and binding to DNA, RNA or protein (Kuroki and Heidelberger, 1971). An examination of the acid stability of *syn-* and *anti*-diol epoxide–DNA adducts which are present after treatment of mouse embryo cells with 7,12-DMBA has shown that the *syn*-diol epoxide–deoxyadenosine adducts in DNA are the most sensitive to acid (Dipple *et al.*, 1985), though the relevance of these observations on the persistence of such adducts *in vivo* is not known.

Hamster embryo cells in culture
The types of DNA adducts isolated after treatment of hamster embryo cells with 7,12-DMBA have not been as well characterized as those occurring in mouse embryo cells. Comparisons have been made between the DNA binding of 7,12-DMBA in low-passage hamster embryo cells and a human hepatoma cell line; much higher levels of binding were found in the hamster embryo cell line, though the pattern of DNA adducts on HPLC was very similar (DiGiovanni *et al.*, 1984). This higher level of DNA binding was also reflected in cell-mediated mutation assays where hamster embryo cells were much more effective. This is

not due to greater overall metabolism, which was about equal in the two cell systems, but rather, the authors concluded, was due to differences in the metabolic pathways leading to a marked reduction in DNA-binding metabolites in the human hepatoma cell line compared with the hamster embryo cells (DiGiovanni *et al.*, 1984). Characterization of the types of adducts present has not yet been carried out.

The introduction of a fluorine atom at the 5-position of 7,12-DMBA causes a reduction in the carcinogenic potency of 7,12-DMBA. In Syrian hamster embryo cells both 7,12-DMBA and 5-fluoro-7,12-DMBA are converted to water-soluble metabolites at equal rates, but 7,12-DMBA binds to DNA to a greater extent (three-fold) (Daniel *et al.*, 1979). This difference in hydrocarbon binding to DNA, however, does not seem sufficient to account for the comparatively large difference (100-fold) in carcinogenic activity. Studies carried out on differences in DNA repair levels suggested that carcinogenic activity may be related to the specific types of adducts entering DNA replication (D'Ambrosio *et al.*, 1979), but much more work needs to be done before the effect on DNA binding of fluorine substitution at the 5-position of 7,12-DMBA can be understood.

Human embryo and tumour cells in culture
The binding of 7,12-DMBA to DNA has been examined in human embryo cells; binding of 7,12-DMBA to DNA, RNA and protein was of the same order of magnitude as that of B[a]P, but was lower than that observed in mouse embryo cells. There did not seem to be significant differences in 7,12-DMBA DNA binding between human embryo cells and human tumour cells (HeLa) (Brookes and Duncan, 1971).

9.4.2 *Reaction of 7,12-dimethylbenz[a]anthracene 5,6-epoxide with DNA*
Probably the most well characterized 7,12-DMBA adduct is that resulting from the reaction of 7,12-DMBA 5,6-epoxide with guanine. The K-region epoxide reacts preferentially with guanine, when compared with the other purine and pyrimidines available, to form four major adducts separable on HPLC (Blobstein *et al.*, 1975; Jeffrey *et al.*, 1976*a*). With poly(A) only two major adducts are found (Jeffrey *et al.*, 1976*a*). The four guanosine adducts formed by the direct reaction of 7,12-DMBA 5,6-epoxide have been characterized by their ultraviolet, circular dichroism, mass and proton magnetic resonance spectra (Jeffrey *et al.*, 1976*b*). Reaction occurs between the epoxide group at either C-5 or C-6 and the N-2 amino group of guanine (Fig. 9.9), there being four

possible isomers. When the K-region epoxide is reacted with guanosine under conditions of high pH, adducts formed at the 2′-hydroxyl group of the ribose moiety (Fig. 9.10) (Kasai *et al.*, 1977), or at the C-8 of guanosine (Nakanishi *et al.*, 1980), are isolated.

Although the majority of evidence indicates that in mouse skin and embryo cells (Moschel *et al.*, 1977; Bigger *et al.*, 1978), hamster embryo cells (Ivanovic *et al.*, 1978), or mouse fibroblasts (Marquardt *et al.*, 1976) binding of 7,12-DMBA to DNA involves carbons C-1 to C-4 of 7,12-DMBA, there are often unidentified 7,12-DMBA intermediates detected that bind to the DNA of mouse skin (Cooper *et al.*, 1980*e*). Similarly, recent experiments with fluorinated derivatives of 7,12-DMBA suggest that both bay- and K-regions are involved in the activation of 7,12-DMBA to mutagenic and carcinogenic metabolites in mouse skin (Huberman and Slaga, 1979*b*). The rat liver microsomal incubation of 7,12-DMBA with DNA yields adducts generated mainly by the reaction of the K-region epoxide with DNA (Bigger *et al.*, 1978), although other adducts are also present (Jeffrey *et al.*, 1976*a*). Indeed K-region adducts have also been detected in the RNA isolated from rat liver cells treated with [³H]-7,12-DMBA, although they were present at a low level, representing less than 5% of the total nucleoside–7,12-DMBA adducts present (Frenkel *et al.*, 1981). Two of these adducts were from the reaction at either the C-5 or C-6 of 7,12-DMBA 5,6-epoxide with the 2′-hydroxyl group of the ribose molecule and in addition a third adduct was derived from the reaction of the K-region epoxide with C-8 of guanine (Fig. 9.10). Neither type of adduct has been reported for other polycyclic aromatic hydrocarbons, and although the two ribose adducts could not be formed with DNA, the third 7,12-DMBA product which is bound to the C-8 of guanine could possibly be formed with DNA.

9.4.3   *7-Hydroxymethyl-12-methylbenz[a]anthracene*
Studies on the DNA-binding ability of products derived from 7-OHM-12-MBA have been carried out principally to examine the hypothesis that the further metabolism of 7-OHM-12-MBA (a major metabolite of 7,12-DMBA in a number of target tissues) may occur generating species which would yield DNA adducts, and that these adducts would contribute to the overall pattern of 7,12-DMBA adducts observed. It has now been established that monomethylhydroxy-7,12-DMBA–DNA adducts are formed in the liver (Joyce and Daniel, 1982) and in mammary gland (Daniel and Joyce, 1983) after administration of 7,12-DMBA to female Sprague–Dawley rats. In addition the presence of DNA adducts derived from 7-OHM-12-MBA has been demonstrated

in DNA isolated from the epidermis of Sencar mice treated with 7,12-DMBA and when epidermal homogenates were utilized to catalyse the covalent binding of 7,12-DMBA to DNA (DiGiovanni *et al.*, 1983*b*). The high carcinogenicity of the *trans*-3,4-dihydrodiol of 7-OHM-12-MBA suggests the diol epoxide of this metabolite could contribute to the carcinogenicity of 7,12-DMBA (Wislocki *et al.*, 1980, 1981*b*).

9.4.4   *7-Bromomethyl-12-methylbenz[a]anthracene*

The compound 7-bromomethyl-12-methylbenz[a]anthracene (7-BrM-12-MBA) has a carcinogenic potency comparable to that demonstrated by 7,12-DMBA (Dipple and Slade, 1970), and is of much greater potency than 7-bromomethylbenz[a]anthracene (7-BrMBA) (Dipple and Slade, 1970, 1971*b*). This difference in carcinogenic potency between 7-BrMBA and 7-BrM-12-MBA is not reflected in the levels of binding to DNA isolated from mouse skin treated *in vivo* with 7-BrMBA or 7-BrM-12-MBA. Much higher levels of DNA binding are found for the weaker carcinogen 7-BrMBA (Rayman and Dipple, 1973*a*). The inverse relationship between carcinogenic potency and extent of reaction with

Fig. 9.9. Chemical structures elucidated by Jeffrey *et al.* (1976*b*) of the guanosine adducts formed from the *in vitro* reaction of 7,12-DMBA 5,6-epoxide with poly(G).

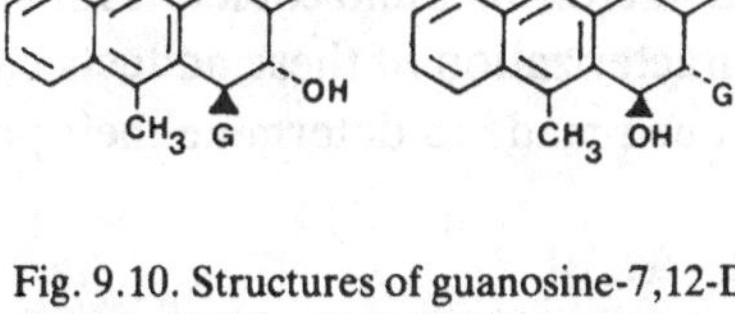

Fig. 9.10. Structures of guanosine-7,12-DMBA 5,6-epoxide adducts isolated from the RNA of 7,12-DMBA treated rat liver cells. From Frenkel *et al.* (1981).

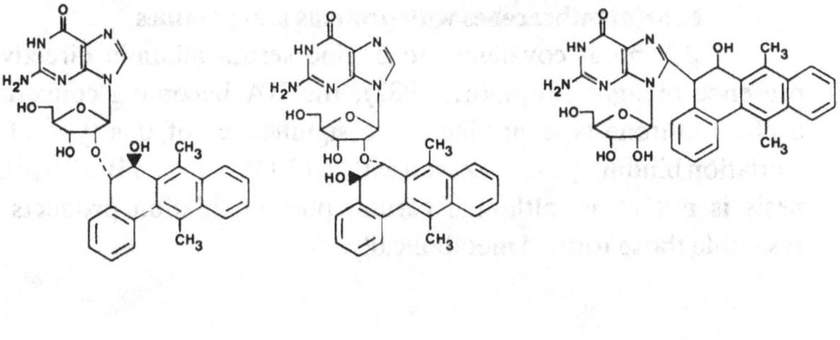

mouse skin DNA indicates that the overall capacity of these compounds to react with DNA cannot be the major determinant of their respective carcinogenic potencies. This is also true when the levels of binding of 7-BrMBA and 7-BrM-12-MBA to DNA *in vitro* have been examined (Rayman and Dipple, 1973*b*), and the levels of modification of individual bases have been determined (Rayman and Dipple, 1973*b*). By analogy with the characterized DNA adducts formed by 7-BrMBA (Dipple *et al.*, 1971*a*), it would be expected that 7-BrM-12-MBA would bind to the amino groups of guanine and adenine. Recently Carrell *et al.* (1981) have used X-ray crystallography to determine that the adduct formed between 2'-deoxyadenosine and 7-BrM-12-MBA is N⁶-(12-methyl-benz[a]anthracenyl-7-methyl)deoxyadenosine.

9.5   Binding of trisubstituted benz[a]anthracenes to DNA and RNA
9.5.1   *Fluorine-substituted 7,12-dimethylbenz[a]anthracene*
The substitution of a fluorine atom at the C-5 of 7,12-DMBA produces a compound which is only weakly carcinogenic (Daniel *et al.*, 1979). Examination of the DNA binding of 7,12-DMBA and its 5-fluoro analogue in Syrian hamster embryo cells, using liver microsome preparations, shows this difference in carcinogenicity to be reflected in the amounts of the hydrocarbon being bound to DNA, i.e. there is an approximately three-fold higher level of 7,12-DMBA binding to DNA, compared with the 5-fluoro analogue (Daniel *et al.*, 1979). In order to pursue the hypothesis that 7-OHM-12-MBA is a proximate carcinogen that requires further metabolism to form a reactive ester which would then be a good leaving group, Chien and Flesher (1981) compared the binding to DNA of 5-fluoro-7-OHM-12-MBA and its acetate ester. The latter compound did bind to DNA nonenzymatically, whereas the 5-fluoro-7-OHM-12-MBA required microsomes and cofactors for covalent binding to DNA. No further characterization of these adducts has been reported nor have any attempts been made to determine their presence *in vivo*.

9.6   Interaction of benz[a]anthracene and substituted benz[a]anthracenes with proteins and peptides
BA binds covalently to bovine serum albumin directly in the presence of light (Fujimori, 1982), the BA becoming converted into a phenanthrene-type product. The significance of this type of photo-oxidation binding (also observed with 7,12-DMBA and B[a]P) in oncogenesis is not clear, although certain photo-oxidation products closely resemble those formed metabolically.

The covalent interaction of metabolic forms of BA with certain cellular protein constituents represents a major route of detoxification. Conjugation of dihydrodiols or diol epoxides with the tripeptide glutathione by glutathione-S-transferases results in water-soluble products readily excreted from the cell. Both the BA 8,9-dihydrodiol and BA 8,9-diol 10,11-epoxide can form glutathione conjugates (Booth and Sims, 1974; Cooper *et al.*, 1980*b*) in the presence of rat liver homogenates. There are multiple forms of glutathione-S-transferases, some of which have been purified to homogeneity; the reader is referred to excellent reviews on what is an extensive subject (Chasseaud, 1979; Jakoby and Habig, 1980). Significant differences exist in the rate of glutathione conjugation between the K-region epoxide of BA and a diol epoxide of BA. The K-region epoxide of BA is a much better substrate for a variety of purified glutathione-S-transferases than the 8,9-diol 10,11-epoxide of BA (Glatt *et al.*, 1983). These observations may explain why the K-region epoxide is a major metabolite of BA from rat liver homogenates, but shows very little binding to DNA when compared with the high level of binding to DNA found with the 8,9-diol 10,11-epoxide. Interestingly, at least one form of the glutathione-S-transferase isoenzymes exhibits stereo-selectivity in its interaction with epoxides of PAHs. When BA 5,6-epoxide is used as substrate there is predominant (95%) attack at the oxirane carbon of [R] absolute configuration to give the [S,S] product (Cobb *et al.*, 1983). Similar observations on the stereoselectivity of cytochrome P-450 and epoxide hydrolase enzymes towards epoxides have also been reported.

BA interacts noncovalently with a number of proteins. The metabolism of BA occurs through noncovalent binding to cytochrome P-450, and the epoxide formed is further metabolized to a dihydrodiol by epoxide hydrolase. Another enzyme which is involved in the detoxification of PAHs and which has recently been purified to apparent homogeneity is cytosolic dihydrodiol dehydrogenase (Vogel *et al.*, 1980). This NADP-dependent enzyme converts a dihydrodiol to a catechol group and appears to have a higher specificity for diol epoxides than simple K-region epoxides (Glatt *et al.*, 1982).

BA is a known inducer of certain forms of cytochrome P-450, and the induction process may be mediated by a specific cytosolic receptor protein (Poland *et al.*, 1976) in a manner similar to steroid receptors. Evidence for a specific receptor protein mediating cytochrome P-450 induction has utilized mainly 3-MC and 2,3,7,8-tetrachlorodibenzo-*p*-dioxine (TCDD) as the ligands. Competition studies with BA have shown there to be interactions both with 3-MC (Tierney *et al.*, 1980) and

TCDD (Bigelow and Nebert, 1982) cytosolic-binding species, suggesting this type of specific binding to protein also occurs with BA.

The covalent interactions of 7,12-DMBA with proteins closely resembles those already described for BA. Thus the exposure of 7,12-DMBA to light results in species which readily bind covalently to protein (Fujimori, 1982) including rat mammary tissue proteins, a target tissue for 7,12-DMBA (Grubbs and Wood, 1976). The metabolism of 7,12-DMBA occurs by interaction with cytochrome P-450 (see Chapter 8) and certain of the metabolites formed can be further conjugated enzymatically with species such as glutathione. The covalent binding of 7,12-DMBA or its metabolites to proteins has been described in a number of tissues including mouse skin (Abell and Heidelberger, 1962) where a positive correlation between the carcinogenicity of a PAH and binding to a particular soluble protein fraction was observed. Such observations, however, possibly provide too simple an explanation for the complex biological changes involved in converting a normal cell into a malignant cell. Thus a lack of correlation was observed between the level of protein binding of 7,12-DMBA and the expressed tumourgenicity in studies showing TCDD to be a potent inhibitor of skin tumour initiation by 7,12-DMBA (DiGiovanni *et al.*, 1979*a*).

The interaction of 7,12-DMBA with adrenal components has been a subject of special interest, due to the selective effect of adrenal necrosis caused by administration of 7,12-DMBA to certain species (Huggins and Morii, 1961). Adrenal cytosolic and microsomal proteins interact with PAHs (Mankowitz *et al.*, 1981: Montelius *et al.*, 1982) and indeed one of the cytosolic proteins appears to have a unique specificity for 7,12-DMBA, the 7,12-DMBA not being displaced by other PAHs such as 3-MC and B[a]P (Mankowitz *et al.*, 1981). The authors suggest such protein binding may have a role in the toxic effects of 7,12-DMBA in the adrenal gland, although the way in which this may occur has not yet been demonstrated.

The similarity between the molecular structure of 7,12-DMBA and progesterone has led one group to consider the effects of 7,12-DMBA on steroid binding (Barlow *et al.*, 1978). These studies have additional interest because the carcinogenic action of 7,12-DMBA in the mammary gland is known to have a marked hormone dependence; ovariectomy plus adrenalectomy, or simply ovariectomy alone result in complete tumour regression (Jabara and Harcourt, 1971). Barlow's group found that 7,12-DMBA treatment leads to a ten-fold increase in progesterone (but not oestradiol or dexamethasone) binding to cytosolic proteins which had been prepared from mammary gland parenchyma of adrenalectomized, ovariectomized rats. However, such enhanced binding is not necessarily restricted to specific steroid-binding proteins such as the progesterone receptor; 7,12-DMBA also considerably enhanced the binding of progesterone to bovine serum albumin, ovalbumin, catalase and rat plasma. This marked positive co-operativity effect may well, *in vivo*, alter the balance of protein-bound versus free steroid, and therefore result in inappropriate signals being received by responsive tissues and possibly such changes could affect the initiation or promotion stages of neoplasia.

The binding of 7,12-DMBA (or its metabolites) with nuclear proteins has revealed some interesting, specific, interactions. One of the earliest studies was conducted by Jungmann and Schweppe (1972); they injected [^{3}H]-7,12-DMBA into rats and examined the PAH binding to histones and acidic proteins isolated from rat liver nuclei. Preferential binding of [^{3}H]-7,12-DMBA was observed to histones H1 and H2B, this binding being specific; excess non-radioactive 7,12-DMBA caused a reduction in the tritium labelled 7,12-DMBA binding. Later studies (Kootstra *et al.*, 1982), using hamster embryo cells, again observed binding of 7,12-DMBA to specific histones, but the major target for 7,12-DMBA was a nuclear protein with a molecular weight of 32 000 daltons. Other PAHs such as B[a]P and 3-MC also bound to this nuclear protein, whose function is, as yet, unknown.

10

Mutagenicity

10.1 Introduction

Chemical carcinogenesis is currently believed to result from the interaction of a carcinogen with the DNA of a target tissue. The mutational events which occur due to this DNA adduct formation may possibly lead to malignant transformation of the cell and to subsequent tumour development. Mutagenicity test systems therefore provide a quick, cheap and reliable method for examining various aspects of the cellular interactions of chemical carcinogens such as: pathways of metabolic activation, the ability of various cell types to produce mutagenic species, and the screening of potentially hazardous chemicals for mutagenic activity. These mutational events may provide clues to the mechanism of chemical carcinogenesis in animals and humans.

The types of mutational test systems available can be divided broadly into two groups, bacterial and mammalian, and some require the addition of an activating system, such as a liver homogenate or a particular cell line, to 'activate' the chemical. In addition mammalian cells may undergo malignant transformation by a chemical carcinogen: a direct link between the cell transformation and cancer being shown by the injection of such cells into an animal and the development of tumours. There have been several extensive reviews on short-term mutagenicity test systems (Brookes, 1977; Hollstein et al., 1979) to which the reader is referred for further information.

10.2 Mutagenicity of benz[a]anthracene

Benz[a]anthracene is mutagenic in a number of short-term mutagenicity testing systems, these include the widely used Ames bacterial system employing *Salmonella typhimurium* strain TA98 (McCann et al., 1975) or TA100 (Norpoth et al., 1984). A comparison between five different strains of *S. typhimurium* showed that strain TA100 gives the highest mutagenic activity; consistent with a frameshift mechanism (Petrilli *et al.*, 1980). Mutagenic activity of BA has been demonstrated in insects; alterations in gene expression being observed in *Drosophila* (Fahmy and Fahmy, 1980). Mutational events also occur in mammalian cell systems such as Chinese hamster V79 cells treated with BA (Huberman and Sachs, 1976; Slaga *et al.*, 1978) and Syrian hamster embryo cells undergo malignant transformation (Pienta *et al.*, 1977). The mutagenic activity of BA may contribute in part to the observed mutagenic activity of environmental samples such as used crankcase oils (Payne *et al.*, 1978), creosote (Bos *et al.*, 1984) and soot (Kaden *et al.*, 1979) which contain BA as a minor component of their composition.

10.3   Mutagenicity of dihydrodiols and diol epoxides of benz[a]anthracene

Examination of the mutagenicity and transforming abilities of various potential metabolites of BA has allowed the quick initial evaluation of the potential role such metabolites may have in the initiation of cancer. Thus the formation of a BA K-region epoxide results in a species with increased mutagenicity in the Ames test (Ames *et al.*, 1972), and mutations in *Drosophila* (Fahmy and Fahmy, 1973) indicating the possible role of K-region epoxides in the mutagenic metabolic activation of BA.

Another route of metabolic activation of BA involves the formation of bay-region diol epoxides; exceptionally high mutagenic activity (Fig. 10.1) was associated with BA 3,4-dihydrodiol (the precursor to the bay-region diol epoxides) in *S. typhimurium* strain TA100 (Wood *et al.*, 1976). This may be contrasted with the relatively low activity of the other dihydrodiols although the mutagenic activity of the 8,9-dihydrodiol is higher than that of the parent hydrocarbon (Malaveille *et al.*, 1975). Similar high levels of mutagenic activity of the 3,4-dihydrodiol of BA are found in Chinese hamster V79 cells (Slaga *et al.*, 1978; Marquardt *et al.*, 1979*b*). The above reports on the mutagenicity of dihydrodiols have required that some sort of activating system, involving cytochrome P-450, be present before mutagenic activity can be expressed. That the high mutagenic activity observed with BA 3,4-dihydrodiol was related to the metabolic formation of a bay-region epoxide at the 1,2-position was confirmed by Wood and co-workers (Wood *et al.*, 1977*a*). BA 3,4-diol 1,2-epoxide was found to be uniquely mutagenic and cytotoxic in both bacterial and mammalian cells; these experiments were performed in the absence of an added activation system and the compounds were therefore 'direct acting'. Further studies have been carried out to determine which of the four possible isomers of the bay-region 3,4-diol 1,2-epoxide[(−)-*anti*; (+)-*anti*; (−)-*syn*; (+)-*syn*] may make the major contribution to the observed mutagenicity of BA (Fig. 10.2). The (+)-*anti* isomer had the highest activity in the bacterial TA100 and mammalian V79 cell test systems whereas the (−)-*anti* isomer was the most mutagenic in the TA98 strain of bacteria (Wood *et al.*, 1983).

A close correlation exists between the microsome-mediated mutagenicities in *S. typhimurium* TA100 of dihydrodiols capable of yielding bay-region diol epoxides and (a) the extents of reaction with DNA in hydrocarbon-treated mouse skin and (b) the carcinogenic potencies of the parent hydrocarbons (Bartsch *et al.*, 1979).

The inhibition of the mutagenic activity of various metabolic products of BA by certain species has suggested possible ways of inactivating

Fig. 10.1. Effect of cytochrome P-448 concentration on the metabolic activation of BA and BA dihydrodiols. From Wood *et al.* (1976).

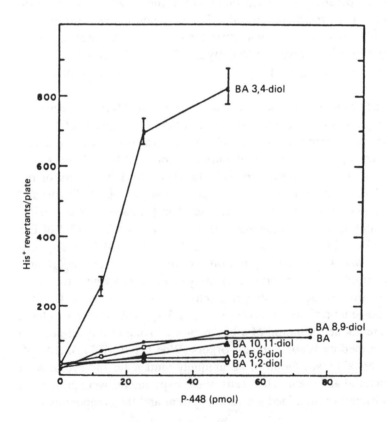

Fig. 10.2. Mutagenicity of the four bay-region diol epoxide isomers (1 refers to the *syn* and 2 to the *anti* isomer) in *S. typhimurium* (a and b) and Chinese hamster V79 cells (c). From Wood *et al.* (1983).

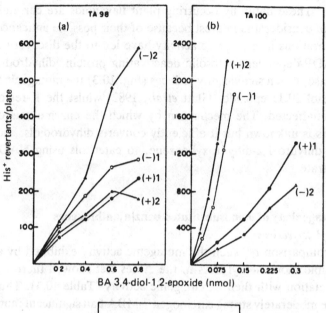

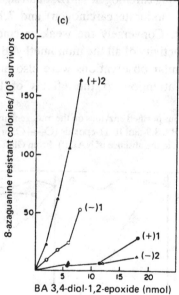

148   Biology

and detoxifying BA. Thus inhibition of BA mutagenicity has been observed with phenolic plant flavanoids (Huang *et al.*, 1983), the effect being possibly the result of direct interaction of the flavanoid with the diol epoxide. These naturally occurring plant flavanoids are currently the subject of considerable interest because of their possible anticancer activity. Alterations in mutagenic activity have led to the discovery of a novel NADP-dependent cytosolic deactivating protein, dihydrodiol dehydrogenase, which significantly reduces (Fig. 10.3) the mutagenicity of BA 8,9-diol 10,11-epoxide (Glatt *et al.*, 1982) whilst the K-region epoxide is unaffected. The mechanism by which the enzyme acts on diol epoxides is unknown but it efficiently converts dihydrodiols, such as *trans*-1,2-dihydro-1,2-dihydroxybenzene, to catechols using NADP as a co-substrate.

10.4   Mutagenicity of monosubstituted benz[a]anthracenes
10.4.1   *Alkyl derivatives*

A comparison between the mutagenic activity exhibited by all twelve possible monomethyl BAs in the Ames test showed there was a poor correlation with their carcinogenic activity (Table 10.1). Thus, although the moderately strong carcinogen 7-MBA had significant mutagenic activity, 12-MBA (a moderate carcinogen) and 7,12-DMBA (a strong carcinogen) did not. Conversely the weak carcinogen 4-MBA had the highest mutagenic activity of all the monomethyl BAs examined (Coombs *et al.*, 1976). Similar observations were also made by Glatt *et al.* (1981) who drew attention to the effects of liver enzyme

Fig. 10.3. Effect of various purified enzymes on the mutagenicity of BA 5,6-epoxide, ●——●, and BA 8,9-diol 10,11-epoxide (○——○, in the presence of NADP, and □——□, in the absence of NADP). From Glatt *et al.* (1982).

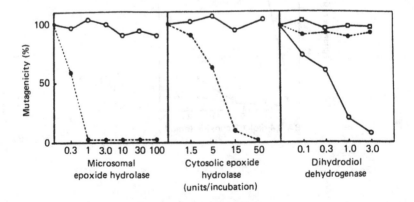

Table 10.1 *Carcinogenic (C) and mutagenic activities (M) of monomethyl BAs*

Compound	C	M (A)	(B)
Benz[a]anthracenes			
Benz[a]anthracene	Weak	994/20	11.3
1-Methylbenz[a]anthracene	±	500/20	6.0
2-Methylbenz[a]anthracene	±	313/10	7.6
3-Methylbenz[a]anthracene	Inactive	194/5	9.4
4-Methylbenz[a]anthracene	Weak	2492/20	30.2
5-Methylbenz[a]anthracene	Weak	699/10	16.9
6-Methylbenz[a]anthracene	Weak	318/10	7.7
7-Methylbenz[a]anthracene	Strong	1275/20	15.4
8-Methylbenz[a]anthracene	Moderate	330/20	4.0
9-Methylbenz[a]anthracene	Weak	348/20	4.4
10-Methylbenz[a]anthracene	Weak	122/10	3.0
11-Methylbenz[a]anthracene	Weak	464/50	2.3
12-Methylbenz[a]anthracene	Moderate	460/20	5.7
7,12-Dimethylbenz[a]anthracene	Very strong	437/20	5.6

(A) Number of revertant colonies per μg of compound incorporated in the plate.
(B) Number of revertant colonies per nmol.
From Coombs *et al.* (1976).

inducers, such as PB, 3-MC or Aroclor 1254, on the observed mutagenic activity, presumably due to alterations in the metabolic pathways.

Mutagenicity of metabolites of methyl-substituted benz[a]anthracene
The mutagenic activity of the various metabolites formed by methyl-substituted BAs may suggest pathways involved in the metabolic activation and the detoxification of these compounds. The relative mutagenic activities observed in the Ames test for metabolites isolated from 6-MBA were 3,4-dihydrodiol > 8,9-dihydrodiol > 6-MBA > 10,11-dihydrodiol > 4-hydroxy-6-MBA (Mushtaq *et al.*, 1985) suggesting that the formation of the bay-region diol epoxide was a major determinant in the mutagenic activity of the parent compound, although, in addition, a significant contribution may be made by the 8,9-dihydrodiol. Examination of the mutagenic activities of 7-MBA metabolites also revealed that the 3,4-dihydrodiol had the highest mutagenic activity of the various dihydrodiols tested in the bacterial Ames system (Malaveille *et al.*, 1977) and in mammalian V79 Chinese hamster cells (Marquardt *et al.*, 1977). In the latter cell line system the 8,9-dihydrodiol of 7-MBA also had higher mutagenic activity than 7-MBA (Table 10.2), thus resembling the dihydrodiols of 6-MBA. The K-region epoxide of 7-MBA could contribute

Table 10.2 In vitro *Malignant transformation in M2 mouse fibroblasts and mutagenesis in V79 Chinese hamster cells induced by dihydrodiols derived from 7-methylbenz[a]anthracene*

Compound	Concentration (μg/ml)	Transformation in M2 cells			Mutagenesis in V79 cells		
		Plating efficiency (%)	Transformed foci/No. treated dishes	Transformed foci/10^3 survivors	Plating efficiency (%)	Azaguanine resistant colonies per dish	per 10^3 survivors
Dimethylsulphoxide	0.5%	42	0/12	0	99	2.8	2.1
N-Methyl-N'-nitro-N-nitrosoguanidine	0.2	21	8/10	3.8	55	59.4	72
	0.4	16	12/8	9.4	41	91.8	149.2
7-Methylbenz[a]anthracene	1.0	38	2/12	0.4	70	2.4	2.3
	10.0	28	8/12	2.4	65	8.4	8.6
Trans-1,2-dihydro-1,2-dihydroxy-7-methylbenz[a]anthracene	1.0	42	0/12	0	67	4.0	4.0
	5.0	38	0/10	0	68	3.8	3.7
	10.0	27	2/12	0.6	64	4.0	4.2
Trans-3,4-dihydro-3,4-dihydroxy-7-methylbenz[a]anthracene	1.0	39	18/12	3.8	59	30.4	31.4
	5.0	16	28/12	14.6	38	17.9	34.4
	10.0	2.5	4/12	13.3	5	5.8	77.3
Trans-5,6-dihydro-5,6-dihydroxy-7-methylbenz[a]anthracene	1.0	39	0/12	0	59	2.9	3.3
	5.0	31	0/12	0	51	2.4	3.1
	10.0	19	0/12	0	46	4.3	5.1
Trans-8,9-dihydro-8,9-dihydroxy-7-methylbenz[a]anthracene	1.0	38	12/12	2.6	80	10.9	9.1
	5.0	22	18/12	7.6	78	9.7	8.3
	10.0	16	2/12	1.0	55	9.9	10.2

From Marquardt *et al.* (1977).

to the observed mutagenic activity of 7-MBA, the epoxide being mutagenic in bacterial (Ames *et al.*, 1972) and mammalian cells (Huberman *et al.*, 1971), though it is less active in inducing malignant transformation of mammalian cells *in vitro* (Marquardt *et al.*, 1972) than the parent hydrocarbon. Hydroxylation of the methyl group of 7-MBA results in a lowering of mutagenicity, relative to the parent hydrocarbon, and may therefore represent part of a detoxification pathway (Wettstein *et al.*, 1979).

10.4.2 *Halogen derivatives*
Although 7-fluoroBA is a much less potent carcinogen than 7-MBA, they have similar levels of mutagenic activity in *S. typhimurium* TA100 (Chiu *et al.*, 1984). Of those potential metabolites which may be formed *in vivo*, high mutagenic activity was observed for the *trans*-3,4-dihydrodiol, as would be predicted by the bay-region theory; however, the *trans*-10,11-dihydrodiol of 7-fluoroBA also exhibited significant mutagenic activity (Chiu *et al.*, 1984). The substitution of a bromine atom into the methyl group of 7-MBA results in a complete loss of the transforming ability of 7-MBA in mouse prostate cells (Marquardt *et al.*, 1972).

10.4.3 *Nitro derivatives*
A number of nitro-PAHs are potent direct acting mutagens in the *Salmonella* reversion assay. 7-NitroBA and BA have been examined in the Ames test to determine the effect of light (White *et al.*, 1985) on the mutagenicity of these compounds. Neither of the compounds produced a positive mutagenic response in the absence of sunlight and only the nitro-BA was activated to a mutagen by exposure to sunlight. The mechanism for such a transformation is, as yet, unclear.

10.4.4 *Oxy derivatives*
A comparison between 7-acetoxymethylBA (7-AcMBA), 7-hydroxymethylBA (7-OHMBA), 7-formylBA (7-CHOBA), 7-methoxymethylBA (7-MOMBA) and 7-MBA revealed all five compounds to be mutagenic in the presence of S-9 to *S. typhimurium* TA98 and TA100, the latter strain showing greater sensitivity. Only 7-AcMBA was an ultimate mutagen requiring no enzymic activation in either bacterial strain (Wettstein *et al.*, 1979). The rank order of mutagenicity in TA100 with S-9 was 7-AcMBA > 7-CHOBA = 7-MBA > 7-OHMBA > 7-MOMBA.

10.5   Mutagenicity of disubstituted benz[a]anthracenes

10.5.1   *Alkyl derivatives*

The potent carcinogen 7,12-DMBA is mutagenic in a number of bacterial and mammalian test systems; these include *Salmonella typhimurium* (McCann *et al.*, 1975), *Drosophila melanogaster* (Fahmy and Fahmy, 1970, 1973; Zijlstra and Vogel, 1984), Chinese hamster cells (Huberman and Sachs, 1976), and mouse lymphoma cells (Thornton *et al.*, 1982). Also, the malignant transformation of cells by 7,12-DMBA has been described in mouse prostate cells (Marquardt *et al.*, 1972), mouse fibroblasts (Marquardt *et al.*, 1979*b*) and mouse epidermal keratinocytes (Indo and Miyaji, 1985).

There is a poor correlation between the observed mutagenicity of BA, 7-MBA and 7,12-DMBA in *S. typhimurium* TA100, and their carcinogenic potential (Bartsch *et al.*, 1979), 7,12-DMBA being less mutagenic than either BA or 7-MBA in this test system (Table 10.3). This may be due either to metabolic differences which occur between *in vivo* and *in vitro* pathways or to metabolic differences between liver (which is most commonly used in the Ames assay) and a target tissue. A much closer correlation between carcinogenic activity and mutagenicity was observed when the bay-region dihydrodiols were employed (Bartsch *et al.*, 1979).

Although it will not be dealt with exhaustively here, the inhibition of 7,12-DMBA-induced mutagenicity by certain compounds often correlates with an observed *in vivo* reduction in tumour yield when such compounds are used, and thus such mutagenicity studies on potential tumour inhibitors are very useful both from a predictive point of view and as indicators of the type of mechanisms which may be involved in one or more of the steps in the carcinogenic process. For instance a particular copper co-ordination compound significantly reduces the mutagenicity of 7,12-DMBA in a mouse keratinocyte-mediated Chinese hamster V79 cell system and reduces the number of tumours by over 50% in a 7,12-DMBA initiation–promotion mouse skin experiment (Solanki *et al.*, 1984). The copper complex is known to have superoxide dismutase activity, suggesting that free-radical formation may play a part in some stage of the carcinogenic process in skin. Certain dietary constituents (sometimes from the most unlikely source) can protect against tumour occurrence (Wattenberg, 1983), e.g. brown seaweed is a common food in Japan and animal model systems suggest that it can inhibit breast cancer. Mutagenicity studies also indicate that organic extracts of brown seaweed significantly inhibit the mutagenic action of 7,12-DMBA in *S. typhimurium* strains TA98 and TA100 (Reddy *et al.*, 1984).

Table 10.3 *Relationships between the mutagenicity of polycyclic hydrocarbons and of certain related dihydrodiols in microsome-mediated assays with S. typhimurium TA100 and the extents of reaction with DNA, tumour initiation and carcinogenesis in mouse skin treated with polycyclic hydrocarbons*

	Polycyclic hydrocarbons				Related dihydrodiols[a]
	Mutagenicity (his^+ revertants/nmol)	Extent of reaction with DNA in mouse skin (pmol/mg DNA)	Tumour initiation on mouse skin (tumours/µmol)	Carcinogenicity[b]	Mutagenicity (his^+ revertants/nmol)
Benz[a]anthracene	6	2	0.9	5	8.5
7-Methylbenz[a]anthracene	5	25	1.7	45	33
7,12-Dimethylbenz[a]anthracene	2.4	42	819	95	80
3-Methylcholanthrene	17	26	102	90	35
Benzo[a]pyrene	29	25	25	70	101

[a] *trans*-Dihydrodiols expected to be the metabolic precursors of 'bay-region' vicinal diol-epoxides were used in each case, i.e. the 3,4-diols derived from benz[a]anthracene, 7-methylbenz[a]anthracene and 7,12-dimethylbenz[a]anthracene, the 9,10-diol derived from 3-methylcholanthrene and the 7,8-diol derived from benzo[a]pyrene.
[b] Iball indices for skin tumour formation in mice.
From Bartsch *et al.* (1979).

Mutagenic activity of metabolites of 7,12-dimethylbenz[a]anthracene
One of the ways of investigating the mechanism by which 7,12-DMBA
exerts its mutagenic effect is by isolating metabolites of 7,12-DMBA
and determining whether these have enhanced mutagenic activity. Early
studies concentrated on the mutagenicity of the K-region epoxide;
this was less active than the parent hydrocarbon in causing mutations
in mouse fibroblasts (Marquardt *et al.*, 1974). Of the various dihydrodiol isomers high mutagenic activity of the 3,4-dihydrodiol (the precursor
to the bay-region diol epoxide) in *S. typhimurium* TA100 was reported
(Malaveille *et al.*, 1978), it being six-fold more mutagenic than the
parent hydrocarbon in the presence of microsomes; there was also
some mutagenic activity in the absence of a NADPH-generating
system. The mutagenicity of the various dihydrodiols of 7,12-DMBA
in V79 Chinese hamster cells and M2 mouse fibroblasts (Table 10.4)
again showed the *trans*-3,4-dihydrodiol to have exceptionally high
mutagenic activity in the V79 cells and to cause malignant transformation of M2 mouse fibroblasts (Marquardt *et al.*, 1978, 1979*b*);
considerable activity was also observed with the *trans*-8,9-dihydro-
diol.

The metabolic formation of a phenol at either the 2-, 3-, 4- or 5-position
in 7,12-DMBA does not result in a compound with significant mutagenic
activity (Slaga *et al.*, 1979*b*). The hydroxylation of either the 7-methyl
group or the 12-methyl group, or both methyl groups, of the *trans*-3,4-
dihydrodiol of 7,12-DMBA (Table 10.5) produces species with lower
mutagenic activity (Wislocki *et al.*, 1980). Several other dihydrodiol and
phenolic compounds, as well as hydroxyl, formyl and carboxylic acid
derivatives at the 7- and 12-positions of 7,12-DMBA were also examined
and found to be without mutagenic activity.

Thus the evidence seems to support strongly activation involving the
1-, 2-, 3- and 4-positions of 7,12-DMBA for the expression of mutagenic
activity by 7,12-DMBA (Bartsch *et al.*, 1979). However, Inbasekaran
et al. (1980) report that saturation, or partial saturation, of the angular
benzene ring of 7,12-DMBA, producing 1,2,3,4-tetrahydro-7,12-DMBA
or 1,2-dihydro-7,12-DMBA, does not result in compounds that
are non-mutagenic. Both the 1,2-dihydro- and the 1,2,3,4-tetrahydro-
analogues have appreciable dose-dependent activity in *S. typhimurium*
in the presence of microsomes, with the tetrahydro derivative exhibiting
mutagenic activity in strain TA98 which is similar to that of 7,12-DMBA
under the same conditions (Table 10.6). In addition, the 1,2-dihydro-
and 1,2,3,4-tetrahydro derivatives were also potent mutagens in the
absence of microsomal activation. In a mammalian cell system

Table 10.4 Induction of malignant transformation and mutagenesis in mammalian cells by dihydrodiols derived from 7,12-dimethylbenz[a]anthracene[a]

Compound	Concentration (µg/ml)	Transformation in M2 cells[b]			Mutagenesis in V79 cells[c]	
		Plating efficiency (%)	Transformed foci per number of dishes treated	Transformed foci 10^3 survivors	Plating efficiency (%)	8-Azaguanine-resistant colonies/10^5 survivors
Dimethylsulphoxide	0.5%	31	0/9	0	84	2.7
N-Methyl-N'-nitro-N-nitrosoguanidine	0.4	21	10/9	5.3	31	294.1
7,12-Dimethylbenz[a]anthracene	0.25	26	9/8	4.3	63	3.0
	1.0	24	19/11	7.2	39	4.4
trans-3,4-Dihydro-3,4-dihydroxy-7,12-dimethyl-benz[a]anthracene	0.12	31	3/5	1.9	67	5.7
	0.25	26	9/10	3.5	58	19.8
	0.5	25	26/8	13.0	50	29.8
	1.0	15	20/9	14.3	43	44.1
trans-5,6-Dihydro-5,6-dihydroxy-7,12-dimethyl-benz[a]anthracene	1.0	28	0/10	0	80	2.0
	5.0	28	0/10	0	73	0.9
	10.0	20	0/10	0	57	0
trans-8,9-Dihydro-8,9-dihydroxy-7,12-dimethyl-benz[a]anthracene	0.25	26	4/4	3.8	62	1.9
	0.5	22	15/5	13.6	45	20.5
	1.0	7	11/6	26.2	32	42.5
trans-10,11-Dihydro-10,11-dihydroxy-7,12-dimethylbenz[a]anthracene	0.25	30	0/8	0	76	6.3
	0.5	26	0/12	0	68	5.6
	1.0	11	0/11	0	44	4.9

[a] Composite results from two separate experiments.
[b] Cells were grown in medium containing the test compounds for 24 h.
[c] Cells were grown in medium containing the test compounds for 3 h.
From Marquardt et al. (1978).

Table 10.5 *Mutagenicity of 7,12-DMBA, its hydroxymethylated derivatives, and their 3,4-diols in strain TA100*

	Histidine revertants/plate[a]					
Compound	3 nmol/ plate	5 nmol/ plate	10 nmol/ plate	20 nmol/ plate	35 nmol/ plate	50 nmol/ plate
7,12-DMBA	—[b]	20	20	101	287	388
7,12-DMBA 3,4-diol	230	309	438	376	—	—
7-OHM-12-MBA	—	0	47	77	396	448
7-OHM-12-MBA 3,4-diol	133	196	427	1194	2096	2713
7-M-12-OHMBA	—	48	65	52	34	52
7-M-12-OHMBA 3,4-diol	—	0	12	176	281	344
7,12-diOHMBA	—	25	7	57	5	29
7,12-diOHMBA 3,4-diol	—	10	0	100	168	285

[a] The background of 170 revertants/plate has been subtracted from the numbers. Each number represents the average of three plates. Each experiment was done at least twice with similar results. The compounds were added to the plate in 100 μl of dimethyl sulphoxide.
[b] —, compound was not tested at this dose level.
From Wislocki *et al.* (1980).

Table 10.6 *Mutagenic activity of 7,12-DMBA and derivatives*

	Net revertant colonies/10 μg of compound with each strain					
	TA1537		TA98		TA100	
Compound	−S9	+S9	−S9	+S9	−S9	+S9
1,2-Dihydro derivative	—	—	146	25	58	69
1,2,3,4-Tetrahydro derivative	42	7	47	78	173	270
7,12-DMBA	—	15	—	58	—	489

From Inbasekaran *et al.* (1980). − = no mutagenic response.

(Chinese hamster V79 cells) the tetrahydro derivative again exhibited mutagenic activity, and also has been shown to be tumourigenic in mice, having a tumour-initiating activity higher than that of B[a]P and 3-MC, although one-tenth that of 7,12-DMBA itself (DiGiovanni *et al.*, 1982*a*). These observations suggest that there are alternative routes of metabolic activation, other than a bay-region diol epoxide, for 7,12-DMBA.

Mammary cell-mediated mutagenicity of 7,12-dimethylbenz[a]anthracene
The development of cell-mediated mutagenicity assays has allowed comparisons to be made on the role particular cell populations may have

in producing mutagenic species. The ability of mammary cells to act as an activating system for the potent breast carcinogen 7,12-DMBA in mutagenicity tests has been reported for mammary cells derived from both rat (Gould, 1980) and human tissue (Gould *et al.*, 1982*b*). Subtle differences are shown by virgin rat mammary cells on the activation to mutagens of 7,12-DMBA (a potent mammary carcinogen), B[a]P (a weak mammary carcinogen) and aflatoxin B_1 (a strong hepato-carcinogen but not a mammary carcinogen). Thus 7,12-DMBA is efficiently activated to a mutagen by both mammary stromal and parenchymal cells, B[a]P by only stromal cells, and aflatoxin B_1 was not activated at all by either cell type (Gould, 1982*a*), suggesting intra-organ cell specificity of carcinogen activation. Organ-specific activation has also been reported for 7,12-DMBA in the lung (Langenbach *et al.*, 1981), another target tissue for 7,12-DMBA.

Using a mammalian cell-mediated V79 mutagenicity assay Moore *et al.* (1983) compared mammary cells derived from various rat strains which differ in their susceptibility to mammary carcinogenesis. Similar levels of mutagenic activity were observed with mammary cells derived from Sprague–Dawley and Wistar/Furth rats (highly susceptible to 7,12-DMBA mammary carcinogenesis) and Long Evans and F344 strain rats (relatively resistant to tumourigenesis). These findings suggest that the mammary cells from the highly susceptible rat strains do not perform unique activation steps at the metabolic level (Moore *et al.*, 1983). In contrast modifications in mammary tumour susceptibility caused by various physiological states may be related, in part, to an altered ability to activate chemical carcinogens in the mammary gland. Kellen (1973) has shown that pregnant rats are more resistant to the effects of 7,12-DMBA than virgin rats. When mammary cells from virgin and pregnant rats were used in a cell-mediated mutagenicity assay, mammary cells from pregnant rats produced 7,12-DMBA mutation levels half that produced by mammary cells from virgin rats (Moore and Gould, 1984). These effects may well reflect the lower metabolizing capability of mammary cells from pregnant rats, suggesting that the lower carcinogenic susceptibility of pregnant rats may be due to lack of metabolic activation.

10.6   Mutagenicity of trisubstituted benz[a]anthracenes

The 1-, 2-, 5- and 11-fluoro derivatives of 7,12-DMBA have all been examined for mutagenic activity in Chinese hamster V79 cells using hamster embryo cells to activate the PAH (Huberman and Slaga, 1979*b*). Both 7,12-DMBA and its 11-fluoro analogue had comparable

Table 10.7 *Mutagenicity of 7,12-DMBA and its fluorinated derivatives*

Hydrocarbon	Concentration (μM)	Cloning efficiency (%)	No. of ouabain-resistant mutants/10^4 survivors
None		76	0.7
7,12-DMBA	0.01	56	7
	0.04	45	24
	0.13	18	52
	0.4	2	69
1-Fluoro-DMBA	3.8	80	1
	12	62	3
	38	59	6
2-Fluoro-DMBA	3.8	67	0.9
	12	71	0.7
	38	66	1.0
5-Fluoro-DMBA	3.8	59	2
	12	55	4
	38	43	10
11-Fluoro-DMBA	0.01	66	5
	0.04	36	19
	0.12	8	37

7,12-DMBA and its derivatives were added 5 h after 3×10^5 V79 cells were seeded on 2×10^4 irradiated embryonic golden hamster cells. Two days after treatment, the cells were dissociated and seeded to determine the cloning efficiency of the V79 cells and the frequency of ouabain-resistant mutants. At the time when the cells were seeded for cloning efficiency and selection of mutation, there were in the control and in the hydrocarbon-treated cultures from 0.9 to 3.0×10^4 V79 cells/Petri dish.
From Huberman and Slaga (1979b).

mutagenic activity; substitution of a fluorine atom at the 1-, 2- or 5-position produced compounds which were either inactive or required a 1000-fold higher dose to induce mutagenic activity comparable to that of 7,12-DMBA (Table 10.7). Similar results were observed in tumour-initiation experiments (Slaga *et al.*, 1979b; Huberman and Slaga, 1979b), suggesting that the 1-, 2- and 5-positions may be involved in the metabolic activation of 7,12-DMBA. When human hepatoma cells were used as the activating system (Diamond *et al.*, 1984), substitution of fluorine in the angular benzene ring (at C-1 and C-4) again resulted in a decrease in mutagenic activity compared with 7,12-DMBA. Interestingly, substitution of fluorine at C-10 gave a six-fold increase in mutagenic activity. These findings are paralleled in skin tumour initiation assays (Di-Giovanni *et al.*, 1983a). Introduction of a hydroxyl group at the 2-, 3-,

4- or 5-positions of 7,12-DMBA produced compounds with very little mutagenic activity (Slaga *et al.*, 1979*b*). It should be noted that for B[a]P, in which the 7-, 8-, 9- and 10-positions are important for metabolic activation, that all of the possible phenols, except for the 2- and 11-hydroxybenzopyrenes, have no tumourigenic activity (Kapitulnik *et al.*, 1976; Wislocki *et al.*, 1977). This makes suspect interpretations of structure/ activity relationships involving 'blocking' by hydroxyl groups of ring positions required for biological activation.

11

Carcinogenicity

11.1   Introduction

'There is only one unambiguous experimental method to determine carcinogenicity; it is to ascertain if your compound produces cancer in animals.' (Quoted from Huggins, 1979.) Cancer induction is a complex process, still not completely understood, and the experimental demonstration of a chemical's carcinogenic properties is dependent on a number of variables such as the dose administered, the species, age and sex of the animal employed, the mode of administration, the use of cocarcinogens or promotors, the time period of experimental observation and ensuring that sufficient numbers of animals survive the experiment for adequate statistical analyses to be performed. Conflicting data are occasionally reported from laboratories in which different procedures are employed. Also difficulties arise when attempts are made to compare the relative potency of various chemicals as carcinogens. Iball (1939) proposed that there are two measurable parameters involved in determining the potency of carcinogenic compounds; one is the percentage incidence of tumours, the other is the average latent period for the appearance of tumours. Giving equal weight to both these factors, Iball constructed an index of carcinogenic potency for various chemical carcinogens; 7,12-DMBA was by far the most potent chemical tested. An additional indicator of carcinogenic potential, which is often reported from skin-painting experiments, is the number of tumours per animal. Comprehensive tables on the carcinogenicity of benz[a]anthracene and its derivatives have been reported by Dipple *et al.* (1984*a*).

11.2   Carcinogenicity of benz[a]anthracene

Early studies showed that the administration of BA to rats, mice and rabbits by painting on the skin or by subcutaneous injection resulted in only one epithelioma in a mouse following skin painting (Barry *et al.*, 1935; Hartwell, 1951). Intravenous injection of an aqueous dispersion of BA into mice did not result in an increased incidence of lung tumours (Andervont and Shimkin, 1940), neither did the painting of mice in the presence of the promoting substance, croton resin, produce tumours (Berenblum, 1941). Shear and Leiter (1941), after careful testing by subcutaneous injection into mice without obtaining tumours concluded that BA was of negligible carcinogenic potency. In contrast to these early papers on the very weak carcinogenic properties of BA, White and Eschenbrenner (1945) reported that after administration of BA in the food of rats, liver tumours were readily formed in two of the six animals used, though this study is marred by the limited number of animals employed. Steiner and Edgcombe (1952) also suggested that BA was a moderate carcinogen when a significant number of mice developed sarcomas after subcutaneous injection of BA. Use of the two-stage initiation–promotion mouse skin model (Friedewald and Rous, 1944; Berenblum and Shubik, 1947) demonstrated that BA is a very weak tumour initiator (Roe and Salaman, 1955; Van Duuren *et al.*, 1970; Scribner, 1973), being about 500 to 1000 times less active than 7,12-DMBA (Slaga *et al.*, 1974). BA does not act as a tumour promotor (Klein, 1952).

11.3   Carcinogenicity of metabolites of benz[a]anthracene

Tumourigenicity studies which have employed BA metabolites, particularly dihydrodiols and diol epoxides, have provided important information regarding the mechanism of metabolic activation of PAHs. The suggestion of Boyland (1950) that epoxides are formed as intermediates in the metabolism of PAHs, and that these intermediates may be the active species responsible for the carcinogenic activity of these hydrocarbons led to the experimental examination of such compounds. Initially the 'K-region' epoxide of BA was tested for carcinogenicity by subcutaneous injection into rodents (Boyland and Sims, 1967*a*); this epoxide was virtually inactive in inducing tumours. In a two-stage carcinogenicity test on mouse skin Miller and Miller (1967) observed that BA 5,6-epoxide was only marginally more active than BA itself.

The carcinogenic activity of both the K-region and non-K-region dihydrodiols has recently been examined in mouse skin and exceptional activity (Table 11.1) of the BA 3,4-dihydrodiol (10- to 20-fold more active than the parent hydrocarbon or any of the other BA dihydrodiols) was observed (Wood *et al.*, 1977*b*). This finding provides strong support

Table 11.1 *Tumour induction by benz[a]anthracene (BA) and BA dihydrodiols after 20 weeks of promotion with TPA*

Compound	Dose (μmol)	Surviving animals (a)	Tumour animals (b)	Total tumours (c)	c/a
Control	—	30	1	1	0.03
BA	0.4	28	4	4	0.14
	1.0	30	6	9	0.30
	2.0	30	7	9	0.30
BA 1,2-dihydrodiol	0.4	28	1	1	0.04
	1.0	29	3	3	0.10
	2.0	30	2	2	0.07
BA 3,4-dihydrodiol	0.4	30	23	73	2.4
	1.0	29	23	103	3.6
	2.0	30	24	144	4.8
BA 5,6-dihydrodiol	0.4	30	2	2	0.07
	1.0	30	1	1	0.03
	2.0	30	6	6	0.20
BA 8,9-dihydrodiol	0.4	30	2	3	0.10
	1.0	28	2	2	0.07
	2.0	29	5	6	0.21
BA 10,11-dihydrodiol	0.4	30	4	4	0.13
	1.0	29	3	3	0.10
	2.0	29	4	4	0.14

The indicated dose of hydrocarbon was applied once, and 18 days later TPA was administered twice weekly.
From Wood *et al.* (1977*b*).

for the bay-region theory which would predict that the BA 3,4-diol 1,2-epoxide would have the greatest carcinogenic activity. Similar high carcinogenic activity of the BA 3,4-dihydrodiol was present after injection i.p. into newborn mice, when compared with the activity of BA and the other metabolically possible *trans*-dihydrodiols (Wislocki *et al.*, 1978). Mice injected with BA 3,4-dihydrodiol developed malignant lymphomas and pulmonary adenomas (6- and 35-fold, respectively, more than mice treated with BA alone) whilst none of the other *trans*-dihydrodiols exhibited carcinogenic activity.

Evidence which confirms the bay-region epoxide as the ultimate carcinogenic metabolite of BA was obtained by determining the tumourigenicity of the BA 3,4-diol 1,2-epoxide by topical application on mouse skin. It was 10- to 40-fold more tumourigenic than the parent hydrocarbon (Levin *et al.*, 1978); these reports represent the first instance of a proximate and ultimate form of a PAH which has more activity than the parent hydrocarbon. There are two possible structural isomers

Table 11.2 *Tumour-initiating activity of benzo-ring derivatives of BA on mouse skin*

Initiator	Dose (μmol)	% of mice with tumours	Tumours/ mouse
None		3	0.03
BA	0.4	7	0.07
	2.0	21	0.4
1,2-H₂BA	0.4	7	0.07
	2.0	35	0.5
3,4-H₂BA	0.4	86	4.5
(±)-BA 3,4-dihydrodiol	0.4	45	1.3
(+)-BA 3,4-dihydrodiol	0.1	3	0.07
	0.4	20	0.4
(−)-BA 3,4-dihydrodiol	0.1	43	1.0
	0.4	50	1.8
(±)-Diol-epoxide-1	0.4	43	0.6
(±)-Diol-epoxide-2	0.4	70	1.9

The indicated dose of hydrocarbon was applied once, and 7 days later 12-*O*-tetra-decanoylphorbol-13-acetate was administered twice weekly for 20 weeks. From Levin *et al.* (1978).

of BA 3,4-diol 1,2-epoxide: using the terminology of Levin *et al.* (1978), the BA 3,4-diol 1,2-epoxide-*1* has the benzylic hydroxyl and the epoxide group *cis* whereas in BA 3,4-diol 1,2-epoxide-*2* the benzylic hydroxyl and the epoxide group are *trans* (Fig. 11.1). The diol epoxide which has the *trans* configuration (diol epoxide-*2*) is more tumourigenic (Table 11.2) on topical application on mouse skin (Levin *et al.*, 1978) and when injected into newborn mice (Wislocki *et al.*, 1979) than the isomer with the *cis* configuration (diol epoxide-*1*); both isomers, however, had greater activity than BA.

Observations on marked differences in tumourigenic potential have also been made in relation to the various optical isomers of BA dihydro-diols and diol-epoxides. Only the BA 3,4-dihydrodiol having a [3R,4R] configuration (the (−)isomer) showed significant tumourigenic activity (Table 11.2) on mouse skin (Levin *et al.*, 1978) and in newborn mice (Wislocki *et al.*, 1979). The diol epoxides-1 and -2 can also each exist in two enantiomeric forms making a total of four possible optical isomers (Fig. 11.1). These have been examined for carcinogenic activity on mouse skin and in newborn mice (Levin *et al.*, 1984). In initiation–promotion experiments on mouse skin only (+)-[IR,2S,3S,4R]-BA 3,4-diol 1,2-

epoxide-*2* and (+)-[IR,2S,3S,4S]-BA 3,4-diol 1,2-epoxide-*1* had significant tumour activity, with the former compound being approximately
four-fold more active (Table 11.3). Similar results were obtained using
the newborn mice tumour model, (+)-diol epoxide-*2* being 60-fold more
active than (+)-diol epoxide-*1*. (+)-Diol epoxide-*2* produced a significant number of hepatic tumours in male mice. The absolute configuration
of these ultimate carcinogens is the same as that reported for benzo[a]-
pyrene and chrysene bay-region diol epoxides (Levin *et al.*, 1984).

The remarkable series of experiments described above have demonstrated the pivotal role in carcinogenesis which the absolute configuration
of a metabolite has. The [R,R] absolute configuration of the BA 3,4-
dihydrodiol, precursor to the bay-region diol epoxide, has the highest
tumourigenic activity of all the dihydrodiol enantiomers. This dihydrodiol is then stereoselectively converted to the bay-region diol epoxide
with [R,S,S,R] absolute configuration, which is also the most tumourigenic of the possible optical isomers.

11.4   Carcinogenicity of monosubstituted benz[a]anthracenes
11.4.1   *Alkyl derivatives*

Although BA itself is a weak carcinogen, the introduction of
particular substituents at certain positions on the BA nucleus can considerably enhance the carcinogenic activity. This was recognized early
on in the study of chemical carcinogenesis; experiments on mouse skin
and by subcutaneous injection into mice of all 12 possible isomeric mono-
methylBA derivatives revealed that the introduction of a methyl group
at positions C-7, -8 or -12 (particularly C-7) resulted in a marked increase
in carcinogenic activity (reviewed in Fieser, 1938; Cook and Kennaway,

Fig. 11.1. Absolute configuration of the four optical isomers of the
diastereomeric bay-region diol epoxides of BA.

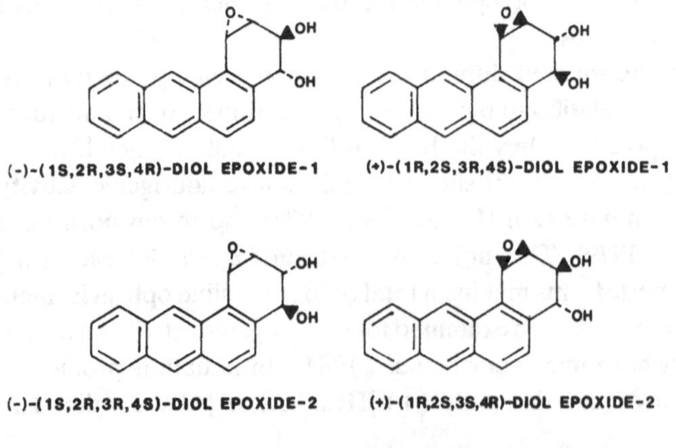

(-)-(1S,2R,3S,4R)-DIOL EPOXIDE-1   (+)-(1R,2S,3R,4S)-DIOL EPOXIDE-1

(-)-(1S,2R,3R,4S)-DIOL EPOXIDE-2   (+)-(1R,2S,3S,4R)-DIOL EPOXIDE-2

Table 11.3 *Tumour-initiating activity of BA and the enantiomers of the diastereomeric bay-region BA 3,4-diol-1,2-epoxides on the skin of CD-1 mice after 25 weeks of promotion*

Initiator	Dose (μmol)	% of mice with tumours	Tumours/mouse
Acetone		7	0.07 ± 0.05^a
BA	0.4	14	0.14 ± 0.07
	2.5	36	0.64 ± 0.20
(−)-BA 3,4-diol-1,2-epoxide-1	0.1	7	0.07 ± 0.05
	0.4	17	0.17 ± 0.07
(+)-BA 3,4-diol-1,2-epoxide-1	0.1	21	0.39 ± 0.17
	0.4	47	0.73 ± 0.27
(−)-BA 3,4-diol-1,2-epoxide-2	0.1	10	0.13 ± 0.08
	0.4	14	0.14 ± 0.07
(+)-BA 3,4-diol-1,2-epoxide-2	0.1	55	1.28 ± 0.28
	0.4	90	3.35 ± 0.60
(±)-BA 3,4-diol-1,2-epoxide-1	0.4	19	0.36 ± 0.11
(±)-BA 3,4-diol-1,2-epoxide-2	0.4	50	1.63 ± 0.31

The indicated dose of compound was applied once, and 16 nmol of 12-*O*-tetra-decanoylphorbol-13-acetate were administered topically twice weekly for 25 weeks beginning 14 days after initiation. Each treatment group contained 30 mice, and at least 27 mice in each group survived to termination of the study.
[a] Mean ± S.E.
From Levin *et al.* (1984).

1940; Badger *et al.*, 1940). These findings have subsequently been confirmed by subcutaneous injection into rats (Dunning and Curtis, 1960; Huggins *et al.*, 1967), by either chronic topical application to mouse skin or by subcutaneous injection into mice (Stevenson and Von Haam, 1965) and in the two-stage initiation–promotion tumour model system (Table 11.4) on mouse skin (Wislocki *et al.*, 1982). From these experiments there is general agreement that the tumourigenic activity of mono-methylBAs is in the order 7- > 8- = 12- > 6- = 9- > BA = 1- > 2-, 3-, 4-, 5-, 10- and 11-methylBA, the latter group of compounds having no significant tumourigenic activity when compared with control (untreated) animals. There has not yet been a satisfactory answer as to why the introduction of a methyl group at these various positions cause such marked changes in the observed carcinogenicity.

The biological data available on monosubstituted BAs with alkyl groups larger than a methyl group are not as extensive as those available

Table 11.4 *Tumour-initiating activity of the twelve MBAs*

Compound	Dose (nmol)	% Mice with papillomas	No. of papillomas per mouse
I. Acetone	—	3	0.03
BA	400	23	0.3
1-MBA	400	27	0.3
2-MBA	400	7	0.07
3-MBA	400	13	0.2
4-MBA	400	10	0.1
5-MBA	400	17	0.23
6-MBA	30	27	0.3
	100	10	0.27
	400	33	0.6
7-MBA	30	28	0.55
	100	70	1.6
	400	77	4.9
8-MBA	30	17	0.23
	100	23	0.73
	400	40	1.03
9-MBA	400	28	0.55
10-MBA	400	13	0.23
11-MBA	400	10	0.1
12-MBA	30	23	0.3
	100	17	0.27
	400	52	1.03
7,12-DMBA	9	97	8.14

Groups of 30 seven-week-old female mice were initiated with the indicated dose of hydrocarbon in 200 μl of acetone and treated with 10 μg of TPA in 200 μl of acetone twice weekly for the duration of the experiment. From Wislocki *et al.* (1982).

for the methyl derivatives. Substitution at the 7-position of BA by either an ethyl, propyl, isopropyl, allyl, butyl or aryl group has resulted in compounds which, unlike 7-MBA, all lack carcinogenic activity, except for 7-ethylBA which is a weak carcinogen (Shear *et al.*, 1940). It would appear that substitution at the 8-position with bulkier alkyl groups than a methyl group has a much less-marked effect. Epithelial tumours have been produced by 8-ethyl, 8-propyl, 8-butyl and 8-hexyl derivatives of BA in skin-painting experiments on mice (Badger *et al.*, 1940).

Attempts have been made to ascertain the metabolic route which may lead to ultimate carcinogenic forms of 7-MBA and 8-MBA. The hydroxylation of the methyl group in 7-MBA lowers tumourigenic activity relative to 7-MBA after injection into mice (Badger *et al.*, 1940). The K-region oxide of 7-MBA is less active as a carcinogen than 7-MBA itself (Miller and Miller, 1967; Van Duuren *et al.*, 1967; Boyland and Sims, 1967*a*). The carcinogenic activity exhibited by various dihydrodiol derivatives of 7-MBA on mouse skin has revealed that the 3,4-dihydrodiol of 7-MBA is the most active (Fig. 11.2), being even more active than the parent hydrocarbon (Chouroulinkov *et al.*, 1977). These observations on the carcinogenic activity of the various dihydrodiols of 7-MBA have been confirmed by Slaga *et al.* (1980); the 3,4-diol 1,2-epoxide of 7-MBA was also examined in this study and, surprisingly, shown to have only weak tumour-initiating activity. When various possible metabolic species of 8-MBA were tested for carcinogenic activity on mouse skin, the 3,4-dihydrodiol of 8-MBA was the most active, and the 8-hydroxymethylBA was less active, as was its 3,4-dihydrodiol (Wislocki *et al.*, 1981*a*). These results in general support the concept that the ultimate carcinogen *in vivo* of both 7- and 8-MBA is a bay-region diol epoxide.

Fig. 11.2. The initiation of tumours on mouse skin by 7-MBA (△——△) and the related 1,2- (●——●), 3,4- (□——□), 5,6- (▲——▲), and 8,9- (○——○) dihydrodiols. From Chouroulinkov *et al.* (1977).

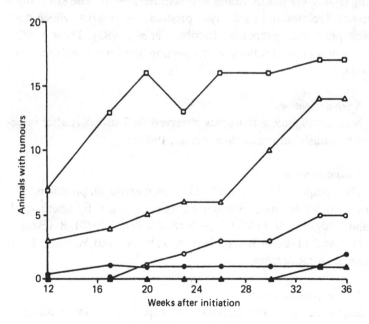

11.4.2   *Halogen derivatives*
Whilst 3-fluoroBA is virtually inactive as a carcinogen, 4-fluoro-BA has considerable activity as a subcutaneous carcinogen in the rat: 93% of treated rats developing sarcomas. Only low tumourigenic activity was observed in mice (Miller and Miller, 1963) after subcutaneous injection although when it was applied to the uterine cervix of mice significant tumour activity was also expressed in this tissue (Stevenson and Haam, 1965). The compound 4-fluoroBA was highly toxic to both rats and mice (Miller and Miller, 1963). Comparison of the skin tumour-initiating activity of 7- and 12-fluoroBA in mice revealed that they were several-fold more active than BA, although the activity was much less than that of their methyl-substituted analogues (Wood *et al.*, 1982).

Introduction of a chlorine atom into the methyl group of 7-MBA results in a compound with very little carcinogenic activity (Shear *et al.*, 1940). Similarly substitution of a bromine atom into the methyl group of 7-MBA reduces the tumourigenic activity after subcutaneous injection into rats (Dipple and Slade, 1970) and mice (Roe *et al.*, 1972). In mouse skin 7-BrMBA is of comparable potency to dibenz[a,c]anthracene as an initiating agent, however 7-BrMBA also has powerful skin tumour-promoting characteristics (Scribner and Scribner, 1980). The effect does not seem to be related to its solvolysis product, 7-OHMBA, which does not exhibit promoting properties (Scribner *et al.*, 1983). These studies have led to a new model for tumour progression being proposed (Scribner *et al.*, 1983).

11.4.3   *Nitro derivatives*
No carcinogenic activity was observed for 7-nitroBA after injection subcutaneously into mice (Shear *et al.*, 1940).

11.4.4   *Amino derivatives*
The compound 7-aminoBA is a weak carcinogen producing sarcomas in 2 out of 60 mice in experiments carried out by Shear *et al.* (1940) and Badger *et al.* (1940). The 5- (Shear *et al.*, 1940), 8- (Badger *et al.*, 1940) and 11-aminoBA derivatives (Dunlap and Warren, 1946) had no carcinogenic activity.

11.4.5   *Hydroxyl derivatives*
Slight carcinogenic activity was reported in mice using 5-hydroxyBA (Shear *et al.*, 1940) whereas no activity was observed for 7- (Shear *et al.*, 1940) and 11-hydroxyBA (Dunlap and Warren, 1946).

11.4.6 *Oxo derivatives*

Weak carcinogenicity has been noted for 7-formylBA (Shear *et al.*, 1940) on subcutaneous injection into mice.

11.4.7 *Carboxy derivatives*

No carcinogenic activity has been observed for BA 8-acetic acid, whereas BA 7-acetic acid is slightly active in mice.

11.4.8 *Thiol derivatives*

In mice slight carcinogenic activity was found with BA 7-mercaptan (Dunlap and Warren, 1946). Substitution of a sulphur atom into the methyl group of 7-MBA to give BA 7-methylmercapten caused a marked reduction in carcinogenic activity compared with the parent compound (Dunlap and Warren, 1946).

11.5 Carcinogenicity of disubstituted benz[a]anthracenes

11.5.1 *Alkyl derivatives*

There are 66 possible isomeric dimethylbenz[a]anthracenes, of which 21 have been tested for carcinogenic activity (Table 11.5). Dimethyl substituents at the 6-, 7-, 8- and 12- positions are compounds which exhibit high levels of carcinogenic activity (the so-called triangle of carcinogenicity), and indeed 7,12-DMBA is one of the most potent chemical carcinogens ever synthesized. This compound is considered separately at the end of this section. Methyl substituents at the 1-, 2-, 3- and 4- positions result in compounds without carcinogenic activity (Table 11.5).

Substitution of groups larger than a methyl group into the 7-position of BA generally produces compounds with reduced carcinogenicity when compared with the methyl analogue. Thus Huggins *et al.* (1967) found that substitution of the 7-methyl group of 7,12-DMBA by either an ethyl, propyl or *n*-butyl group yielded compounds with decreasing carcinogenic potency (the latter being inactive). Similarly 7,12-diethyl-benz[a]anthracene (Badger *et al.*, 1940; Huggins *et al.*, 1967), 7,12-di-*n*-propylbenz[a]anthracene (Bradbury *et al.*, 1941), and 7,12-diphenyl-benz[a]anthracene (Barry *et al.*, 1935), are completely devoid of carcinogenic activity. These observations suggest that molecular thickness may be an important factor in determining the carcinogenic potency of a compound, so that a dialkyl derivative of BA would be active only if the thickness of either the convex side of the molecule (positions 6, 7, 8) or the concave side (positions 11,12, 1) did not exceed 4Å,

Table 11.5 *Carcinogenicity of dimethylbenz[a]anthracenes*[a]

Position of substituent	Species	Number of animals	Total dose (mg)	Mode of administration	Duration of experiment (months)	Number with tumours	References
1,7	mice	40	5.0	SC	15	0	Shear et al., 1940
1,12	rats	8	2.5	IM	9	0	Pataki and Huggins, 1969
2,9	mice	10	b	SP	12	0	Barry et al., 1935
	mice	15	2.0	IM	12	0	Barry et al., 1935
	mice	15	0.15	SP	11	2(pap)	Heidelberger et al., 1962
2,10	mice	10	b	SP	12	0	Barry et al., 1935
3,9	mice	10	b	SP	12	0	Barry et al., 1935
	rats	10	2.0	IM	6	0	Huggins et al., 1964
	rats	8	2.5	IM	9	0	Pataki and Huggins, 1969
3,10	mice	10	b	SP	12	0	Barry et al., 1935
4,7	rats	8	2.5	IM	9	0	Pataki et al., 1971
4,12	rats	8	2.5	IM	9	0	Pataki et al., 1971
5,12	mice	20	2.0	SC	13	0	Shear and Leiter, 1941
	rats	8	2.5	IM	9	0	Pataki et al., 1971
6,7	mice	20	1.0	SC	14	7	Shear et al., 1940
	rats	8	2.5	IM	9	8(iss)	Pataki and Huggins, 1969
6,8	rats	8	2.0	IM	6	8(s)	Huggins et al., 1964
	rats	8	2.5	IM	9	8(iss)	Pataki and Huggins, 1969
6,12	mice	30	0.25–0.6	SP	5	18(pap)	Levin et al., 1983
	mice	20	2.0	SC	12	9	Shear and Leiter, 1941
	rats	8	2.5	IM	9	8(iss)	Pataki and Huggins, 1969
7,8	mice	15	10	SC	4	7	Fieser and Newman, 1936
	mice	16	10	SC	4	9	Shear, 1938
	rats	8	2.5	IM	9	8(iss)	Pataki and Huggins, 1969

Table 11.5 (*Contd*)

Position of substituent	Species	Number of animals	Total dose (mg)	Mode of administration	Duration of experiment (months)	Number with tumours	References
7,11	mice	15	1–5	SC	6	6	Dunlap and Warren, 1946
	rats	7	2.5	IM	9	7(iss)	Pataki *et al.*, 1971
7,12	mice	20	b	SP	6	8(e), 5(pap)	Bachmann *et al.*, 1938
	mice	20	0.1	SC	4	6	Shear, 1938
8,9	mice	20	b	SP	12	16(e)	Barry *et al.*, 1935
8,11	mice	25	1.0	SC	6	2(pa)	Dunlap and Warren, 1946
8,12	mice	20	1.0	SC	4	18	Shear, 1938
	rats	8	2.5	IM	9	8(iss)	Pataki and Huggins, 1969
9,10	mice	20	b	SP	12	2(pap)	Barry *et al.*, 1935
	rats	8	2.5	IM	9	1(iss)	Pataki and Huggins, 1969

[a] Abbreviations used: SC, subcutaneous; SP, skin painting; IM, intermuscular; pap, papillomas; iss, injection site sarcoma; s, sarcoma; e, epitheliomas; pa, pulmonary adenoma; b, one drop of a 0.3% solution of the PAH in benzene applied twice weekly.

that is, the thickness of a methyl group (Huggins *et al.*, 1967). So far experimental data have failed to support the concept that thickness of a molecule is a critical requirement for carcinogenicity (Pataki and Balick, 1972), indeed in contrast to the lack of carcinogenicity of 7,12-diethylBA after intramuscular injection into rats, 6,7-diethylBA is a highly potent carcinogen.

Carcinogenicity of 7,12-dimethylbenz[a]anthracene
Since the original observation that 7,12-DMBA causes cancer when applied to the skin of mice (Bachmann *et al.*, 1938) there has been extensive use of this carcinogen in various model systems. Its extreme potency was recognized very early (Iball, 1939), it being carcinogenic on application to the skin of mice, rabbits, rat and guinea pig (the latter species generally being refractory to skin painting of carcinogens) and the mouse, rat and guinea pig were equally responsive to tumour formation after subcutaneous injection (Berenblum, 1949a).

Depending on the mode of application of 7,12-DMBA various types of cancer may be evoked in a particular species. A single 'flash' exposure to 7,12-DMBA by intravenous injection elicits mammary cancer, multiple doses will evoke leukaemia in rat and mouse, injection of 7,12-DMBA intramuscularly or subcutaneously will evoke the development of a fibrosarcoma at the site of injection (see Huggins, 1979, for a fuller discussion).

Skin carcinogenesis with 7,12-dimethylbenz[a]anthracene
In a limited study in which 7,12-DMBA was applied daily for one week to the skin of a man, an eczematous reaction occurred, but no tumours were reported over the time period (two months) of observation (Williams, 1958). Using a more acceptable experimental procedure, human skin has been transplanted onto nude mice, and then treated with 7,12-DMBA and a promotor: epidermal hyperplasia occurred, and those tumours which did appear (located mainly in the graft border region) were of murine rather than human origin (Graem, 1986). When applied topically to mouse skin, 7,12-DMBA is rapidly absorbed and excreted, predominantly in the faeces, less than 18% of the applied 7,12-DMBA remaining at the application site after 24 hours (Sanders *et al.*, 1984). There are marked histological changes to the mouse skin occurring in the first few weeks after application of the carcinogen, by the third week there are firm, nodular, tumour-like growths in some animals (Levy *et al.*, 1951).

Initially the experimental induction of skin cancer was demonstrated by repeated application of a chemical carcinogen to the target site. Berenblum (1941), Berenblum and Shubik (1947) and Mottram (1944) introduced the concept of a two-stage mechanism of skin carcinogenesis in which a subthreshhold dose of a carcinogen is applied (initiation phase) followed by repetitive treatment of a noncarcinogenic promotor. The initiation phase requires only a single application of the carcinogen and is essentially an irreversible step; the promotion phase is considered to be reversible initially and later becomes irreversible. The most common promotors used are phorbol esters derived from croton oil, in particular 12-O-tetradecanoylphorbol-13-acetate(TPA). Saffiotti and Shubik (1956) and Slaga *et al.* (1974) have reported a 'summation effect' when the initiating carcinogen is applied at repeated low doses. This would indicate that there is no threshhold dose below which a carcinogen can be considered harmless, since these agents have a cumulative effect and the smallest dose, given often enough, will result in tumours. Mouse skin carcinogenesis was dependent also on the dose and duration of the applied promotor (Verma and Boutwell, 1980); there being a good correlation between the induction of ornithine decarboxylase activity and formation of skin tumours by various doses of TPA.

The majority of studies examining two-stage skin carcinogenesis with 7,12-DMBA have employed mice as the target species (different strains of which can vary in their susceptibility; DiGiovanni *et al.*, 1980*a*); however, other species such as the rat (Schweizer *et al.*, 1982), the rabbit (Goerttler *et al.*, 1982) and the Syrian golden hamster (Goerttler *et al.*, 1980*b*) also are susceptible to this type of treatment. In the rat a relatively broad spectrum of tumours of epidermal origin were observed (neoplastic epidermal cysts, papillomas, basaliomas, squamous cell carcinomas), comprising also benign and malignant lesions of the epidermal appendages (sebaceous gland adenomas and carcinomas). In the mouse the tumour spectrum consists mainly of papillomas and squamous cell carcinomas. There also occurred in the rat a high incidence of tumours of the connective tissue (Schweizer *et al.*, 1982).

The crucial requirement for the initiating event is believed to be the binding of the chemical carcinogen to DNA. Much less is known about how the promotional stage of skin carcinogenesis develops. Boutwell (1964) has suggested that in mouse skin the process of promotion itself consists of two different stages, involving the conversion of initiated cells into dormant tumour cells, followed by their propagation, involving activation and clonal expansion of the dormant tumour cells. The results of experiments using incomplete promotors, such as 12-retinoylphorbol-13-acetate or the diterpene ester mezerein, have supported the concept of stage 1 of promotion being brought about by a single treatment with a so-called complete promotor such as TPA, and stage 2 using an incomplete promotor over a long period. Although it was generally thought that stage 1 was persistent and stage 2 reversible, recent evidence (Furstenberger *et al.*, 1985) has revealed that stage 1 effects are slowly reversible and that they are independent of whether the stage 1 of promotion occurs before or after the initiating event. The authors believe these findings may still be accommodated within Boutwell's concept but that it is unimportant whether an epidermal cell is initiated first and then converted into a dormant tumour cell or is converted into a state in which treatment with a carcinogen immediately results in the formation of a dormant tumour cell.

One of the main areas of current investigation, using mouse skin carcinogenesis as a model system, is into ways of inhibiting tumour formation. Surprisingly certain PAHs inhibit 7,12-DMBA-induced skin carcinogenesis (Slaga and Boutwell, 1977*a*; Slaga *et al.*, 1979*c*). This effect may be related to an increased induction of the cytochrome P-450 monooxygenase system and indeed compounds which are potent inducers of this system, such as TCDD, also exhibit strong anticarcinogenic effects on tumour initiation by 7,12-DMBA (DiGiovanni *et al.*, 1979*a*; Cohen *et al.*, 1979). Immunization with a noncarcinogenic fluorinated 7,12-DMBA analogue can provide protection against 7,12-DMBA induced carcinogenicity (Moolten *et al.*, 1981); the previous studies on this subject which suggested that immunization had no effect were carried out with too high a dose of the carcinogen for the effect to be observed (Moolten *et al.*, 1981).

As well as using the technique of skin painting on the backs of test animals to produce skin cancers, 7,12-DMBA has also been applied to the hamster cheek pouch to provide an extremely reliable model for the production of oral mucosal epidermoid carcinoma (Silberman and Shklar, 1963). Another technique recently employed by Goerttler *et al.* (1980*a*) induced tumours in mice by the intravaginal administration of 7,12-DMBA followed by promotion with TPA using small tampons. Papillomas, carcinomas and sarcomas located in the vaginal area were observed as well as tumours of the lung and forestomach.

Mammary carcinogenesis with 7,12-dimethylbenz[a]anthracene
The induction of mammary cancer by 7,12-DMBA has been reviewed by Huggins (1979) and will be considered only briefly here. Mammary

carcinoma can be induced in rats by a single intravenous injection of 7,12-DMBA, or by a single feeding of a large amount of 7,12-DMBA. The development and yield of tumours are precise and reproducible events under stipulated laboratory conditions. This has made 7,12-DMBA-induced mammary cancer a widely used model system, particularly as it bears a close resemblance to hormone-dependent human breast cancer (Russo and Russo, 1978). As in humans where an early full-term pregnancy protects against the development of breast cancer (Valaoras *et al.*, 1969), the incidence of mammary tumours induced by 7,12-DMBA in rats is also reduced by pregnancy and lactation (Huggins, 1979). Mammary cancer rarely arises in rats deprived of their ovaries, and the development of tumours is dependent on the presence of hormones such as estrogen and prolactin (Meites, 1972; Huggins, 1979) and insulin.

The way in which pregnancy and lactation protect against 7,12-DMBA-induced mammary cancer is not fully understood although attention has been drawn to the change which occurs in undifferentiated terminal end buds and terminal ducts (which are believed to be the site at which rat mammary carcinomas originate) present in glands of virgin rats to the more differentiated alveolar buds and lobules following pregnancy and lactation. It should be noted, however, that repeated multiple doses of 7,12-DMBA will also induce mammary cancer in male rats. Mice are also susceptible to 7,12-DMBA-induced mammary cancer (Engelbreth-Holm and Lefevre, 1941; Medina and Warner, 1976) and the mouse model mammary tumour system is unique in having a discrete morphological lesion, preneoplastic alveolar and ductal hyperplasias, which is a precursor to mammary tumour formation. Of those metabolites formed from 7,12-DMBA by mammary cells (see Chapter 8) only the hydroxymethyl derivatives have been tested for carcinogenic activity; they do not have potent mammary tumour-inducing properties (Boyland *et al.*, 1965c; Wheatley and Inglis, 1968) and probably represent routes of detoxification.

Inhibition of 7,12-DMBA-induced mammary cancer can occur after treatment with compounds as diverse as: sodium selenite (Thompson *et al.*, 1984; Welsch *et al.*, 1981); antioxidants (McCormick *et al.*, 1984); the monoterpene, d-limonene (Elegbede *et al.*, 1984); an inhibitor of β-glucuronidase, D-glucaro-1,4-lactone (Walaszek *et al.*, 1984); retinoids (Moon *et al.*, 1976); and even sodium cyanate (Wattenberg, 1980). Some of these compounds affect the initiating activity of 7,12-DMBA, some alter the promotional stage of the development of this cancer.

The mammary cancer model system has also been used to examine the effect of dietary constituents such as carbohydrates; of those rats fed diets containing either sucrose, lactose or corn starch only those which were fed lactose had a significantly lower incidence of 7,12-DMBA-induced mammary tumours (Klurfeld *et al.*, 1984). High dietary fat intake significantly enhances mammary tumourigenesis in rats (Carroll and Khor, 1970; Welsch and Aylsworth, 1983) and there is a similar correlation between the incidence and mortality of breast cancer in women and high intake of dietary fat (Armstrong and Doll, 1975; Gray *et al.*, 1979; Hems, 1978). Whilst the type of fatty acids, whether *cis* or *trans*, do not seem to affect the number of mammary tumours which develop, it does appear that polyunsaturated fats are more effective in promoting mammary carcinogenesis than mono-unsaturated or saturated fats (Selenskas *et al.*, 1984), possibly by inhibition of intercellular communication (Aylsworth *et al.*, 1984). Selenskas *et al.* (1984) also noted that the fatty acid content of the mammary pad generally reflected the dietary fatty acid intake. The current evidence strongly suggests that dietary fat exerts its influence at the promotional stage of carcinogenesis (Carroll and Khor, 1970; Aylsworth *et al.*, 1984). Other suggested mechanisms involved in the inhibition of 7,12-DMBA-induced mammary cancer include changes in the endocrine system, resulting in higher levels of estrogen and prolactin (Ip *et al.*, 1980), and also that alterations in the immune system may play a part (Wagner *et al.*, 1982).

Other carcinogenic effects of 7,12-dimethylbenz[a]anthracene
When given to pregnant rats 7,12-DMBA exerts transplacental carcinogenic effects with the nervous system as the principal target organ (Napalkov and Alexandrov, 1974; Rice *et al.*, 1978), there being tumours of the nervous system in up to 60% of the offspring. This may be contrasted with the transplacental carcinogenic effects produced in mice in which epidermal tumours predominate (Goerttler *et al.*, 1980c), tumours of the lung and liver could also be detected (Goerttler *et al.*, 1981). The latter studies are interesting in that the pregnant mice were given the initiating dose of 7,12-DMBA and the offspring were treated with the promoter. Such studies (which up to now have been limited in number) may help to estimate the risk to babies from mothers who smoke.

The induction of leukaemia in rats by 7,12-DMBA has been reviewed (Huggins, 1979). The formation of tumours by 7,12-DMBA in the lungs of mice has been described (Walters, 1966), as well as on the forestomach (Goerttler *et al.*, 1979) and in liver (Wislocki *et al.*, 1981b) of mice. The induction of melanomas, with complete unresponsiveness of the dorsal epithelium, by 7,12-DMBA in the Syrian golden hamster has been reported (Goerttler *et al.*, 1980b).

Metabolic activation involving the aromatic nucleus of 7,12-dimethylbenz[a]anthracene

The subcutaneous injection of the K-region epoxide of 7,12-DMBA into rats failed to produce any sarcomas (Flesher *et al.*, 1976). In contrast the 3,4-dihydrodiol of 7,12-DMBA on mouse skin (using the classical two-stage initiation–promotion system) had higher levels of carcinogenic activity than 7,12-DMBA itself, the 5,6-, 8,9- and 10,11-dihydrodiols being inactive as tumour initiators (Slaga *et al.*, 1979a; Wislocki *et al.*, 1980). The 8,9-diol 10,11-epoxide had weak tumour-initiating properties (Slaga *et al.*, 1979b). When the dihydrodiols of 7,12-DMBA were examined in the newborn mouse lung adenoma system, the 3,4-dihydrodiol again exhibiting the highest tumourigenicity (Wislocki *et al.*, 1981b); in this study liver tumours, predominantly in male mice, were also observed.

Rather than compare the carcinogenicity of various possible metabolites involved in the metabolic activation of 7,12-DMBA, an alternative approach is to 'block' various positions on the aromatic nucleus to metabolic attack by the introduction of particular substituents. If the position that is blocked is involved in the metabolic activation of 7,12-DMBA then there will be a reduction in carcinogenic activity of that compound. This approach generally ignores any electronic effects on the aromatic nucleus that the introduction of the blocking substituent may have. Also metabolic studies by Yang *et al.* (1979a) indicate that the presence of a methyl group at a particular position does not necessarily inhibit the formation of an epoxide by cytochrome P-450 at that position.

Using the mouse skin initiation–promotion system Slaga *et al.* (1979b) found that the introduction of a methyl group at positions C-1, C-2 and to a lesser extent at C-5 into 7,12-DMBA, resulted in compounds with reduced carcinogenicity relative to that of 7,12-DMBA (Table 11.6). The introduction of a hydroxyl group at positions C-1, -2, -3, -4 or -5 into 7,12-DMBA abolished tumourigenic activity (Slaga *et al.*, 1979b). Similarly the presence of a fluorine atom at positions C-1, C-2 and C-5, and to a lesser extent at position C-4 of 7,12-DMBA almost completely blocked skin tumour-initiating activity (Slaga *et al.*, 1979b; Huberman and Slaga, 1979b; DiGiovanni *et al.*, 1982a, 1983a). There was no reduction of carcinogenic activity when 9- and 11-fluoro-7,12-DMBA (Huberman and Slaga, 1979b; DiGiovanni *et al.*, 1983a) were employed, whilst there was an increase in carcinogenic activity when 7,12-DMBA was substituted at C-10 by fluorine (DiGiovanni *et al.*, 1983a). This represents the first example of a fluorine substituent leading to an increase in

Table 11.6 *Skin tumour-initiating activities of various DMBA derivatives after TPA promotion*[a]

DMBA derivative	No. of mice[b]	Papillomas/ mouse[c]	Mice with tumours (%)[d]
Control (only DMBA initiation)[e]	30	0	0
Control (only TPA promotion)[f]	29	0.10	6
DMBA	28	9.10	100
1-OHDMBA	29	0.10	10
2-OHDMBA	30	0.07	7
3-OHDMBA	30	0.14	14
4-OHDMBA	28	0.17	14
5-OHDMBA	29	0.10	10
9-OHDMBA	30	0.40	24
10-OHDMBA	30	0.47	30
DMBA 5,6-diol	29	0.10	10
DMBA 8,9-diol	29	0.21	18
DMBA 8,9-diol-10,11-epoxide	28	0.30	20
1-CH$_3$-DMBA	30	0.03	3
2-CH$_3$-DMBA	30	0.10	7
5-CH$_3$-DMBA	29	0.40	34
1-F-DMBA	30	0.03	3
2-F-DMBA	29	0.10	10
5-F-DMBA	28	0.20	15
11-F-DMBA	29	8.20	100

[a] DMBA and derivatives were applied at a dose of 200 nmol and were followed 1 week later by twice-weekly applications of 10 μg of TPA.
[b] Surviving at the 30th week after promotion.
[c] Total number papillomas divided by total number of surviving mice.
[d] Percentage of surviving mice with tumours.
[e] These mice were only initiated with 200 nmol of DMBA.
[f] These mice were only promoted twice weekly with 10 μg of TPA for 30 weeks.
From Slaga *et al.* (1979*b*).

carcinogenic activity relative to that of the parent compound. Experiments in which bromine and methoxy groups (Lijinsky *et al.*, 1983) have been used as substituents generally confirm the findings that positions C-1, -2, -3 and -5 may be involved in the metabolic activation of 7,12-DMBA in skin.

When substituted 7,12-DMBA compounds were examined as complete carcinogens in the rat, 5-fluoro-7,12-DMBA was virtually inactive (Newman *et al.*, 1978), 1- and 2-fluoro- and 2- and 3-methyl-7,12-DMBA had very little carcinogenic activity, whereas 4-, 8- and 11-fluoro- and 4-methyl-7,12-DMBA showed high levels of carcinogenic activity (Harvey and Dunne, 1978). The lack of carcinogenic activity of 2-fluoro-7,12-DMBA has been confirmed (Newman and Tuncay, 1980). The C-4 position of 7,12-DMBA can thus be blocked and yet metabolic activation still occurs; this might not be expected if the formation of a bay-region 3,4-diol 1,2-epoxide is a necessary step in the metabolic activation of 7,12-DMBA (it is interesting that 4-fluoroBA also has high carcinogenic activity: Miller and Miller, 1963). Similarly, the high carcinogenic activity of 1,2,3,4-tetrahydro-7,12-DMBA (which although approximately one-tenth that of 7,12-DMBA, is still slightly more active than 3-MC and three times more active than B[a]P as a tumour initiator) cannot be explained by metabolism to a bay-region diol epoxide (DiGiovanni *et al.*, 1982*a*; Lijinsky *et al.*, 1983). It thus appears that for 7,12-DMBA there are alternate metabolic pathways available in the formation of ultimate carcinogens.

Metabolic activation involving the aliphatic side chain of 7,12-dimethylbenz[a]anthracene
The methyl groups at positions C-7 and C-12 on the BA nucleus can be metabolically hydroxylated. Experiments have shown that hydroxylation at either the 7-methyl, 12-methyl or both methyl groups of 7,12-DMBA results in compounds with reduced carcinogenic activity when compared with that of 7,12-DMBA (Pataki and Huggins, 1969; Flesher and Sydnor, 1971; DiGiovanni *et al.*, 1978; Wislocki *et al.*, 1980, 1981*b*) suggesting aliphatic hydroxylation is not involved in the metabolic activation of 7,12-DMBA. However, various hydroxymethyl dihydrodiols of 7,12-DMBA do exhibit significant carcinogenic activity, thus the 3,4-dihydrodiol of 7-OHM-12-MBA has a higher carcinogenic activity on mouse skin (Wislocki *et al.*, 1980) and in newborn mice (Wislocki *et al.*, 1981*b*) than 7-OHM-12-MBA itself, indicative of the 3,4-dihydrodiol being a proximate carcinogen for the hydroxymethyl derivative, and may therefore also contribute to some of the carcinogenicity observed for 7,12-DMBA.

Biological effects of 7,12-dimethylbenz[a]anthracene in other tissues
The effect of 7,12-DMBA in the adrenal cortex and testis has been reviewed (Huggins, 1979) and will be considered only briefly here. 7,12-DMBA-induced immunotoxicity has also been reviewed recently (Dean *et al.*, 1985) and will not be discussed further here.

In the adrenal cortex, 7,12-DMBA is unique amongst PAHs in 'invariably, selectively and totally destroying two zones, the zona fasciculata and zona reticularis, and giving rise to the induction of adrenal apoplexy' (Huggins and Morii, 1961). The effect is not observed in young rats (Morii and Huggins, 1962), and it is not observed in other species such as hamsters, guinea pigs or mice (Cefis and Goodall, 1965). Adrenal necrosis can be blocked by pretreatment of the animal with certain PAHs (including small doses of 7,12-DMBA itself), particularly those with 4 or 5 benzene rings (Dao, 1964). Rats with impaired liver function are protected against adrenal necrosis caused by 7,12-DMBA (Wheatley et al., 1966b), as are animals treated with chemicals known to induce rat-liver microsomal enzymes (Dao, 1964; Dao and Varela, 1966). These observations have led to suggestions that the active agent may be a hepatic metabolite of 7,12-DMBA and indeed one particular metabolite, 7-OHM-12-MBA, is more potent than 7,12-DMBA itself in causing adrenal necrosis (Boyland et al., 1965c) (see Chapter 8). Immature or hypophysectomized rats may be made susceptible to the effects of 7,12-DMBA by administration of an adrenocorticotrophic hormone (ACTH) (Morii and Huggins, 1962). Other steroids have been shown either to decrease the adrenocorticolytic effect, as with spironolactone and ethylestrenol, or to aggravate the lesion, as with estradiol and methylandrostenediol (Somogyi and Kovacs, 1970) in mature rats.

The specific interactions of 7,12-DMBA with adrenal cellular macromolecules which cause adrenal necrosis are not known. Whether 7-OHM-12-MBA is an obligatory intermediate in the generation of reactive intermediates or whether other metabolites, such as diol epoxides, are necessary is not known. Extensive binding to adrenal proteins has been reported (Montelius et al., 1982; Swallow et al., 1983) and one particular adrenal protein, which is highly specific for 7,12-DMBA has been partially characterized (Mankowitz et al., 1981).

In testes of rats which had been injected intravenously with 3-MC or B[a]P, no damage was detected, whereas damage was severe in rats injected with 7,12-DMBA. The primary site of damage caused by 7,12-DMBA was a bed of seminiferous cells near the basement membrane of the tubule (Ford and Huggins, 1963); this type of damage was also accompanied by enzyme changes in the testes (Ahlquist, 1966).

11.5.2 Halogen derivatives
Halogen substituted in the side chain
The higher carcinogenic activity of 7,12-DMBA compared with 7-MBA is reflected in the higher carcinogenic activity of 7-BrM-12-MBA compared with the virtually inactive 7-Br-MBA with regard to induction of injection site sarcomas in adult rats (Dipple and Slade, 1970), skin papillomas in mice (Dipple and Slade, 1971b) and tumours at the injection site and in the lung and liver of newborn mice (Roe et al., 1972). The replacement of a hydrogen atom by either chlorine, bromine or

iodine at the 7-methyl group of 7,12-DMBA produces compounds capable of acting as complete carcinogens (Flesher and Sydnor, 1971). These compounds containing a halogen atom in the alkyl side arm are able to alkylate directly cellular macromolecules such as DNA; therefore metabolic activation may not be required, although the mixed function oxidase inhibitor 7,8-benzoflavone can partially reduce their carcinogenic activity (DiGiovanni *et al.*, 1978).

Halogen substituted in the nucleus
The effect on carcinogenicity, by the presence of fluorine at various ring positions of 7-MBA, has been studied in mouse skin and in the subcutaneous tissues of rats and mice. Substitution of fluorine into the C-5 position of 7-MBA virtually abolished the carcinogenic activity of 7-MBA (Miller and Miller, 1960; Stevenson and Von Haam, 1965; Wood *et al.*, 1982) whereas substitution of fluorine at the C-6 position had little effect (Miller and Miller, 1963). Each of the 2-, 3-, 6-, 9- and 10-fluoro- derivatives of 7-MBA had considerable carcinogenic activity in either the skin or subcutaneous tissue of rats and mice suggesting that these regions are not involved in the metabolic activation of 7-MBA to an ultimate carcinogen (Miller and Miller, 1960, 1963; Harvey and Dunne, 1978). The reason for the suppression of carcinogenic activity by the introduction of a fluorine atom at position C-5 in 7-MBA is not completely understood, though a fluorine atom *peri* to a dihydrodiol (i.e. the 3,4-dihydrodiol) may cause such a dihydrodiol to adopt a *quasi*-diaxial conformation and inhibit the formation of a bay-region diol epoxide. Alternatively the fluorine atom will introduce electronic effects, such as ring deactivation or *ortho/para* directing influences, which may cause alterations in the routes of metabolic activation. The insertion of fluorine into the C-4 position of 7-MBA produces a compound highly toxic to rats and mice. The 4-fluoro derivative does have moderate activity as a skin tumour initiator, but is so toxic that it has proved impossible to test its carcinogenicity adequately (Miller and Miller, 1960). Similar results were found when this compound was applied to the uterine cervix of mice (Stevenson and Von Haam, 1965). The corresponding compound without the 7-methyl group, 4-fluoro-BA, again exhibited some toxicity, but had considerable activity as a subcutaneous carcinogen in the rat (Miller and Miller, 1963). The substitution of either chlorine or bromine at the C-4 position of 7-MBA produces compounds without carcinogenic activity (Newman and Venkateswaran, 1967).

Replacement of either methyl group of 7,12-DMBA with a fluorine

182 Biology

Table 11.7 Sarcoma at site of injection in Sprague–Dawley female rats

No. of rats	Benz[a]anthracene derivative	Rats with sarcoma	Tumour induction time (days) (mean ± S.E.)	No. of tumours (Mean ± S.E.)
12	7,12-Dimethyl-	12/12	96.8 ± 6.7	4.0 ± 1.1
11	7-Benzoyloxymethyl-12-methyl-	11/11	97.9 ± 3.1	3.0 ± 0.2
11	7-Formyl-12-methyl-	10/11	137.7 ± 12.1	1.6 ± 0.3
12	7-Bromomethyl-12-methyl-	6/12	149.0 ± 15.5	1.0
12	7-Hydroxymethyl-12-methyl-	3/12	173.0	1.0
11	7-Iodomethyl-12-methyl-	4/11	149.0	1.1
10	7-Methoxymethyl-12-methyl-	0/10		
10	5-Methoxy-7,12-dimethyl-	0/10		
10	4-Methoxy-7,12-dimethyl-	0/10		
10	4-Hydroxy-7,12-dimethyl-	0/10		
10	Sesame oil	0/10		

A 100 μg dose of the test compound was given by s.c. injection in 0.1 ml of sesame oil on alternate days for 20 doses beginning at 30 days of age. Observation period was 200 days. From Flesher and Sydnor (1971).

atom lowers the carcinogenic activity; however, 7-methyl-12-fluoro- and 7-fluoro-12-methyl-BA are two to three times more active than 7-MBA. Thus fluorine substitution at the C-7 and/or C-12 position enhances tumourigenic activity relative to the unfluorinated compound but not as much as a methyl substituent would (Wood et al., 1982), 7,12-difluoroBA being far less active than 7,12-DMBA.

Halogen substituted in both side chain and nucleus
Very little carcinogenic activity is associated with 4-chloro-7-BrMBA after subcutaneous injection into newborn mice (Roe et al., 1972). Using topical application to the backs of mice followed by promotion, Dipple and Slade (1971b) observed that 6-fluoro-7-BrMBA was more carcinogenic than 7-BrMBA, whereas the 4-chloro- and 4-bromo-7-BrMBAs were virtually inactive. The reason for the high carcinogenic activity of the 6-fluoro derivative is not known.

11.5.3 Other carcinogenic disubstituted derivatives of benz[a]anthracene
    Whereas Badger et al. (1940) found that 7-cyano-12-MBA was a weak skin carcinogen, Shear et al. (1940) tested 8-cyano- and 10-cyano-7-MBA by subcutaneous injection into mice and reported that they were potent carcinogens, the hydrolysis product of the 8-cyano derivative also having potent carcinogenic activity. Flesher and Sydnor (1971) examined a series of 7- and 12-substituted BA derivatives at two dose levels in the rat for carcinogenic activity. The results of the lower dose are given in Table 11.7. Whilst 7-benzoyloxymethyl-12-MBA and 7-formyl-

12-MBA have comparable carcinogenic activities to that of 7,12-DMBA, the introduction of other substituents results in a loss of carcinogenic activity. Dunlap and Warren (1946) had previously reported that 7-methyl-8-methoxy-, 7-ethoxymethyl-12-methyl- and 7-methoxy-12-methyl-BA all exhibited carcinogenic activity in mice after the compounds had been administered by subcutaneous injection. Similar results have been found in the rat for 7-methoxymethyl-12-methyl-, 7-ethoxymethyl-12-methyl-, 7,12-dimethoxy-, and 7-formyl-12-methyl-BA (Pataki and Huggins, 1969). The 7-methoxy- and 7-ethoxy-12-methyl-BA compounds are carcinogenic in the rat (Huggins *et al.*, 1967) although in this study no carcinogenic activity was observed for 7-methoxymethyl-12-methyl-BA (see also Table 11.7). The skin tumour-initiating activities in mice of 7- and 12- substituted derivatives of 7,12-DMBA were investigated by DiGiovanni *et al.* (1978). Thus 12-MBA-7-aldehyde, 7-MBA-12-aldehyde and BA-7,12-dialdehyde all exhibited tumour-initiating activity although considerably higher doses were required to give tumourigenicity levels comparable to that of 7,12-DMBA.

11.6 Carcinogenicity of trisubstituted benz[a]anthracenes
11.6.1 *Alkyl derivatives*
There are 220 isomeric trimethyl BA derivatives theoretically possible, and of these 12 have been examined for carcinogenic activity mainly by injection rather than skin painting (Table 11.8). It is clear that the addition of a methyl group at positions C-1, -2 and -3 of 7,12-DMBA results in the complete loss of carcinogenic activity as might be expected if metabolic activation proceeds via a bay-region diol epoxide. However, the high level of carcinogenicity of 4,7,12-trimethylBA and the lack of carcinogenicity of 5,7,12-trimethylBA cannot be explained in these terms. When a series of trimethyl-substituted BAs was tested, under the same conditions, for carcinogenic activity, the 4,7,12-, 6,8,12-, 7,9,12-, and 7,10,12-trimethylBAs were of equal potency to 7,12-DMBA in terms of the number of sarcomas produced (100%) and in the mean latent period for the appearance of tumours (Pataki and Huggins, 1969; Pataki *et al.*, 1971). As only a single dose was used in these studies, lower doses may reveal more information on the potency of these compounds.

In one of the few skin-painting tumourigenicity studies employing trimethyl BAs Levin *et al.* (1983), compared the carcinogenic activity of 7,11,12-trimethylBA with that of 7,12-DMBA on mouse skin, it being proposed that if steric strain is responsible for the high carcinogenic activity of 7,12-DMBA then 7,11,12-trimethylBA should be even more

Table 11.8 *Carcinogenicity of trimethylbenz[a]anthracenes[a]*

Position of substituent	Species	Number of animals	Total dose (mg)	Mode of administration	Duration of experiment (months)	Number with tumours	References
1,7,12	rat	18	0.5	SC	15	0	Newman and Hung, 1977
2,7,12	rat	12	2.3	SC	18	0	Newman and Hung, 1977
	rat	16	2.5	IM	9	0	Pataki et al., 1971
3,7,12	rat	8	2.5	IM	9	0	Pataki et al., 1971
4,7,12	rat	8	2.5	IM	9	8(iss)	Pataki et al., 1971
5,7,12	rat	8	2.5	IM	9	1(iss)	Pataki et al., 1971
	rat	10	b	IV	4	0	Huggins et al., 1970
6,7,8	rat	54	4.0	SC	6	53(iss)	Dunning et al., 1968
	rat	7	2.5	IM	9	7(iss)	Pataki and Huggins, 1969
6,7,12	rat	8	b	IV	4	0	Huggins et al., 1970
	rat	8	2.5	IM	9	8(iss)	Pataki and Huggins, 1969
6,8,12	rat	9	b	IV	4	2(l)	Huggins et al., 1970
	rat	8	2.5	IM	9	8(iss)	Pataki and Huggins, 1969
7,8,12	mice	26	c	SP	6	7(pap), 10(e)	Badger et al., 1940
	mice	20	d	SP	4	5(pap)	Bachmann et al., 1938
	rat	20	6	IV	4	20(mt)	Pataki and Huggins, 1969
	rat	8	2.5	IM	9	8(iss)	Pataki and Huggins, 1969
7,9,12	mice	20	d	SP	6	3(pap), 8(e)	Badger et al., 1940
	rat	14	b	IV	4	1(l)	Huggins et al., 1970
	rat	8	2.5	IM	9	8(iss)	Pataki et al., 1971
7,10,12	rat	7	2.5	IM	9	7(iss)	Pataki et al., 1971
	mice	383	0.1–0.4	BI	21	91(bs)	Janisch, 1966
	rat	189	0.1–0.4	BI	21	67(bs)	Janisch, 1966
7,11,12	rat	16	1.0	SC	8	15(s)	Newman, 1983a
	mice	30	0.01	SP	5	14(pap)	Levin et al., 1983

[a] Abbreviations as in Table 11.5, together with: IV, intravenous; BI, brain implantation; mt, mammary tumours; l, leukaemia; bs, brain sarcoma; b, 35 ml/kg of 0.5% solution; c, 1 drop of 0.6% solution in benzene applied twice weekly; d, as (c) with 0.3% solution.

carcinogenic. This was found not to be the case; 7,11,12-trimethylBA was at least 20-fold less active than 7,12-DMBA as a tumour initiator.

11.6.2 *Halogen derivatives*

The effect of halogen substitution on 7,12-DMBA carcinogenicity has been discussed in the section 'routes of metabolic activation of 7,12-DMBA'. Briefly, substitution of fluorine at the C-1, -2 and -5 positions of 7,12-DMBA completely blocks tumourigenicity. This effect is less marked when position C-4 is substituted, and there is comparable carcinogenicity with 9- and 11-fluoro-7,12-DMBA relative to 7,12-DMBA. Substitution of fluorine into position C-10 of 7,12-DMBA increases the carcinogenic activity. In order to determine whether the latter observation is due to resonance properties Newman and Veeraraghavan (1983*b*) examined the carcinogenicity of 9- and 10-CF$_3$-7,12-DMBA. The CF$_3$ group is electron withdrawing and it was proposed that both compounds should be less active than 7,12-DMBA. Although 10-CF$_3$-7,12-DMBA is inactive, this was not so for 9-CF$_3$-7,12-DMBA; 50% of rats developed sarcomas in 8 months. Studies using bromine rather than fluorine have confirmed the importance of positions C-1, -2, -3 and -5 in the metabolic activation of 7,12-DMBA.

Modification of the 7-methyl group by acetylation or hydroxylation of 5-fluoro-7,12-DMBA, does not enhance the observed tumourigenic activity significantly, indicating that oxygenation of the 7-methyl group may not be a pathway of metabolic activation (Newman *et al.*, 1978).

11.6.3 *Other trisubstituted derivatives*

The 1-, 2-, 3-, 4- and 5-phenols of 7,12-DMBA appear to be without tumour-initiating activity, whereas the 9- and 10-phenols have weak tumour-initiating activity on mouse skin (Slaga *et al.*, 1979*b*). Neither the 4-phenol nor the 4- or 5-methoxy derivatives of 7,12-DMBA had significant carcinogenic activity when injected subcutaneously into rats (Flesher and Sydnor, 1971). An examination of the initiating activity of 2-, 3- and 4-methoxy- and 2-, 3- and 4-bromo-7,12-DMBA on mouse skin revealed that 2-methoxy- and 4-bromo-7,12-DMBA have moderate tumour-initiating activity, the former compound producing mainly squamous cell carcinomas and the latter, neurosarcomas. The other compounds were only very weakly active (Lijinsky *et al.*, 1983). The 8-bromo- and 8-cyano-7,12-DMBA compounds are potent carcinogens on subcutaneous injection into mice (Dunlap and Warren, 1946).

11.7   Carcinogenicity of tetrasubstituted benz[a]anthracene
7,8,9,12-TetramethylBA shows moderate activity as a skin carcinogen; of 20 mice treated, eight developed epitheliomas and one, a papilloma. After subcutaneous injection of 10 mice, one developed a sarcoma (Badger *et al.*, 1940).

12

References to Part 2

Reference titles contain original nomenclature.

Abell, C. W. & Heidelberger, C. (1962). Binding of tritium-labelled hydrocarbons to the soluble proteins of mouse skin. *Cancer Res.*, 22, 931–46.

Ahlquist, K. A. (1966). Enzyme changes in rat testis produced by the administration of busulphan and of 7,12-dimethylbenz[a]anthracene. *J. Reprod. Fertil.*, 12, 377–9.

Allen, J. A. & Coombs, M. M. (1980). Covalent binding of polycyclic aromatic compounds to mitochondrial and nuclear DNA. *Nature*, 287, 244–5.

Ames, B. N., Sims, P. & Grover, P. L. (1972). Epoxides of carcinogenic polycyclic hydrocarbons are frameshift mutagens. *Science*, 176, 47–9.

Andervont, H. B. & Shimkin, M. B. (1940). Biologic testing of carcinogens. II. Pulmonary-tumour-induction technique. *J. Nat. Cancer Inst.*, 1, 225–39.

Arcos, J. C. & Argus, M. F. (1968). Molecular geometry and carcinogenic activity of aromatic compounds. *Adv. Cancer Res.*, 11, 305–471.

Armstrong, B. & Doll, R. (1975). Environmental factors and cancer incidence mortality in different countries, with special reference to dietary practices. *Int. J. Cancer*, 15, 617–31.

Aylsworth, C. F., Jone, C., Trosko, J. E., Meites, J. & Welsch, C. W. (1984). Promotion of 7,12-dimethylbenz[a]anthracene-induced mammary tumorigenesis by high dietary fat in the rat: possible role of intercellular communication. *J. Nat. Cancer Inst.*, 72, 637–45.

Bachmann, W. E., Kennaway, E. L. & Kennaway, N. M. (1938). The rapid production of tumours by two new hydrocarbons. *Yale J. Biol. & Med.*, 11, 97–102.

Badger, G. M., Cook, J. W., Hewett, C. L., Kennaway, E. L., Kennaway, N. M., Martin, R. H. & Robinson, A. M. (1940). The production of cancer by pure hydrocarbons. V. *Proc. Roy. Soc. Lond. B*, 129, 439–67.

Badger, G. M. (1954). Chemical constitution and carcinogenic activity. *Adv. Cancer Res.*, 2, 73–127.

Baird, W. M. & Brookes, P. (1973a). Isolation of the hydrocarbon–deoxyribonucleoside products from the DNA of mouse embryo cells treated in culture with 7-methyl-benz[a]anthracene. *Cancer Res.*, 33, 2378–85.

Baird, W. M., Dipple, A., Grover, P. L., Sims, P. & Brookes, P. (1973b). Studies on the formation of hydrocarbon deoxyribonucleoside products by the binding of derivatives of 7-methylbenz[a]anthracene to DNA in aqueous solution and in mouse embryo cells in culture. *Cancer Res.*, 33, 2386–92.

Baird, W. M., Grover, P. L., Sims, P. & Brookes, P. (1976). Comparison of the products of the reaction of 7-methylbenz[a]anthracene 5,6-oxide and RNA, with those formed in 7-methylbenz[a]anthracene treated cells. *Cancer Res.*, 36, 2306–11.

Baird, W. M. & Dipple, A. (1977). Photosensitivity of DNA-bound 7,12-dimethyl-benz[a]anthracene. *Int. J. Cancer*, 20, 427–31.

Baird, W. M. (1978a). Effect of light on the hydrocarbon–DNA adducts formed in hamster embryo cells. *Int J. Cancer*, **22**, 292–7.

Baird, W. M., Chemerys, R., Chern, C. J. & Diamond, L. (1978b). Formation of glucuronic acid conjugates of 7,12-dimethylbenz[a]anthracene phenols in 7,12-dimethylbenz[a]anthracene-treated hamster embryo cells. *Cancer Res.*, **38**, 3432–7.

Baird, W. M., Salmon, C. P. & Diamond, L. (1984). Benzo[e]pyrene-induced alterations in the metabolic activation of benzo[e]pyrene and 7,12-dimethylbenz[a]anthracene by hamster embryo cells. *Cancer Res.*, **44**, 1445–52.

Balani, S. K., Yeh, H. C., Ryan, D. E., Thomas, P. E., Levin, W. & Jerina, D. M. (1985). Absolute configuration of the 5,6-oxide formed from 7,12-dimethyl-benz[a]anthracene by cytochrome P-450c. *Biochem. Biophys. Res. Commun.*, **130**, 610–16.

Balmain, A. & Pragnell, I. B. (1983). Mouse skin carcinomas induced *in vivo* by chemical carcinogens have a transforming Harvey-*ras* oncogene. *Nature*, **303**, 72–4.

Balmain, A., Ramsden, M., Bowden, G. T. & Smith, G. (1984). Activation of the mouse cellular Harvey-*ras* gene in chemically induced benign skin papillomas. *Nature*, **307**, 658–60.

Barlow, J. W., Minasian, L. C. & Funder, J. W. (1978). Potentiation of steroid binding to proteins by 7,12-dimethylbenz[a]anthracene. *J. Steroid Biochem.*, **9**, 1027–32.

Barrett, J. C. & Ts'o, P. O. P. (1978). Relationship between somatic mutation and neoplastic transformation. *Proc. Nat. Acad. Sci. U.S.A.*, **75**, 3297–301.

Barry, G., Cook, J. W., Haslewood, G., Hewett, C. L., Hieger, I. & Kennaway, E. L. (1935). The production of cancer by pure hydrocarbons. Part III. *Proc. Roy. Soc. Lond. B*, **117**, 318–51.

Bartsch, H., Malaveille, C., Tierney, B., Grover, P. L. & Sims, P. (1979). The association of bacterial mutagenicity of hydrocarbon-derived 'bay region' dihydrodiols with the Iball indices for carcinogenicity and with the extents of DNA-binding on mouse skin of the parent hydrocarbons. *Chem. Biol. Interact.*, **26**, 185–96.

Berenblum, I. (1941). The mechanism of carcinogenesis. A study of the significance of cocarcinogenic action and related phenomena. *Cancer Res.*, **1**, 807–14.

Berenblum, I. & Schoental, R. (1943). The metabolism of 1,2-benzanthracene in mice and rats. *Cancer Res.*, **3**, 686–8.

Berenblum, I. & Shubik, P. (1947). A new quantitative approach to the study of chemical carcinogenesis in the mouses skin. *Br. J. Cancer*, **1**, 383–91.

Berenblum, I. (1949a). The carcinogenic action of 9,10-dimethyl-1,2-benz[a]anthracene on the skin and subcutaneous tissues of the mouse, rabbit, rat and guinea pig. *J. Nat. Cancer Inst.*, **10**, 167–74.

Berenblum, I. & Shubik, P. (1949b). The persistence of latent tumour cells induced in the mouses skin by a single application of 9,10-dimethyl-1,2-benzanthracene. *Br. J. Cancer*, **3**, 384–6.

Bigelow, S. W. & Nebert, D. W. (1982). The Ah regulatory gene product. Survey of 19 polycyclic aromatic compounds and 15 benzo[a]pyrene metabolites capability to bind to the cytosolic receptor. *Toxicol. Lett.*, **10**, 109–18.

Bigger, C. A. H., Tomaszewski, J. E. & Dipple, A. (1978). Differences between products of binding of 7,12-dimethylbenz[a]anthracene to DNA in mouse skin and in a rat liver microsomal system. *Biochem. Biophys. Res. Commun.*, **80**, 229–35.

Bigger, C. A. H., Tomaszewski, J. E., Andrews, A. W. & Dipple, A. (1980a). Evaluation of metabolic activation of 7,12-dimethylbenz[a]anthracene *in vitro* by Aroclor 1254-induced rat liver S-9 fraction. *Cancer Res.*, **40**, 655–61.

Bigger, C. A. H., Tomaszewski, J. E. & Dipple, A. (1980b). Variation in route of microsomal activation of 7,12-dimethylbenz[a]anthracene with substrate concentration. *Carcinogenesis*, **1**, 15–20.

Bigger, C. A. H., Sawicki, J. T., Blake, D. M., Raymond, L. G. & Dipple, A. (1983).

Products of binding of 7,12-dimethylbenz[a]anthracene to DNA in mouse skin. *Cancer Res.*, **43**, 5647–51.

Blobstein, S. H., Weinstein, I. B., Grunberger, D., Weisgras, J. & Harvey, R. G. (1975). Products obtained after *in vitro* reaction of 7,12-dimethylbenz[a]anthracene 5,6-oxide with nucleic acids. *Biochemistry*, **14**, 3451–8.

Booth, J. & Sims, P. (1974). 8,9-Dihydro-8,9-dihydroxybenz[a]anthracene 10,11-oxide: a new type of polycyclic aromatic hydrocarbon metabolite. *FEBS Lett.*, **47**, 30–3.

Bos, R. P., Theuws, J. L. G., Leijdekkers, C. M. & Henderson, P. T. (1984). The presence of the mutagenic polycyclic aromatic hydrocarbons benzo[a]pyrene and benz[a]anthracene in creosote PI. *Mutation Res.*, **130**, 153–8.

Boutwell, R. K. (1964). Some biological aspects of skin carcinogenesis. *Prog. Exp. Tumor Res.*, **4**, 207–50.

Boyland, E. (1950). The biological significance of metabolism of polycyclic compounds. *Biochem. Soc. Symp.*, **5**, 40–54.

Boyland, E., Kimura, M. & Sims, P. (1964a). Metabolism of polycyclic compounds 26. The hydroxylation of some aromatic hydrocarbons by the ascorbic acid model hydroxylating system and by rat liver microsomes. *Biochem. J.*, **92**, 631–8.

Boyland, E. & Sims, P. (1964b). The metabolism of polycyclic compounds 24. The metabolism of benz[a]anthracene. *Biochem. J.*, **91**, 493–506.

Boyland, E. & Sims, P. (1965a). The metabolism of benz[a]anthracene and dibenz[ah]anthracene and their 5,6-epoxy-5,6-dihydro-derivatives by rat-liver homogenates. *Biochem. J.*, **97**, 7–16.

Boyland, E. & Sims, P. (1965b). The metabolism of 7,12-dimethylbenz[a]anthracene by rat-liver homogenates. *Biochem. J.*, **95**, 780–7.

Boyland, E., Sims, P. & Huggins, C. H. (1965c). Induction of adrenal damage and cancer with metabolites of 7,12-dimethylbenz[a]anthracene. *Nature*, **207**, 816–17.

Boyland, E. & Sims, P. (1967a). The carcinogenic activities in mice of compounds related to benz[a]anthracene. *Int. J. Cancer*, **2**, 500–4.

Boyland, E. & Sims, P. (1967b). The effect of pretreatment with adrenal-protecting compounds on the metabolism of 7,12-dimethylbenz[a]anthracene and related compounds by rat-liver homogenates. *Biochem. J.*, **104**, 394–403.

Bradbury, J. T., Bachmann, W. E. & Lewisohn, M. G. (1941). The production of cancer by some new chemical compounds. *Cancer Res.*, **1**, 685–94.

Breathnach, R. & Chambron, P. (1981). Organisation and expression of eucaryotic split genes coding for proteins. *Ann. Rev. Biochem.*, **50**, 349–83.

Brookes, P. & Lawley, P. D. (1964). Evidence for the binding of polynuclear aromatic hydrocarbons to the nucleic acids of mouse skin: relation between carcinogenic power of hydrocarbons and their binding to deoxyribonucleic acid. *Nature*, **202**, 781–4.

Brookes, P. & Duncan, M. E. (1971). Carcinogenic hydrocarbons and human cells in culture. *Nature*, **234**, 40–2.

Brookes, P. (1977). Mutagenicity of polycyclic aromatic hydrocarbons. *Mutation Res.*, **39**, 257–84.

Bun-Hoi, N. P. (1964). New developments in chemical carcinogenesis by polycyclic hydrocarbons and related heterocycles. *Cancer Res.*, **24**, 1511–23.

Carrell, H. L., Glusker, J. P., Moschel, R. C., Hudgins, W. R. & Dipple, A. (1981). Crystal structure of a carcinogen:nucleoside adduct. *Cancer Res.*, **41**, 2230–4.

Carroll, K. K. & Khor, H. T. (1970). Effects of dietary fat and dose level of 7,12-dimethyl-benz[a]anthracene on mammary tumour incidence in rats. *Cancer Res.*, **30**, 2260–4.

Cary, P. D., Turner, C. H., Cooper, C. S., Ribeiro, O., Grover, P. L. & Sims, P. (1980). Metabolic activation of benz[a]anthracene in hamster embryo cells: the structure of a guanosine–*anti*-BA-8,9-diol 10,11-oxide adduct. *Carcinogenesis*, **1**, 505–12.

Cefis, F. & Goodall, C. M. (1965). Distribution and species limitation of the adrenal lesions induced by 7,12-dimethylbenz[a]anthracene. *Am. J. Path.*, **46**, 227–43.

Cerniglia, C. E., Fu, P. P. & Yang, S. K. (1982). Metabolism of 7-methyl-benz[a]anthracene and 7-hydroxymethylbenz[a]anthracene by *Cunninghamella-elegans*. *Appl. Environ. Microbiol.*, **44**, 682–9.

Cerniglia, C. E., Fu, P. P. & Yang, S. K. (1983). Regio- and stereo- selective metabolism of 4-methylbenz[a]anthracene by the fungus *Cunninghamella-elegans*. *Biochem. J.*, **216**, 377–84.

Chasseaud, L. F. (1979). The role of glutathione and glutathione-S-transferases in the metabolism of chemical carcinogens and other electrophilic agents. *Adv. Cancer Res.*, **29**, 175–274.

Chen, C. & Tu, M. H. (1976). Transannular dioxygenation of 9,10-dimethyl-1,2-benz-anthracene by cytochrome P-450 oxygenase of rat liver. *Biochem. J.*, **160**, 805–8.

Chien, M. & Flesher, J. W. (1981). Binding of the carcinogens 5-fluoro-7-hydroxy-methyl-12-methylbenz[a]anthracene and its acetate ester to DNA *in vitro*. *Life Sciences*, **28**, 1175–81.

Chiu, P. L., Fu, P. P. & Yang, S. K. (1982). Effect of a *peri* fluoro substituent on the conformation of dihydrodiol derivatives of polycyclic aromatic hydrocarbons. *Biochem. Biophys. Res. Commun.*, **106**, 1405–11.

Chiu, P. L., Fu, P. P. & Yang, S. K. (1984). Stereoselectivity of rat liver microsomal enzymes in the metabolism of 7-fluorobenz[a]anthracene and mutagenicity of metabolites. *Cancer Res.*, **44**, 562–70.

Cho-Chung, Y. S., Clair, T. & Shepheard, C. (1983). Anticarcinogenic effect of N^6,O^2-dibutyl cyclic adenosine 3',5'-monophosphate on 7,12-dimethylbenz[a]anthracene mammary tumour induction in the rat and its relationship to cyclic adenosine 3',5'-monophosphate metabolism and protein kinase. *Cancer Res.*, **43**, 2736–40.

Chou, M. W. & Yang, S. K. (1978). Identification of four *trans*-3,4-dihydrodiol metabolites of 7,12-dimethylbenz[a]anthracene and their *in vitro* DNA binding activities upon further metabolism. *Proc. Nat. Acad. Sci. U.S.A.*, **75**, 5466–70.

Chou, M. W., Easton, G. D. & Yang, S. K. (1979a). Metabolism of 7,12-dimethyl-benz[a]anthracene and its methyl-hydroxylated metabolites: formation of phenolic metabolites at the 2-positions. *Biochem. Biophys. Res. Commun.*, **88**, 1085–91.

Chou, M. W. & Yang, S. K. (1979b). Combined reverse-phase and normal-phase high performance liquid chromatography in the purification of 7,12-dimethyl-benz[a]anthracene metabolites. *J. Chromatography*, **185**, 635–54.

Chou, M. W., Yang, S. K., Sydor, W. & Yang, C. S. (1981). Metabolism of 7,12-dimethylbenz[a]anthracene and 7-hydroxymethyl-12-methylbenz[a]anthracene by rat liver nuclei and microsomes. *Cancer Res.*, **41**, 1559–64.

Chou, M. W., Chiu, P. L., Fu, P. P. & Yang, S. K. (1983). The effect of enzyme induction on the stereoselective metabolism of optically pure (−)1R,2R- and (+)1S,2S-dihydroxy-1,2-dihydrobenz[a]anthracene to vicinal 1,2-dihydrodiol 3,4-epoxides by rat liver microsomes. *Carcinogenesis*, **4**, 629–38.

Chouroulinkov, I., Gentil, A., Tierney, B., Grover, P. L. & Sims, P. (1977). The metabolic activation of 7-methylbenz[a]anthracene in mouse skin: high tumour initiating activity of the 3,4-dihydrodiol. *Cancer Lett.*, **3**, 247–53.

Christou, M., Wilson, N. M. & Jefcoate, C. R. (1984). The role of secondary metabolism in the metabolic activation of 7,12-dimethylbenz[a]anthracene by rat liver microsomes. *Carcinogenesis*, **5**, 1239–47.

Cobb, D., Boehlert, C., Lewis, D. & Armstrong, R. N. (1983). Stereoselectivity of Isozyme C of glutathione-S-transferase toward arene and azoarene oxides. *Biochemistry*, **22**, 805–12.

Cohen, G. M., Bracken, W. M., Iyar, R. P., Berry, D. L., Selkirk, J. K. & Slaga, T. J. (1979). Anticarcinogenic effects of 2,3,7,8-tetrachlorodibenzo-*p*-dioxin on benzo[a]pyrene and 7,12-dimethylbenz[a]anthracene tumour initiation and its relationship to DNA binding. *Cancer Res.*, **39**, 4027–33.

Cook, J. W. & Kennaway, E. L. (1940). Chemical compounds as carcinogenic agents. *Am. J. Cancer*, **39**, 381–428.

Coombs, M. M., Dixon, C. & Kissonerghis, A. (1976). Evaluation of the mutagenicity of compounds of known carcinogenicity, belonging to the benz[a]anthracene, chrysene and cyclopenta[a]phenanthrene series, using Ames test. *Cancer Res.*, **36**, 4525–9.

Cooper, C. S., Hewer, A., MacNicoll, A. D., Ribeiro, O., Grover, P. L. & Sims, P. (1980a). The metabolism of the 10,11-dihydrodiol of benz[a]anthracene to a vicinal diol epoxide that is not involved in metabolic activation. *Carcinogenesis*, **1**, 937–43.

Cooper, C. S., Hewer, A., Ribeiro, O., Grover, P. L. & Sims, P. (1980b). The enzyme-catalysed conversion of a non-'bay-region' diol-epoxide of benz[a]anthracene into a glutathione conjugate. *FEBS Lett.*, **118**, 39–42.

Cooper, C. S., MacNicoll, A. D., Ribeiro, O., Gervasi, P. G., Hewer, A., Walsh C., Pal, K., Grover, P. L. & Sims, P. (1980c). The involvement of a non-'bay-region' diol epoxide in the metabolic activation of benz[a]anthracene in hamster embryo cells. *Cancer Lett.*, **9**, 53–9.

Cooper, C. S., Ribeiro, O., Farmer, P. B., Hewer, A., Walsh, C., Pal, K., Grover, P. L. & Sims, P. (1980d). The metabolic activation of benz[a]anthracene in hamster embryo cells, evidence that diol epoxides react with guanosine, deoxyguanosine and adenosine in nucleic acids. *Chem. Biol. Interact.*, **32**, 209–31.

Cooper, C. S., Ribeiro, O., Hewer, A., Walsh, C., Grover, P. L. & Sims, P. (1980e). Additional evidence for the involvement of the 3,4-diol 1,2-epoxides in the metabolic activation of 7,12-dimethylbenz[a]anthracene in mouse skin. *Chem. Biol. Interact.*, **29**, 357–67.

Cooper, C. S., Ribeiro, O., Hewer, A., Walsh, C., Pal, K., Grover, P. L. & Sims, P. (1980f). The involvement of a 'bay-region' and a non-'bay-region' diol-epoxide in the metabolic activation of benz[a]anthracene in mouse skin and in hamster embryo cells. *Carcinogenesis*, **1**, 233–43.

Cooper, C. S., Pal, K., Hewer, A., Grover, P. L. & Sims, P. (1982). The metabolism and activation of polycyclic aromatic hydrocarbons in epithelial cell aggregates and fibroblasts prepared from rat mammary tissue. *Carcinogenesis*, **3**, 203–10.

Cooper, C. S., Gerwin, B. I. & Scheiner, L. A. (1983). Sites of single strand breaks in DNA treated with a diol-epoxide of benz[a]anthracene. *Carcinogenesis*, **4**, 1645–9.

Cooper, G. M. (1982). Cellular transforming genes. *Science*, **217**, 801–6.

D'Ambrosio, S. M., Daniel, F. B., Hart, R. W., Cazer, F. D. & Witiak, D. T. (1979). DNA repair in Syrian hamster embryo cells treated with 7,12-dimethyl-benz[a]anthracene and its weakly carcinogenic 5-fluoro analog. *Cancer Lett.*, **6**, 255–61.

Daniel, F. B., Cazer, F. D., D'Ambrosio, S. M., Hart, R. W., Kim, W. H. & Witiak, D. T. (1979). Comparative metabolism and DNA binding of 7,12-dimethyl-benz[a]anthracene and its weakly carcinogenic 5-fluoro analog. *Cancer Lett.*, **6**, 263–72.

Daniel, F. B. & Joyce, N. J. (1983). DNA adduct formation by 7,12-dimethyl-benz[a]anthracene and its noncarcinogenic 2-fluoro analogue in female Sprague–Dawley rats. *J. Nat. Cancer Inst.*, **70**, 111–18.

Daniel, F. B. & Joyce, N. J. (1984). 7,12-Dimethylbenz[a]anthracene–DNA adducts in Sprague–Dawley and Long–Evans female rats: the relationship of DNA adducts to mammary cancer. *Carcinogenesis*, **5**, 1021–6.

Dao, T. L. (1964). Some considerations on molecular structures of polynuclear hydrocarbons and inhibition of adrenal necrosis in rats. *Cancer Res.*, **24**, 1238–42.

Dao, T. L. & Varela, R. M. (1966). On the mechanism of inducing protection of the adrenal cortex against injury from 7,12-dimethylbenz[a]anthracene. *Cancer Res.*, **26**, 1015–21.

Dean, J. H., Ward, E., Murray, M. J., Lauer, L. D. & House, R. V. (1985). Mechanism of dimethylbenzanthracene-induced immunotoxicity. *Clin. Physiol. Biochem.*, **3**, 98–110.

Demple, B. & Linn, S. (1982). On the recognition and cleavage mechanism of *Escherichia coli* endodeoxyribonuclease V, a possible DNA repair-enzyme. *J. Biol. Chem.*, **257**, 2848–55.

Diamond, L. (1971). Metabolism of polycyclic hydrocarbons in mammalian cell cultures. *Int. J. Cancer*, **8**, 451–62.

Diamond, L., Cherian, K., Harvey, R. G. & DiGiovanni, J. (1984). Mutagenic activity of methyl- and fluoro-substituted derivatives of polycyclic aromatic hydrocarbons in a human hepatoma (Hep G2) cell-mediated assay. *Mutation Res.*, **136**, 65–72.

Dickens, F. (1945). Studies related to the metabolism of carcinogenic hydrocarbons. *Report Br. Empire Cancer Campaign*, **22**, 55.

DiGiovanni, J., Slaga, T. J., Berry, D. L. & Juchau, M. R. (1977). Metabolism of 7,12-dimethylbenz[a]anthracene in mouse skin homogenates analysed with high-pressure liquid chromatography. *Drug Met. Dispos.*, **5**, 295–301.

DiGiovanni, J., Slaga, T. J., Viaje, A., Berry, D. L., Harvey, R. G. & Juchau, M. R. (1978). Effects of 7,8-benzoflavone on skin tumour-initiating activities of various 7- and 12- substituted derivatives of 7,12-dimethylbenz[a]anthracene in mice. *J. Nat. Cancer Inst.*, **61**, 135–40.

DiGiovanni, J., Berry, D. L., Juchau, M. R. & Slaga, T. J. (1979*a*). TCDD: potent anticarcinogenic activity in CD-1 mice. *Biochem. Biophys. Res. Commun.*, **86**, 577–84.

DiGiovanni, J., Romson, J. R., Linville, D. & Juchau, M. R. (1979*b*). Covalent binding of polycyclic aromatic hydrocarbons to adenine correlates with tumorigenesis in mouse skin. *Cancer Lett.*, **8**, 39–43.

DiGiovanni, J., Slaga, T. J. & Boutwell, R. K. (1980*a*). Comparison of the tumour initiating activity of 7,12-dimethylbenz[a]anthracene and of benzo[a]pyrene in female SENCAR and CD-1 mice. *Carcinogenesis*, **1**, 381–9.

DiGiovanni, J., Viaje, A., Fisher, S., Slaga, T. J. & Boutwell, R. K. (1980*b*). Biotransformation of 7,12-dimethylbenz[a]anthracene by mouse epidermal cells in culture. *Carcinogenesis*, **1**, 41–9.

DiGiovanni, J., Diamond, L., Singer, J. M., Daniel, F. B., Witiak, D. T. & Slaga, T. J. (1982*a*). Tumour-initiating activity of 4-fluoro-7,12-dimethylbenz[a]anthracene and 1,2,3,4-tetrahydro-7,12-dimethylbenz[a]anthracene in female SENCAR mice. *Carcinogenesis*, **3**, 651–5.

DiGiovanni, J., Rymer, J., Slaga, T. J. & Boutwell, R. K. (1982*b*). Anticarcinogenic and cocarcinogenic effects of benzo[e]pyrene and dibenz[a,c]anthracene on skin tumor initiation by polycyclic hydrocarbons. *Carcinogenesis*, **3**, 371–5.

DiGiovanni, J., Decina, P. C. & Diamond, L. (1983*a*). Tumour initiating activity of 9- and 10-fluoro-7,12-dimethylbenz[a]anthracene and the effect of 2,3,7,8-tetrachloro-dibenzo-*p*-dioxin on tumour initiation by monofluoro-derivatives of DMBA in SENCAR mice. *Carcinogenesis*, **4**, 1045–9.

DiGiovanni, J., Nebzydoski, A. P. & Decina, P. C. (1983*b*). Formation of 7-hydroxy-methyl-12-methylbenz[a]anthracene in mouse epidermis. *Cancer Res.*, **43**, 4221–6.

DiGiovanni, J., Sina, J. F., Ashurst, S. W., Singer, J. M. & Diamond, L. (1983*c*). Benzo[a]pyrene and 7,12-dimethylbenz[a]anthracene metabolism and DNA adduct formation in primary cultures of hamster epidermal cells. *Cancer Res.*, **43**, 163–70.

DiGiovanni, J., Singer, J. M. & Diamond, L. (1984). Comparison of the metabolic activation of 7,12-dimethylbenz[a]anthracene by a human hepatoma cell line (Hep G2) and low passage hamster embryo cells. *Cancer Res.*, **44**, 2878–84.

DiGiovanni, J., Fisher, E. P., Aalfs, K. K. & Krichett, W. P. (1985). Covalent binding of 7,12-dimethylbenz[a]anthracene and 10-fluoro-7,12-dimethylbenz[a]anthracene to mouse epidermal DNA and its relationship to tumour-initiating activity. *Cancer Res.*, **45**, 591–7.

Dipple, A. & Slade, T. A. (1970). Structure and activity in chemical carcinogenesis:

reactivity and carcinogenicity of 7-bromomethylbenz[a]anthracene and 7-bromomethyl-12-methylbenz[a]anthracene. *Eur. J. Cancer*, **6**, 417–23.

Dipple, A., Brookes, P., Mackintosh, P. S. & Rayman, M. P. (1971a). Reaction of 7-bromomethylbenz[a]anthracene with nucleic acids, polynucleotides and nucleosides. *Biochemistry*, **10**, 4323–30.

Dipple, A. & Slade, T. A. (1971b). Structure and activity in chemical carcinogenesis: studies of variously substituted 7-bromomethylbenz[a]anthracenes. *Eur. J. Cancer*, **7**, 473–6.

Dipple, A. & Roberts, J. J. (1977). Excision of 7-bromomethylbenz[a]anthracene–DNA adducts in replicating mammalian cells. *Biochemistry*, **16**, 1499–503.

Dipple, A. & Nebzydoski, J. A. (1978). Evidence for the involvement of a diol-epoxide in the binding of 7,12-dimethylbenz[a]anthracene to DNA in cells in culture. *Chem. Biol. Interact.*, **20**, 17–26.

Dipple, A. & Hayes, M. E. (1979a). Differential excision of carcinogenic hydrocarbon–DNA adducts in mouse embryo cell cultures. *Biochem. Biophys. Res. Commun.*, **91**, 1225–31.

Dipple, A., Tomaszewski, J. E., Moschel, R. C., Bigger, C. A. H., Nebzydoski, J. A. & Egan, M. (1979b). Comparison of metabolism-mediated binding to DNA of 7-hydroxymethyl-12-methylbenz[a]anthracene and 7,12-dimethylbenz[a]anthracene. *Cancer Res.*, **39**, 1154–8.

Dipple, A., Levy, L. S. & Lawley, P. D. (1981). Comparative carcinogenicity of alkylating agents: comparisons of a series of alkyl and aryl bromides of differing chemical reactivities as inducers of sarcoma at the site of a single injection in the rat. *Carcinogenesis*, **2**, 103–7.

Dipple, A., Pigott, M., Moschel, R. C. & Constantino, N. (1983). Evidence that binding of 7,12-dimethylbenz[a]anthracene to DNA in mouse embryo cell cultures results in extensive substitution of both adenine and guanine residues. *Cancer Res.*, **43**, 4132–5.

Dipple, A., Moschel, R. C. & Bigger, C. A. H. (1984a). Polynuclear aromatic carcinogens. In: *Chemical Carcinogens*, vol. 1, ed. C. E. Searle, pp. 41–126. Washington, D.C.: American Chemical Society.

Dipple, A., Pigott, M. A., Bigger, C. A. H. & Blake, D. M. (1984b). 7,12-Dimethyl benz[a]anthracene–DNA binding in mouse skin: response of different mouse strains and effects of various modifiers of carcinogenesis. *Carcinogenesis*, **5**, 1087–90.

Dipple, A., Moschel, R. C., Pigott, M. A. & Tondeur, Y. (1985). Acid lability of the hydrocarbon–deoxyribonucleoside linkages in 7,12-dimethylbenz[a]anthracene-modified deoxyribonucleic acid. *Biochemistry*, **24**, 2291–8.

Dunlap, C. E. & Warren, S. (1946). The carcinogenic activity of some new derivatives of aromatic hydrocarbons. *Cancer Res.*, **6**, 454–65.

Dunning, W. F. & Curtis, M. R. (1960). Relative carcinogenic activity of monomethyl derivatives of benz[a]anthracene in Fischer Line 344 rats. *J. Nat. Cancer Inst.*, **25**, 387–91.

Dunning, W. F., Curtis, M. R. & Stevens, M. (1968). Comparative carcinogenic activity of dimethyl and trimethyl derivatives of benz[a]anthracene in Fischer Line 344 rats. *Proc. Soc. Exp. Biol. Med.*, **128**, 720–2.

Elegbede, J. A., Elson, C. E., Qureshi, A., Tanner, M. A. & Gould, M. N. (1984). Inhibition of DMBA-induced mammary cancer by the monoterpene d-limonene. *Carcinogenesis*, **5**, 661–4.

Engelbreth-Holm, J. & Lefevre, H. (1941). Acceleration of the development of leukemias and mammary carcinomas in mice by 9,10-dimethyl-1,2-benzanthracene. *Cancer Res.*, **1**, 102–8.

Fahmy, O. G. & Fahmy, M. J. (1970). Genetic deletions at specific loci by polycyclic hydrocarbons in relation to carcinogenesis. *Int. J. Cancer*, **6**, 250–60.

194   *Biology*

Fahmy, O. G. & Fahmy, M. J. (1973). Oxidative activation of benz[a]anthracene and methylated derivatives in mutagenesis and carcinogenesis. *Cancer Res.*, **33**, 2354–61.

Fahmy, M. J. & Fahmy, O. G. (1980). Intervening DNA insertions and the alteration of gene expression by carcinogens. *Cancer Res.*, **40**, 3374–82.

Fieser, L. F. & Newman, M. S. (1936). The synthesis of 1,2-benzanthracene derivatives related to cholanthrene. *J. Am. Chem. Soc.*, **58**, 2376–82.

Fieser, L. F. (1938). Carcinogenic activity, structure, and chemical reactivity of polynuclear aromatic hydrocarbons. *Am. J. Cancer*, **34**, 37–124.

Flesher, J. W., Soedigdo, S. & Kelley, D. R. (1967). Synthesis of metabolites of 7,12-dimethylbenz[a]anthracene: 4-hydroxy-7,12-dimethylbenz[a]anthracene, 7-hydroxymethyl-12-methylbenz[a]anthracene, their methyl ethers and acetoxy derivatives. *J. Med. Chem.*, **10**, 932–6.

Flesher, J. W. & Sydnor, K. (1971). Carcinogenicity of derivatives of 7,12-dimethylbenz[a]anthracene. *Cancer Res.*, **31**, 1951–4.

Flesher, J. W., Harvey, R. G. & Sydnor, K. L. (1976). Oncogenicity of K-region epoxides of benzo[a]pyrene and 7,12-dimethylbenz[a]anthracene. *Int. J. Cancer*, **18**, 351–3.

Flesher, J. W., Myers, S. R. & Blake, J. W. (1984). Biosynthesis of the potent carcinogen 7,12-dimethylbenz[a]anthracene. *Cancer Lett.*, **24**, 335–43.

Flesher, J. W. & Myers, S. R. (1985). Oxidative metabolism of 7-methylbenz[a]anthracene, 12-methylbenz[a]anthracene and 7,12-dimethylbenz[a]anthracene by rat liver cytosol. *Cancer Lett.*, **26**, 83–8.

Ford, E. & Huggins, C. (1963). Selective destruction in testis induced by 7,12-dimethylbenz[a]anthracene. *J. Exp. Med.*, **118**, 27–40.

Frenkel, K., Grunberger, D., Kasai, H., Komura, H. & Nakanishi, K. (1981). Identification of novel 7,12-dimethylbenz[a]anthracene adducts in cellular ribonucleic acid. *Biochemistry*, **20**, 4377–81.

Friedewald, W. F. & Rous, P. (1944). The initiating and promoting elements in tumour production. *J. Exp. Med.*, **80**, 101–44.

Fu, P. P., Chou, M. W. & Yang, S. K. (1982). *In vitro* metabolism of 12-methylbenz[a]anthracene: effect of the methyl group on the stereochemistry of a 5,6-dihydrodiol metabolite. *Biochem. Biophys. Res. Commun.*, **106**, 940–6.

Fu, P. P. & Yang, S. K. (1983a). Stereoselective metabolism of 7-bromobenz[a]anthracene by rat liver microsomes: absolute configurations of *trans*-dihydrodiol metabolites. *Carcinogenesis*, **4**, 979–84.

Fu, P. P. & Yang, S. K. (1983b). Stereoselective metabolism of 7-nitrobenz[a]anthracene to 3,4- and 8,9- *trans*-dihydrodiols. *Biochem. Biophys. Res. Commun.*, **115**, 123–9.

Fujimori, E. (1982). Covalent binding of photo-oxidized benz[a]anthracene and related carcinogenic hydrocarbons to protein. *Cancer Lett.*, **16**, 219–25.

Furstenberger, G., Kinzel, V., Schwarz, M. & Marks, F. (1985). Partial inversion of the initiation–promotion sequence of multistage tumorigenesis in the skin of NMRI mice. *Science*, **230**, 76–8.

Gentil, A., Lasne, C. & Chouroulinkov, I. (1974). Metabolism of 7,12-dimethylbenz[a]anthracene by hamster liver homogenates. *Xenobiotica*, **4**, 537–48.

Gentil, A., Lasne, C. & Chouroulinkov, I. (1977). Metabolism and cytotoxicity of 7,12-dimethylbenz[a]anthracene by hamster, rat and rabbit embryo cell cultures. *Xenobiotica*, **7**, 221–33.

Glatt, H., Vogel, K., Bentley, P., Sims, P. & Oesch, F. (1981). Large differences in metabolic activation and inactivation of chemically closely related compounds: effects of pure enzymes and enzyme induction on the mutagenicity of the twelve monomethylated benz[a]anthracenes, 7,12-dimethylbenz[a]anthracene and benz[a]anthracene in the Ames test. *Carcinogenesis*, **2**, 813–21.

Glatt, H. R., Cooper, C. S., Grover, P. L., Sims, P., Bentley, P., Merdes, M., Waechter, F., Vogel, K., Guenthner, T. M. & Oesch, F. (1982). Inactivation of a diol epoxide by dihydrodiol dehydrogenase, but not by two epoxide hydrolases. *Science*, **215**, 1507–9.

Glatt, H., Friedberg, T., Grover, P. L., Sims, P. & Oesch, F. (1983). Inactivation of a diol-epoxide and a K-region epoxide with high efficiency by glutathione transferase X. *Cancer Res.*, **43**, 5713–17.

Goerttler, K., Loehrke, H., Schweizer, J. & Hesse, B. (1979). Systemic 2-stage carcinogenesis in female Sprague–Dawley rats using DMBA as initiator and TPA as promoter. *Cancer Res.*, **39**, 1293–7.

Goerttler, K., Loehrke, H. & Hesse, B. (1980a). Two-stage carcinogenesis on NMRI mice. *Carcinogenesis*, **1**, 707–13.

Goerttler, K., Loehrke, H., Schweizer, J. & Hesse, B. (1980b). Two-stage tumourigenesis of dermal melanocytes in the back skin of the Syrian golden hamster. *Cancer Res.*, **40**, 155–61.

Goerttler, K., Loehrke, H., Schweizer, J. & Hesse, B. (1980c). Two-stage skin carcinogenesis by systemic initiation of pregnant mice with 7,12-DMBA. *J. Cancer Res. Clin. Oncol.*, **98**, 267–75.

Goerttler, K., Loehrke, H., Hesse, B., Milz, A. & Schweizer, J. (1981). Displacental initiation of NMRI mice with 7,12-dimethylbenz[a]anthracene during gestation days 6-20 and postnatal treatment of the F1-generation with the phorbol ester 12-O-tetradecanoylphorbol-13-acetate: tumour incidence in organs other than skin. *Carcinogenesis*, **2**, 1087–94.

Goerttler, K., Loehrke, H., Schweizer, J. & Hesse, B. (1982). Diterpene-ester mediated 2-stage carcinogenesis. In: *Carcinogenesis*, vol. 7, ed. E. Hecker, pp. 75–83. New York: Raven Press.

Gould, M. N. (1980). Mammary gland cell-mediated mutagenesis of mammalian cells by organ-specific carcinogens. *Cancer Res.*, **40**, 1836–41.

Gould, M. N. (1982a). Chemical carcinogen activation in the rat mammary gland: intra-organ cell specificity. *Carcinogenesis*, **3**, 667–9.

Gould, M. N., Cathers, L. E. & Moore, C. J. (1982b). Human breast cell-mediated mutagenesis of mammalian cells by polycyclic aromatic hydrocarbons. *Cancer Res.*, **42**, 4619–24.

Graem, N. (1986). Epidermal changes following application of 7,12-dimethyl-benz[a]anthracene and 12-O-tetradecanoylphorbol-13-acetate to human skin transplanted to nude mice studied with histological species markers. *Cancer Res.*, **46**, 278–84.

Gray, G. E., Pike, M. C. & Henderson, B. E. (1979). Breast cancer incidence and mortality rates in different countries in relation to known risk factors and dietary practices. *Br. J. Cancer*, **39**, 1–7.

Grover, P. L., Hewer, A. & Sims, P. (1971). Epoxides as microsomal metabolites of polycyclic hydrocarbons. *FEBS Lett.*, **18**, 76–80.

Grover, P. L., Hewer, A. & Sims, P. (1973). Metabolism of polycyclic hydrocarbons in rat-lung preparations. *Biochem. Pharmacol.*, **23**, 323–32.

Grover, P. L., MacNicoll, A. D., Sims, P., Easty, G. C. & Neville, A. M. (1980). Polycyclic hydrocarbon activation and metabolism in epithelial cell aggregates prepared from human mammary tissues. *Int. J. Cancer*, **26**, 467–75.

Grubbs, C. J. & Wood, J. L. (1976). The binding of benz[a]anthracene derivatives to glyceraldehyde-3-phosphate dehydrogenase and mammary tissue following exposure to laboratory light. *Chem. Biol. Interact.*, **12**, 135–44.

Guenthner, T. M., Nebert, D. W. & Menard, R. H. (1979). Microsomal arylhydrocarbon hydroxylase in rat adrenal regulation by ACTH but not by polycyclic hydrocarbons. *Molec. Pharmacol.*, **15**, 719–28.

Gupta, R. C. (1985). Enhanced sensitivity of ^{32}P-postlabelling analysis of aromatic carcinogen:DNA adducts. *Cancer Res.*, **45**, 5656–62.

Harris, C. C., Autrup, H., Stoner, G., Yang, S. K., Leutz, J. C., Gelboin, H. V., Selkirk, K. J., Conner, R. J., Barrett, L. A., Jones, R. T., McDowell, E. & Trump, B. F. (1977). Metabolism of benzo[a]pyrene and 7,12-dimethylbenz[a]anthracene in cultured human bronchus and pancreatic duct. *Cancer Res*, **37**, 3349–55.

Hartwell, J. L. (1951). Survey of compounds which have been tested for carcinogenic activity. *U.S. Public Health Service*, Bethesda, Md.

Harvey, R. G. & Dunne, F. B. (1978). Multiple regions of metabolic activation of carcinogenic hydrocarbons. *Nature*, **273**, 566–8.

Heidelberger, C., Baumann, M. E., Griesbach, L., Ghobar, A. & Vaughan, T. M. (1962). The carcinogenic activities of various derivatives of dibenzanthracene. *Cancer Res.*, **22**, 78–83.

Hemminki, K., Cooper, C. S., Ribeiro, O., Grover, P. L. & Sims, P. (1980). Reactions of 'bay-region' and non-'bay-region' diol-epoxides of benz[a]anthracene with DNA: evidence indicating that the major products are hydrocarbon-N_2-guanine adducts. *Carcinogenesis*, **1**, 277–86.

Hems, G. (1978). The contributions of diet and childbearing to breast cancer rates. *Br. J. Cancer*, **37**, 974–82.

Hewer, A., Phillips, D. H., Hodgson, R. M. & Grover, P. L. (1984). Microsome mediated reactions of phenols of polycyclic hydrocarbons with DNA. *Cancer Lett.*, **22**, 321–8.

Hieger, I. (1930). The spectra of cancer-producing tars and oils and of related substances. *Biochem. J.*, **24**, 505–11.

Hollstein, M., McCann, J., Angelosanto, F. A. & Nichols, W. W. (1979). Short term tests for carcinogens and mutagens. *Mutation Res.*, **65**, 133–226.

Huang, M. T., Wood, A. W., Newmark, H. L., Sayer, J. M., Yagi, H., Jerina, D. M. & Conney, A. H. (1983). Inhibition of the mutagenicity of bay region diol epoxides of polycyclic aromatic hydrocarbons by phenolic plant flavanoids. *Carcinogenesis*, **4**, 1631–8.

Huang, F. L., Hasuma, T. & Cho-Chung, Y. S. (1984). Relationship between the anticarcinogenic effect of $N^6, O^{2'}$-dibutyl cyclic adenosine $3', 5'$-monophosphate and modulation of gene expression and inhibition of binding of 7,12-dimethyl-benz[a]anthracene to DNA of mammary cells. *Cancer Res.*, **44**, 1595–9.

Huberman, E., Aspiras, L., Heidelberger, C., Grover, P. L. & Sims, P. (1971). Mutagenicity to mammalian cells of epoxides and other derivatives of polycyclic hydrocarbons. *Proc. Nat. Acad. Sci. U.S.A.*, **68**, 3195–9.

Huberman, E. & Sachs, L. (1976). Mutability of different genetic loci in mammalian cells by metabolically activated carcinogenic polycyclic hydrocarbons. *Proc. Nat. Acad. Sci. U.S.A.*, **73**, 188–92.

Huberman, E., Chou, M. W. & Yang, S. K. (1979a). Identification of 7,12-dimethyl-benz[a]anthracene metabolites that lead to mutagenesis in mammalian cells. *Proc. Nat. Acad. Sci. U.S.A.*, **76**, 862–6.

Huberman, E. & Slaga, T. J. (1979b). Mutagenicity and tumour-initiating activity of fluorinated derivatives of 7,12-dimethylbenz[a]anthracene. *Cancer Res.*, **39**, 411–14.

Huggins, C. & Morii, S. (1961). Selective adrenal necrosis and apoplexy induced by 7,12-dimethylbenz[a]anthracene. *J. Exp. Med.*, **114**, 741–60.

Huggins, C. & Fukunishi, R. (1964a). Induced protection of adrenal cortex against 7,12-dimethylbenz[a]anthracene. *J. Exp. Med.*, **119**, 923–30.

Huggins, C., Grand, L. & Fukunishi, R. (1964b). Aromatic influences on the yields of mammary cancers following administration of 7,12-dimethylbenz[a]anthracene. *Proc. Nat. Acad. Sci. U.S.A.*, **51**, 737–42.

Huggins, C., Pataki, J. & Harvey, R. G. (1967). Geometry of carcinogenic polycyclic aromatic hydrocarbons. *Proc. Nat. Acad. Sci. U.S.A.*, **58**, 2253–60.

Huggins, C., Grand, L. & Oka, H. (1970). Hundred day leukaemia: preferential induction in rat by pulse doses of 7,8,12-TMBA. *J. Exp. Med.*, **131**, 321–9.

Huggins, C. H. (1979). *Experimental Leukemia and Mammary Cancer*. Chicago: The University of Chicago Press.

Iball, J. (1939). The relative potency of carcinogenic compounds. *Am. J. Cancer*, **35**, 188–90.

Inbasekaran, M. N., Witiak, D. T., Barone, K. & Loper, J. C. (1980). Synthesis and mutagenicity of A-ring reduced analogues of 7,12-dimethylbenz[a]anthracene. *J. Med. Chem.*, **23**, 278–81.

Indo, K. & Miyaji, H. (1985). Malignant transformation of a cloned, nontumorigenic mouse epidermal keratinocyte cell line MSK-C3H-NU, by 7,12-dimethyl-benz[a]anthracene. *Cancer Res.*, **45**, 774–82.

Ip, C., Yip, P. & Bernardis, L. L. (1980). Role of prolactin in the promotion of dimethyl-benz[a]anthracene-induced mammary tumours by dietary fat. *Cancer Res.*, **40**, 374–8.

Ivanovic, V., Geacintov, N. E., Jeffrey, A. M., Fu, P. P., Harvey, R. G. & Weinstein, I. B. (1978). Cell and microsome mediated binding of 7,12-dimethylbenz[a]anthracene to DNA studied by fluorescence spectroscopy. *Cancer Lett.*, **4**, 131–40.

Jabara, A. G. & Harcourt, A. G. (1971). Effects of progesterone, ovariectomy and adrenalectomy on mammary tumours induced by 7,12-dimethylbenz[a]anthracene in Sprague–Dawley rats. *Pathology*, **3**, 209–14.

Jacob, J., Schmoldt, A. & Grimmer, G. (1981). Time course of oxidative benz[a]anthracene metabolism by liver microsomes of normal and PCB-treated rats. *Carcinogenesis*, **2**, 395–401.

Jakoby, W. B. & Habig, W. H. (1980). *Enzymic Basis of Detoxification*, Vol. II, pp. 63–94. New York: Academic Press.

Janisch, W. (1966). The induction of experimental brain tumours with carcinogenic hydrocarbons. *Z. Krebsforsch.*, **68**, 224–33.

Janss, D. H., Moon, R. C. & Irving, C. C. (1972). The binding of 7,12-dimethyl-benz[a]anthracene to mammary parenchyma DNA and protein *in vivo*. *Cancer Res.*, **32**, 254–8.

Janss, D. H. & Ben, T. L. (1978). Age related modification of 7,12-dimethyl-benz[a]anthracene binding to rat mammary gland DNA. *J. Nat. Cancer Inst.*, **60**, 173–7.

Jeffrey, A. M., Blobstein, S. H., Weinstein, I. B. & Harvey, R. G. (1976a). High pressure liquid chromatography of carcinogen–nucleoside conjugates: separation of 7,12-dimethylbenzanthracene derivatives. *Anal. Biochem.*, **73**, 378–85.

Jeffrey, A. M., Blobstein, S. H., Weinstein, I. B., Beland, F. A., Harvey, R. G., Kasai, H. & Nakanishi, K. (1976b). Structure of 7,12-dimethylbenz[a]anthracene–guanosine adducts. *Proc. Nat. Acad. Sci. U.S.A.*, **73**, 2311–15.

Jellinck, P. H. & Gondy, B. (1966). Protective action of polycyclic hydrocarbons against induction of adrenal necrosis by dimethylbenz[a]anthracene. *Science*, **152**, 1375–6.

Jellinck, P. H., Coles, S. & Garland, M. (1967). Comparative metabolism of dimethyl-benzanthracene-12-^{14}C *in vitro*. *Biochem. Pharmacol.*, **16**, 2449–51.

Jerina, D. M. & Daly, J. W. (1974). Arene oxides: a new aspect of drug metabolism. *Science*, **185**, 573–82.

Jerina, D. M. & Lehr, R. E. (1978). The bay-region theory: a quantum mechanical approach to aromatic hydrocarbon-induced carcinogenicity. In *Microsomes and Drug Oxidations*, ed. V. Ullrich, A. Roots, A. Hildebrandt & R. W. Estabrook, pp. 709–20. New York: Pergamon Press.

Joyce, N. J. & Daniel, F. B. (1982). 7,12-Dimethylbenz[a]anthracene–deoxyribonucleoside adduct formation *in vivo*: evidence for the formation and binding of a mono-hydroxymethyl-DMBA metabolite to rat liver DNA. *Carcinogenesis*, **3**, 297–301.

Jungmann, R. A. & Schweppe, J. S. (1972). Binding of chemical carcinogens to nuclear proteins of rat liver. *Cancer Res.*, **32**, 952–9.

Kaden, D. A., Hites, R. A. & Thilly, W. G. (1979). Mutagenicity of soot and associated polycyclic aromatic hydrocarbons to *Salmonella typhimurium*. *Cancer Res.*, **39**, 4152–9.

Kapitulnik, J., Levin, W., Yagi, H., Jerina, D. M. & Conney, A. H. (1976). Lack of carcinogenicity of 4-, 5-, 6-, 7-, 8-, 9- and 10-hydroxybenzo[a]pyrene on mouse skin. *Cancer Res.*, **36**, 3625–8.

Kasai, H., Nakanishi, K., Frenkel, K. & Grunberger, D. (1977). Structures of 7,12-dimethylbenz[a]anthracene 5,6-oxide derivatives linked to the ribose moiety of guanosine. *J. Am. Chem. Soc.*, **99**, 8500–2.

Kellen, J. A. (1973). Suppression of DMBA-tumour induction in rat mammary glands by pregnancy or chlorotrianisene. *Z. Krebsforsch.*, **79**, 75–7.

Kennaway, E. L. (1930). Further experiments on cancer producing substances. *Biochem. J.*, **24**, 497–504.

Keysell, G. R., Booth, J., Grover, P. L., Hewer, A. & Sims, P. (1973). The formation of 'K-region' epoxides as hepatic microsomal metabolites of 7-methylbenz[a]anthracene and 7,12-dimethylbenz[a]anthracene and their 7-hydroxymethyl derivatives. *Biochem. Pharmacol.*, **22**, 2853–67.

Kinoshita, N. & Gelboin, H. V. (1972). The role of arylhydrocarbon hydroxylase in 7,12-dimethylbenz[a]anthracene skin tumorigenesis: on the mechanism of 7,8-benzoflavone inhibition of tumorigenesis. *Cancer Res.*, **32**, 1329–39.

Klein, M. (1952). The action of methylcholanthrene, croton oil and 1,2-benzanthracene in the induction of skin tumors in strain DBA mice. *Cancer Res.*, **12**, 735–42.

Klurfeld, D. M., Weber, M. M. & Kritchevsky, D. (1984). Comparison of dietary carbohydrates for promotion of DMBA-induced mammary tumorigenesis in rats. *Carcinogenesis*, **5**, 423–5.

Kootstra, A., MacLeod, M. C., Iyer, R., Selkirk, J. K. & Slaga, T. J. (1982). Selective modification of nuclear proteins by polycyclic aromatic hydrocarbons and by benzo[a]pyrene diol epoxides. *Carcinogenesis*, **3**, 821–4.

Kuroki, T. & Heidelberger, C. (1971). The binding of polycyclic aromatic hydrocarbons to the DNA, RNA and proteins of transformable cells in culture. *Cancer Res.*, **31**, 2168–76.

Land, H., Parada, L. F. & Weinberg, R. A. (1983). Cellular oncogenes and multistep carcinogenesis. *Science*, **222**, 771–8.

Langenbach, R., Nesnow, S., Tompa, A., Gingell, R. & Kuszynski, C. (1981). Lung and liver cell-mediated mutagenesis systems: specificities in the activation of chemical carcinogens. *Carcinogenesis*, **2**, 851–8.

Lawley, P. D. (1966). Effects of some chemical mutagens and carcinogens on nucleic acids. *Prog. Nucleic Acid Res. Molec. Biol.*, **5**, 89–131.

Lee, J. P., Suzuki, K., Muktar, H. & Bend, J. R. (1980). Hormonal regulation of cytochrome P-450-dependent monooxygenases activity and epoxide metabolizing enzyme activities in testis of hypophysectomized rats. *Cancer Res.*, **40**, 2486–92.

Lesca, P. (1981). Influence of the rate of 7,12-dimethylbenz[a]anthracene metabolic activation, *in vivo*, on its binding to epidermal DNA and skin carcinogenesis. *Carcinogenesis*, **2**, 199–204.

Levin, W. & Conney, A. H. (1967). Stimulatory effect of polycyclic hydrocarbons and aromatic azo derivatives on the metabolism of 7,12-dimethylbenz[a]anthracene. *Cancer Res.*, **27**, 1931–8.

Levin, W., Thakker, D. R., Wood, A. W., Chang, R. L., Lehr, R. E., Jerina, D. M. & Conney, A. H. (1978). Evidence that benz[a]anthracene 3,4-diol 1,2-epoxide is an ultimate carcinogen on mouse skin. *Cancer Res.*, **38**, 1705–10.

Levin, W., Wood, A. W., Chang, R. L., Newman, M. S., Thakker, D. R., Conney, A. H. & Jerina, D. M. (1983). The effect of steric strain in the bay-region of polycyclic aromatic hydrocarbons: Tumourgenicity of alkyl-substituted benz[a]anthracenes. *Cancer Lett.*, **20**, 139–46.

Levin, W., Chang, R. L., Wood, A. W., Yagi, H., Thakker, D. R., Jerina, D. M. & Conney, A. H. (1984). High stereoselectivity among the optical isomers of the diastereomeric bay-region diol-epoxides of benz[a]anthracene in the expression of tumorigenic activity in murine tumor models. *Cancer Res.*, **44**, 929–33.

Levy, B. M., Gorlin, R. & Gottsegen, R. (1951). Histology of early reactions of skin and mucous membrane of the lip of the mouse to a single application of a carcinogen. *J. Nat. Cancer Inst.*, **12**, 275–8.

Lieberman, M. W. & Dipple, A. (1972). Removal of bound carcinogen during DNA repair in nondividing human lymphocytes. *Cancer Res.*, **32**, 1855–60.

Lijinsky, W., Manning, W. & Andrews, A. (1983). Skin carcinogenesis tests in mice of derivatives of 7,12-dimethylbenz[a]anthracene substituted in the 'A' ring. *Carcinogenesis*, **4**, 1221–4.

MacNicoll, A. D., Burden, P. M., Ribeiro, O., Hewer, A., Grover, P. L. & Sims, P. (1979a). The formation of dihydrodiols by the chemical or enzymic oxidation of 7-hydroxymethyl-12-methylbenz[a]anthracene and the possible role of hydroxymethyl dihydrodiols in the metabolic activation of 7,12-dimethylbenz[a]anthracene. *Chem. Biol. Interact.*, **26**, 121–32.

MacNicoll, A. D., Cooper, C. S., Ribeiro, O., Gervasi, P. G., Hewer, A., Walsh, C., Grover, P. L. & Sims, P. (1979b). The involvement of a non-bay-region diol-epoxide in the formation of benz[a]anthracene–DNA adducts in a rat-liver microsomal system. *Biochem. Biophys. Res. Commun.*, **91**, 490–7.

MacNicoll, A. D., Easty, G. C., Neville, A. M., Grover, P. L. & Sims, P. (1980a). Metabolism and activation of carcinogenic polycyclic hydrocarbons by human mammary cells. *Biochem. Biophys. Res. Commun.*, **95**, 1599–606.

MacNicoll, A. D., Grover, P. L. & Sims, P. (1980b). The metabolism of a series of polycyclic hydrocarbons by mouse skin maintained in short-term organ culture. *Chem. Biol. Interact.*, **29**, 169–88.

MacNicoll, A. D., Cooper, C. S., Ribeiro, O., Pal, K., Hewer, A., Grover, P. L. & Sims, P. (1981). The metabolic activation of benz[a]anthracene in three biological systems. *Cancer Lett.*, **11**, 243–9.

Malaveille, C., Bartsch, H., Grover, P. L. & Sims, P. (1975). Mutagenicity of non-K-region diols and diol-epoxides of benz[a]anthracene and benzo[a]pyrene. *Biochem. Biophys. Res. Commun.*, **66**, 693–700.

Malaveille, C., Tierney, B., Grover, P. L., Sims, P. & Bartsch, H. (1977). High microsome-mediated mutagenicity of the 3,4-dihydrodiol of 7-methylbenz[a]anthracene in *S. typhimurium* TA98. *Biochem. Biophys. Res. Commun.*, **75**, 427–33.

Malaveille, C., Bartsch, H., Tierney, B., Grover, P. L. & Sims, P. (1978). Microsome-mediated mutagenicities of the dihydrodiols of 7,12-dimethylbenz[a]anthracene: high mutagenic activity of the 3,4-dihydrodiol. *Biochem. Biophys. Res. Commun.*, **83**, 1468–73.

Mankowitz, L., Montelius, J. & Rydstrom, J. (1981). Demonstration and partial characterization of a 7,12-dimethylbenz[a]anthracene binding protein in rat adrenal. *Chem. Biol. Interact.*, **37**, 55–65.

Marquardt, E. H., Sternberg, S. S. & Philips, F. S. (1970). 7,12-Dimethyl-benz[a]anthracene and hepatic neoplasia in regenerating rat liver. *Chem. Biol. Interact.*, **2**, 401–3.

Marquardt, H., Kuroki, T., Huberman, E., Selkirk, J. K., Heidelberger, C., Grover, P. L. & Sims, P. (1972). Malignant transformation of cells derived from mouse prostate by epoxides and other derivatives of polycyclic hydrocarbons. *Cancer Res.*, **32**, 716–20.

Marquardt, H., Sodergren, J. E., Sims, P. & Grover, P. L. (1974). Malignant transformation *in vitro* of mouse fibroblasts by 7,12-dimethylbenz[a]anthracene and by their K-region derivatives. *Int. J. Cancer.*, **13**, 304–10.

Marquardt, H., Grover, P. L. & Sims, P. (1976). *In vitro* malignant transformation of mouse fibroblasts by non-K-region dihydrodiols derived from 7-methyl-benz[a]anthracene, 7,12-dimethylbenz[a]anthracene and benzo[a]pyrene. *Cancer Res.*, **36**, 2059–64.

Marquardt, H., Baker, S., Tierney, B., Grover, P. L. & Sims, P. (1977). The metabolic activation of 7-methylbenz[a]anthracene: the induction of malignant transformation and mutation in mammalian cells by non-K-region dihydrodiols. *Int. J. Cancer.*, **19**, 828–33.

Marquardt, H., Baker, S., Tierney, B., Grover, P. L. & Sims, P. (1978). Induction of malignant transformation and mutagenesis by dihydrodiols derived from 7,12-dimethyl-benz[a]anthracene. *Biochem. Biophys. Res. Commun.*, **85**, 357–62.

Marquardt, H. (1979a). DNA – the critical target in carcinogenesis? In *Chemical Carcinogens and DNA*, Vol. 2, ed. P. L. Grover, pp. 159–79. CRC Press, Inc.: Boca Raton, Florida, USA.

Marquardt, H., Baker, S., Tierney, B., Grover, P. L. & Sims, P. (1979b). Comparison of mutagenesis and malignant transformation by dihydrodiols from benz[a]anthracene and 7,12-dimethylbenz[a]anthracene. *Br. J. Cancer*, **39**, 540–7.

Marshall, C. J., Vonsden, K. H. & Phillips, D. H. (1984). Activation of c-Ha-*ras*-1 proto-oncogene by *in vitro* modification with a chemical carcinogen, benzo[a]pyrene diol-epoxide. *Nature*, **310**, 586–9.

McCann, J., Choi, E., Yamasaki, E. & Ames, B. N. (1975). Detection of carcinogens as mutagens in the Salmonella/microsome test: Assay of 300 chemicals. *Proc. Nat. Acad. Sci. U.S.A.*, **72**, 5135–9.

McCaw, B. A., Dipple, A., Young, S. & Roberts, J. J. (1978). Excision of hydrocarbon–DNA adducts and consequent cell survival in normal and repair defective human cells. *Chem. Biol. Interact.*, **22**, 139–51.

McCormick, D. L., Major, N. & Moon, R. C. (1984). Inhibition of 7,12-dimethyl-benz[a]anthracene-induced rat mammary carcinogenesis by concomitant or post-carcinogen antioxidant exposure. *Cancer Res.*, **44**, 2858–63.

Medina, D. & Warner, M. R. (1976). Mammary tumorigenesis in chemical carcinogen treated mice. *J. Nat. Cancer Inst.*, **57**, 331–7.

Meites, J. (1972). Relation of prolactin and estrogen to mammary tumorigenesis in the rat. *J. Nat. Cancer Inst.*, **48**, 1217–24.

Miller, E. C. & Miller, J. A. (1960). The carcinogenicity of fluoro-derivatives of 10-methyl-1,2-benzanthracene. *Cancer Res.*, **20**, 133–7.

Miller, J. A. & Miller, E. C. (1963). The carcinogenicities of fluoro-derivatives of 10-methyl-1,2-benzanthracene. *Cancer Res.*, **23**, 229–39.

Miller, E. C. & Miller, J. A. (1967). Low carcinogenicity of the K-region epoxide of 7-methylbenz[a]anthracene and benz[a]anthracene in the mouse and rat. *Proc. Soc. Exp. Biol. Med.*, **124**, 915–19.

Montelius, J., Papadopoulos, D., Bengtsson, M. & Rydstrom, J. (1982). Metabolism of polycyclic aromatic hydrocarbons and covalent binding of metabolites to protein in rat adrenal gland. *Cancer Res.*, **42**, 1479–86.

Moolten, F. R., Schreiber, B., Rizzone, A., Weiss, A. J. & Boger, E. (1981). Protection of mice against 7,12-dimethylbenz[a]anthracene-induced skin tumours by immunization with a fluorinated analog of the carcinogen. *Cancer Res.*, **41**, 425–9.

Moon, R. C., Grubbs, C. J. & Sporn, M. B. (1976). Inhibition of 7,12-dimethyl-benz[a]anthracene-induced mammary carcinogenesis by retinyl acetate. *Cancer Res.*, **36**, 2626–30.

Moore, C. J., Bachhuber, A. J. & Gould, M. N. (1983). Relationship of mammary tumour susceptibility, mammary cell-mediated mutagenesis and metabolism of polycyclic aromatic hydrocarbons in four types of rats. *J. Nat. Cancer Inst.*, **70**, 777–86.

Moore, C. J. & Gould, M. N. (1984). Differences in mediated mutagenesis and polycyclic aromatic hydrocarbon metabolism in mammary cells from pregnant and virgin rats. *Carcinogenesis*, **5**, 103–8.

Moreau, J., Matyash-Smirniaguina, L. & Scherrer, K. (1981). Systematic punctuation of eucaryotic DNA by A + T rich sequences. *Proc. Nat. Acad. Sci. U.S.A.*, **78**, 1341–5.

Morii, S. & Huggins, C. (1962). Adrenal apoplexy induced by 7,12-dimethyl-benz[a]anthracene related to corticosterone content of adrenal gland. *Endocrinology*, **71**, 972–6.

Moschel, R. C., Baird, W. M. & Dipple, A. (1977). Metabolic activation of the carcinogen 7,12-dimethylbenz[a]anthracene for DNA binding. *Biochem. Biophys. Res. Commun.*, **76**, 1092–8.

Moschel, R. C., Hudgins, W. R. & Dipple, A. (1979). Fluorescence of hydrocarbon-deoxyribonucleoside adducts. *Chem. Biol. Interact.*, **27**, 69–79.

Moschel, R. C., Pigott, M. A., Costantino, N. & Dipple, A. (1983). Chromatographic and fluorescence spectroscopic studies of individual 7,12-dimethylbenz[a]anthracene-deoxyribonucleoside adducts. *Carcinogenesis*, **4**, 1201–4.

Mottram, J. C. (1944). A developing factor in epidermal blastogenesis. *J. Path. Bacter.*, **56**, 181–7.

Mushtaq, M., Weems, H. B. & Yang, S. K. (1984). Resolution and absolute configuration of 7,12-dimethylbenz[a]anthracene 5,6-epoxide enantiomers. *Biochem. Biophys. Res. Commun.*, **125**, 539–45.

Mushtaq, M., Fu, P. P., Miller, D. W. & Yang, S. K. (1985). Metabolism of 6-methyl-benz[a]anthracene by rat liver microsomes and mutagenicity of metabolites. *Cancer Res.*, **45**, 4006–14.

Nagasawa, H. & Yanai, R. (1974). Frequency of mammary cell division in relation to age: its significance in the induction of mammary tumors by carcinogens in rats. *J. Nat. Cancer Inst.*, **52**, 609–10.

Nagasawa, H., Yanai, R. & Taniguchi, H. (1976). Importance of mammary gland DNA synthesis in carcinogen-induced tumorogenesis in rats. *Cancer Res.*, **36**, 2223–6.

Nakanishi, K., Komura, H., Miura, I., Kasai, H., Frenkel, K. & Grunberger, D. (1980). Structure of a 7,12-dimethylbenz[a]anthracene 5,6-oxide derivative bound to C-8 of guanosine. *J. Chem. Soc. Chem. Commun.*, 82–3.

Napalkov, N. P. & Alexandrov, V. A. (1974). Effect of 7,12-DMBA in transplacental carcinogenesis. *J. Nat. Cancer Inst.*, **52**, 1365–6.

Newbold, R. F. & Overall, R. W. (1983). Fibroblast immortality is a prerequisite for transformation by EJC-Ha-*ras* oncogene. *Nature*, **304**, 648–51.

Newman, M. S. & Venkateswaran, N. (1967). The synthesis of 4′-bromo-10-methyl-1,2-benz[a]anthracene and 4′-chloro-10-methyl-1,2-benz[a]anthracene. *J. Med. Chem.*, **10**, 728–9.

Newman, M. S. & Hung, W. M. (1977). Structure–carcinogenic activity relationships in the benz[a]anthracene series. 1,7,12- and 2,7,12-trimethylbenz[a]anthracenes. *J. Med. Chem.*, **20**, 179–81.

Newman, M. S., Fikes, C. E., Hashem, M. M., Kannan, R. & Sankaran, V. (1978). Synthesis and carcinogenic activity of 5-fluoro-7-(oxygenated methyl)-12-methyl-benz[a]anthracenes. *J. Med. Chem.*, **21**, 1076–8.

Newman, M. S. & Tuncay, A. (1980). Synthesis of 2-fluoro-7,12-dimethyl-benz[a]anthracene. *J. Org. Chem.*, **45**, 348–9.

Newman, M. S. (1983a). Synthesis of 7,11,12-trimethylbenz[a]anthracene. *J. Org. Chem.*, **48**, 3249–51.

Newman, M. S. & Veeraraghavan, S. (1983b). Synthesis of 9-(trifluoromethyl)- and 10-(trifluoromethyl)-7,12-DMBA. *J. Org. Chem.*, **48**, 3246–8.

Norpoth, K., Kemena, A., Jacob, J. & Schumann, C. (1984). The influence of 18 environmentally relevant polycyclic aromatic hydrocarbons and Clophen A50, as liver monooxygenase inducers, on the mutagenic activity of benz[a]anthracene in the Ames test. *Carcinogenesis*, **5**, 747–52.

Oravec, C. T., Daniel, F. B. & Wong, L. K. (1983). Comparative metabolism of 7,12-

dimethylbenz[a]anthracene and its non-carcinogenic 2-fluoro analogue by Syrian hamster embryo cells. *Cancer Lett.*, **21**, 43–55.

Pal, K., Tierney, B., Grover, P. L. & Sims, P. (1978). Induction of sister-chromatid exchanges in Chinese hamster ovary cells treated *in vitro* with non-K-region dihydrodiols of 7-methylbenz[a]anthracene and benzo[a]pyrene. *Mutation Res.*, **50**, 367–75.

Palmer, W. G., Allen, T. J. & Tomaszewski, J. E. (1978). Metabolism of 7,12-dimethyl-benz[a]anthracene by macrophages and uptake of macrophage-derived metabolites by respiratory tissues *in vitro. Cancer Res.*, **38**, 1079–84.

Pataki, J. & Huggins, C. (1969). Molecular site of substituents of benz[a]anthracene related to carcinogenicity. *Cancer Res.*, **29**, 506–9.

Pataki, J., Duguid, C., Rabideau, P. W., Huisman, H. & Harvey, R. G. (1971). Carcinogenic and adrenocorticolytic derivatives of benz[a]anthracene. *J. Med. Chem.*, **14**, 940–5.

Pataki, J. & Balick, R. (1972). Relative carcinogenicity of some diethyl-benz[a]anthracenes. *J. Med. Chem.*, **15**, 905–9.

Payne, J. F., Martins, I. & Rahimtular, A. (1978). Crankcase oils: are they a major mutagenic burden in the aquatic environment? *Science*, **200**, 329–30.

Petrilli, F. L., De Renzi, G. P. & De Flora, S. (1980). Interaction between polycyclic aromatic hydrocarbons, crude oil and oil dispersants in the *Salmonella* mutagenesis assay. *Carcinogenesis*, **1**, 51–6.

Phillips, D. H., Grover, P. L. & Sims, P. (1978). Some properties of vicinal diol-epoxides derived from benz[a]anthracene and benzo[a]pyrene. *Chem. Biol. Interact.*, **20**, 63–75.

Phillips, D. H., Grover, P. L. & Sims, P. (1979a). A quantitative determination of the covalent binding of a series of polycyclic hydrocarbons to DNA in mouse skin. *Int. J. Cancer*, **23**, 201–8.

Phillips, D. H. & Sims, P. (1979b). Polycyclic aromatic hydrocarbon metabolites: their reactions with nucleic acids. In *Chemical Carcinogens and DNA*, Vol. 2, ed. P. L. Grover, pp. 29–57. Boca Raton, Florida: CRC Press.

Pienta, R. J., Poiley, J. A. & Lebherz, W. B. (1977). Morphological transformation of early passage golden Syrian hamster embryo cells derived from cryopreserved primary cultures as a reliable *in vitro* bioassay for identifying diverse carcinogens. *Int. J. Cancer*, **19**, 642–55.

Poland, A., Glover, E. & Kende, A. S. (1976). Stereospecific, high affinity binding of TCDD, evidence that the binding species is the receptor for the induction of aryl hydrocarbon hydroxylase. *J. Biol. Chem.*, **251**, 4936–46.

Prodi, G., Rocchi, P. & Sandro, G. (1970). Binding of 7,12-dimethylbenz[a]anthracene and benzo[a]pyrene to nucleic acids and proteins of organs in rats. *Cancer Res.*, **30**, 1020–3.

Pulciani, S., Santos, E., Lauver, A., Long, L., Aaronson, S. & Barbacid, M. (1982). Oncogenes in solid human tumours. *Nature*, **300**, 539–42.

Pullman, B. & Pullman, A. (1952). *Les Théories Électroniques de la Chimie organique*, p. 588. Paris: Masson et Cie.

Randerath, E., Agrawal, H. P., Reddy, M. V. & Randerath, K. (1983). Highly persistent PAH–DNA adducts in mouse skin: detection by ^{32}P-postlabelling analysis. *Cancer Lett.*, **20**, 109–14.

Randerath, K., Agrawal, H. P. & Randerath, E. (1985a). 12-O-Tetradecanoylphorbol-13-acetate-induced rapid loss of persistent 7,12-DMBA–DNA adducts in mouse epidermis and dermis. *Cancer Lett.*, **27**, 35–43.

Randerath, E., Agrawal, H. P., Weaver, J. A., Bordelon, C. B. & Randerath, K. (1985b). ^{32}P-Postlabelling analysis of DNA adducts persisting for up to 42 weeks in the skin, epidermis and dermis of mice treated topically with 7,12-dimethyl-benz[a]anthracene. *Carcinogenesis*, **6**, 1117–26.

Rayman, M. P. & Dipple, A. (1973*a*). Structure and activity in chemical carcinogenesis. Comparison of the reactions of 7-bromomethylbenz[a]anthracene and 7-bromomethyl-12-methylbenz[a]anthracene with mouse skin deoxyribonucleic acid *in vivo*. *Biochemistry*, **12**, 1538–42.

Rayman, M. P. & Dipple, A. (1973*b*). Structure and activity in chemical carcinogenesis. Comparison of the reactions of 7-bromomethylbenz[a]anthracene and 7-bromomethyl-12-methylbenz[a]anthracene with deoxyribonucleic acid *in vitro*. *Biochemistry*, **12**, 1202–7.

Reddy, B. S., Sharma, C. & Mathews, L. (1984). Effect of Japanese seaweed (*Laminana angustata*) extracts on the mutagenicity of 7,12-dimethylbenz[a]anthracene, a breast carcinogen, and of 3,2′-dimethyl-4-aminobiphenyl, a colon and breast carcinogen. *Mutation Res.*, **127**, 113–18.

Rice, J. M., Joshi, S. R., Shenefelt, R. E. & Wenk, M. L. (1978). Transplacental carcinogenic activity of 7,12-DMBA. In: *Polynuclear Aromatic Hydrocarbons; Carcinogenesis*, vol. 3, ed. P. W. Jones & R. I. Freudenthal, pp. 413–22. New York: Raven Press.

Roe, F. J. & Salaman, M. H. (1955). Further studies on incomplete carcinogenesis: triethylene melamine, 1,2-benzanthracene and β-propiolactone, as initiators of skin tumour formation in the mouse. *Br. J. Cancer*, **9**, 117–203.

Roe, F. J., Dipple, A. & Mitchley, B. C. (1972). Carcinogenic activity of some benz[a]anthracene derivatives in newborn mice. *Br. J. Cancer*, **26**, 461–5.

Rosenkranz, H. S. & Mermelstein, R. (1983). Mutagenicity and genotoxicity of nitroarenes: all nitro-containing chemicals were not created equal. *Mutation Res.*, **114**, 217–67.

Rubin, H. (1980). Is somatic mutation the major mechanism of malignant transformation? *J. Nat. Cancer Inst.*, **64**, 995–1000.

Russo, J. & Russo, I. H. (1978). DNA labelling index and structure of the rat mammary gland as determinates of its susceptibility to carcinogenesis. *J. Nat. Cancer Inst.*, **61**, 1451–7.

Saffiotti, U. & Shubik, P. (1956). The effects of low concentrations of carcinogen in epidermal carcinogenesis. A comparison with promoting agents. *J. Nat. Cancer Inst.*, **16**, 961–9.

Sanders, C. L., Skinner, C. & Gelman, R. A. (1984). Percutaneous absorption of [7,10-^{14}C]benzo[a]pyrene and [7,12-^{14}C]dimethylbenz[a]anthracene in mice. *Environmental Res.*, **33**, 353–60.

Sawicki, J. T., Moschel, R. C. & Dipple, A. (1983). Involvement of both *Syn*- and *Anti*-dihydrodiol-epoxides in the binding of 7,12-dimethylbenz[a]anthracene to DNA in mouse embryo cell cultures. *Cancer Res.*, **43**, 3212–18.

Schweizer, J., Loehrke, H., Hesse, B. & Goerttler, K. (1982). 7,12-Dimethyl-benz[a]anthracene/12-O-tetradeconyl-phorbol-13-acetate-mediated skin tumor initiation and promotion in male Sprague–Dawley rats. *Carcinogenesis*, **3**, 785–9.

Scribner, J. D. (1973). Tumor initiation by apparently noncarcinogenic polycyclic aromatic hydrocarbons. *J. Nat. Cancer Inst.*, **50**, 1717–19.

Scribner, N. K. & Scribner, J. D. (1980). Separation of initiating and promoting effects of the skin carcinogen 7-bromomethylbenz[a]anthracene. *Carcinogenesis*, **1**, 97–100.

Scribner, J. D., Scribner, N. K., McKnight, B. & Mottet, N. K. (1983). Evidence for a new model of tumor progression from carcinogenesis and tumor promotion studies with 7-bromomethylbenz[a]anthracene. *Cancer Res.*, **43**, 2034–41.

Selenskas, S. L., Ip, M. M. & Ip, C. (1984). Similarity between *trans* fat and saturated fat in the modification of rat mammary carcinogenesis. *Cancer Res.*, **44**, 1321–6.

Shahbaz, M., Harvey, R. G., Prakash, A. S., Boal, T. R., Zegar, I. S. & LeBreton, P. R. (1983). Fluorescence and photoelectron studies of the intercalative binding of benz[a]anthracene metabolite models to DNA. *Biochem. Biophys. Res. Commun.*, **112**, 1–7.

Shear, M. J. (1938). Methyl derivatives of 1,2-benz[a]anthracene. *Am. J. Cancer*, **33**, 499–537.

Shear, M. J., Leiter, J. & Perrault, A. (1940). Studies in carcinogenesis XIV. 3-substituted and 10-substituted derivatives of 1,2-benzanthracene. *J. Nat. Cancer Inst.*, **1**, 303–36.

Shear, M. J. & Leiter, J. (1941). Studies in carcinogenesis XVI. Production of subcutaneous tumours in mice by miscellaneous polycyclic compounds. *J. Nat. Cancer Inst.*, **2**, 241–58.

Sheikh, Y. M., Hart, R. W. & Witiak, D. T. (1981). A study of steric and electronic factors governing the position of biofunctionalization of the benz[a]anthracene nucleus: metabolism *in vitro* of fluoro- and methyl- substituted analogs. *Bioorganic Chem.*, **10**, 429–42.

Shepherd, R. E. & Bryan, A. H. (1977). Metabolism of 7,12-dimethylbenz[a]anthracene (DMBA) by rat mammary cells *in vitro*. *Proc. Am. Assoc. Cancer Res. Am. Soc. Clin. Oncol.*, **18**, 210.

Shoyab, M. (1978). Dose-dependent preferential binding of polycyclic aromatic hydrocarbons to reiterated DNA of murine skin cells in culture. *Proc. Nat. Acad. Sci.*, **75**, 5841–5.

Silberman, S. & Shklar, G. (1963). The effect of a carcinogen (DMBA) applied to the hamster's buccal pouch in combination with croton oil. *Oral Surg.*, **16**, 1344–55.

Sims, P. (1967a). The metabolism of 7- and 12-methylbenz[a]anthracene and their derivatives. *Biochem. J.*, **105**, 591–8.

Sims, P. & Grover, P. L. (1967b). Variations dependent on age and diet in the metabolism of 7,12-dimethylbenz[a]anthracene by rat liver homogenates. *Nature*, **216**, 77–8.

Sims, P. & Grover, P. L. (1968). Quantitative aspects of the metabolism of 7,12-dimethyl-benz[a]anthracene by liver homogenates from animals of different age, sex and species. *Biochem. Pharmacol.*, **17**, 1751–8.

Sims, P. (1970a). Qualitative and quantitative studies on the metabolism of a series of aromatic hydrocarbons by rat liver preparations. *Biochem. Pharmacol.*, **19**, 795–818.

Sims, P. (1970b). The metabolism of some aromatic hydrocarbons by mouse embryo cell cultures. *Biochem. Pharmacol.*, **19**, 285–97.

Sims, P. (1970c). Studies on the metabolism of 7-methylbenz[a]anthracene and 7,12-dimethylbenz[a]anthracene and its hydroxymethyl derivatives in rat liver and adrenal homogenates. *Biochem. Pharmacol.*, **19**, 2261–75.

Sims, P. (1971). The preparation of benz[a]anthracene 8,9-oxide and 10,11-dihydro-benz[a]anthracene 8,9-oxide and their metabolism by rat-liver preparations. *Biochem. J.*, **125**, 159–68.

Sims, P. (1973). The preparation and metabolism of epoxides related to 7,12-dimethyl-benz[a]anthracene. *Biochem. J.*, **131**, 405–13.

Sinha, D. & Dao, T. L. (1975). Site of origin of mammary tumours induced by 7,12-dimethylbenz[a]anthracene in the rat. *J. Nat. Cancer Inst.*, **54**, 1007–8.

Sinha, D. K. & Dao, T. L. (1980). Induction of mammary tumours in ageing rats by 7,12-dimethylbenz[a]anthracene: role of DNA synthesis during carcinogenesis. *J. Nat. Cancer Inst.*, **64**, 519–21.

Slaga, T. J., Bowden, G. T., Scribner, J. P. & Boutwell, R. K. (1974). Dose–response studies on the ability of 7,12-dimethylbenz[a]anthracene to initiate skin tumors. *J. Nat. Cancer Inst.*, **53**, 1337–40.

Slaga, T. J. & Boutwell, R. K. (1977a). Inhibition of the tumor-initiating ability of the potent carcinogen 7,12-dimethylbenz[a]anthracene by the weak tumor initiator 1,2,3,4-dibenzanthracene. *Cancer Res.*, **37**, 128–33.

Slaga, T. J. & Bracken, W. M. (1977b). The effects of antioxidants on skin tumor initiation and aryl hydrocarbon hydroxylase. *Cancer Res.*, **37**, 1631–5.

Slaga, T. J., Huberman, E., Selkirk, J. K., Harvey, R. G. & Bracken, W. M. (1978). Carcinogenicity and mutagenicity of benz[a]anthracene diols and diol-epoxides. *Cancer Res.*, **38**, 1699–704.

Slaga, T. J., Gleason, G. L., DiGiovanni, J., Sukumaran, K. B. & Harvey, R. G. (1979a). Potent tumor-initiating activity of the 3,4-dihydrodiol of 7,12-dimethyl-benz[a]anthracene in mouse skin. *Cancer Res.*, **39**, 1934–6.

Slaga, T. J., Huberman, E., DiGiovanni, J. & Gleason, G. (1979b). The importance of the 'bay-region' diol epoxide in 7,12-dimethylbenz[a]anthracene skin tumor initiation and mutagenesis. *Cancer Lett.*, **6**, 213–20.

Slaga, T. J., Jecker, L., Bracken, W. M. & Weeks, C. E. (1979c). The effects of weak or non-carcinogenic polycyclic hydrocarbons on 7,12-dimethylbenz[a]anthracene and benzo[a]pyrene skin tumor-initiation. *Cancer Lett.*, **7**, 51–9.

Slaga, T. J., Gleason, G. L., Mills, G., Enald, L., Fu, P. P., Lee, H. M. & Harvey, R. G. (1980). Comparison of the skin tumor-initiating activities of dihydrodiols and diol epoxides of various polycyclic aromatic hydrocarbons. *Cancer Res.*, **40**, 1981–4.

Solanki, V., Yotti, L., Logani, M. K. & Slaga, T. J. (1984). The reduction of tumor initiating activity and cell mediated mutagenicity of dimethylbenz[a]anthracene by a copper coordination compound. *Carcinogenesis*, **5**, 129–31.

Somogyi, A. & Kovacs, K. (1970). Effect of various steroids on the adrenal necrosis induced by 7,12-dimethylbenz[a]anthracene in rats. *Rev. Can. Biol.*, **29**, 169–80.

Steiner, P. E. & Edgcombe, J. H. (1952). Carcinogenicity of 1,2-benzanthracene. *Cancer Res.*, **12**, 657–9.

Stevenson, J. L. & Von Haam, E. (1965). Carcinogenicity of benz[a]anthracene and benzo[c]phenanthrene derivatives. *Am. Ind. Hyg. Assoc. J.*, **26**, 475–8.

Swaisland, A. J., Hewer, A., Pal, K., Keysell, G. R., Booth, J., Grover, P. L. & Sims, P. (1974). Polycyclic hydrocarbon epoxides: the involvement of 8,9-dihydro-8,9-dihydroxybenz[a]anthracene 10,11-oxide in reactions with the DNA of benz[a]anthracene-treated hamster embryo cells. *FEBS Lett.*, **47**, 34–8.

Swallow, W. H., Pal, K., Phillips, D. H., Grover, P. L. & Sims, P. (1983). The metabolism of 7,12-dimethylbenz[a]anthracene and 7-hydroxymethyl-12-methyl-benz[a]anthracene by rat liver and adrenal homogenates and by rat adrenocortical cells. *Chem. Biol. Interact.*, **47**, 347–60.

Tamulski, T. S., Morreal, C. E. & Dao, T. L. (1973). Comparative metabolism of 7,12-dimethylbenz[a]anthracene in liver and mammary tissue. *Cancer Res.*, **33**, 3117–22.

Taparowsky, E., Shimizu, K., Goldfarb, M. & Wigler, M. (1983). Structure and activation of the human N-*ras* gene. *Cell*, **34**, 581–6.

Tay, L. K. & Russo, J. (1981). Formation and removal of 7,12-dimethyl benz[a]anthracene–nucleic acid adducts in rat mammary epithelial cells with different susceptibility to carcinogenesis. *Carcinogenesis*, **2**, 1327–33.

Thakker, D. R., Yagi, H., Lehr, R. E., Levin, W., Buening, M., Lu, A. H. Y., Chang, R. L., Wood, A. W., Conney, A. H. & Jerina, D. M. (1978). Metabolism of *trans*-9,10-dihydroxy-9,10-dihydrobenzo[a]pyrene occurs primarily by aryl hydroxylation rather than formation of a diol epoxide. *Molec. Pharmacol.*, **14**, 502–13.

Thakker, D. R., Levin, W., Yagi, H., Ryan, D., Thomas, P. E., Karle, J. M., Lehr, R. E., Jerina, D. M. & Conney, A. H. (1979a). Metabolism of benzo[a]anthracene to its tumorigenic 3,4-dihydrodiol. *Molec. Pharmacol.*, **15**, 138–53.

Thakker, D. R., Levin, W., Yagi, H., Tada, M., Conney, A. H. & Jerina, D. M. (1979b). Comparative metabolism of dihydrodiols of polycyclic aromatic hydrocarbons to bay-region diol epoxides. In: *Polynuclear Aromatic Hydrocarbons*, ed. A. Bjorseth & A. J. Dennis, p. 267. Columbus, Ohio: Battelle Press.

206   *Biology*

Thakker, D. R., Levin, W., Yagi, H., Turujman, S., Kapadia, D., Conney, A. H. & Jerina, D. M. (1979c). Absolute stereochemistry of the *trans*-dihydrodiols formed from benzo[a]anthracene by liver microsomes. *Chem. Biol. Interact.*, 27, 145–61.

Thakker, D. R., Levin, W., Yagi, H., Tada, M., Ryan, D. E., Thomas, P. G., Conney, A. H. & Jerina, D. M. (1982). Stereoselective metabolism of the (+) and (−)-enantiomers of *trans*-3,4-dihydroxy-3,4-dihydrobenz[a]anthracene by rat liver microsomes and by a purified and reconstituted cytochrome P-450 system. *J. Biol. Chem.*, 257, 5103–10.

Thompson, H. J., Meeker, D. L. & Kokoska, S. (1984). Effect of an inorganic and organic form of dietary selenium on the promotional stage of mammary carcinogenesis in the rat. *Cancer Res.*, 44, 2803–6.

Thornton, S. C., Diamond, L., Hite, M. & Baird, W. M. (1982). The effect of liver homogenate S-20 concentration on polycyclic aromatic hydrocarbon activation and mutation induction in the L-5178 mouse lymphoma mutation assay. *Mutation Res.*, 106, 101–12.

Tierney, B., Hewer, A., Walsh, C., Grover, P. L. & Sims, P. (1977). The metabolic activation of 7-methylbenz[a]anthracene in mouse skin. *Chem. Biol. Interact.*, 18, 179–93.

Tierney, B., Abercrombie, B., Walsh, C., Hewer, A., Grover, P. L. & Sims, P. (1978a). The preparation of dihydrodiols from 7-methylbenz[a]anthracene. *Chem. Biol. Interact.*, 21, 289–98.

Tierney, B., Hewer, A., MacNicoll, A. D., Gervasi, G. P., Rattle, H., Walsh, C., Grover, P. L. & Sims, P. (1978b). The formation of dihydrodiols by the chemical or enzymic oxidation of benz[a]anthracene and 7,12-dimethylbenz[a]anthracene. *Chem. Biol. Interact.*, 23, 243–57.

Tierney, B., Burden, P., Hewer, A., Ribeiro, O., Walsh, C., Rattle, H., Grover, P. L. & Sims, P. (1979). High performance liquid chromatography of isomeric dihydrodiols of polycyclic hydrocarbons: the effect of conformation on elution order. *J. Chromatography*, 176, 329–35.

Tierney, B., Weaver, D., Heintz, N. H., Schaeffer, W. I. & Bresnick, E. (1980). The identity and nuclear uptake of a cytosolic binding protein for 3-methylcholanthrene. *Arch. Biochem. Biophys.*, 200, 513–23.

Valaoras, V. G., MacMahon, B., Trichopoulos, D. & Polychronopoulou, A. (1969). Lactation and reproductive histories of breast cancer patients in greater Athens, 1965–1967. *Int. J. Cancer*, 4, 350–62.

Van Bladeren, P. J., Sayer, J. M., Ryan, D. E., Thomas, P. E., Levin, W. & Jerina, D. M. (1985). Differential stereoselectivity of cytochrome P-450b and P-450c in the formation of naphthalene and anthracene 1,2-oxides. The role of epoxide hydrolase in determining the enantiomer composition of the 1,2-dihydrodiols formed. *J. Biol. Chem.*, 260, 10226–35.

Van Duuren, B. L., Langseth, L., Orris, L., Baden, M. & Kuschner, M. (1967). Carcinogenicity of epoxides, lactones and peroxy compounds. V. Subcutaneous injection into rats. *J. Nat. Cancer Inst.*, 39, 1213–26.

Van Duuren, B. L., Sivak, A. & Goldschmidt, B. M. (1970). Initiating activity of aromatic hydrocarbons in two stage carcinogenesis. *J. Nat. Cancer Inst.*, 44, 1167–73.

Venitt, S. & Tarmy, E. M. (1972). The selective excision of aryl alkylated products from the DNA of *Escherichia coli* treated with the carcinogen 7-bromomethyl-benz[a]anthracene. *Biochim. Biophys. Acta*, 287, 38–51.

Verma, A. K. & Boutwell, R. K. (1980). Effects of dose and duration of treatment with the tumour promoting agent, TPA. *Carcinogenesis*, 1, 271–6.

Vigny, P., Duquesne, M., Coulomb, H., Lacombe, C., Tierney, B., Grover, P. L. & Sims, P. (1977a). Metabolic activation of polycyclic hydrocarbons; fluorescence spectral evidence is consistent with metabolism at the 1,2- and 3,4-double bonds of 7-methyl-benz[a]anthracene. *FEBS Lett.*, **75**, 9–12.

Vigny, P., Duquesne, M., Coulomb, H., Tierney, B., Grover, P. L. & Sims, P. (1977*b*). Fluorescence spectral studies on the metabolic activation of 3-methylcholanthrene and 7,12-dimethylbenz[a]anthracene in mouse skin. *FEBS Lett.*, **82**, 278–82.

Vigny, P., Kindts, M., Duquesne, M., Cooper, C. S., Grover, P. L. & Sims, P. (1980). Metabolic activation of benz[a]anthracene, fluorescence spectral evidence indicates the involvement of a non 'bay-region' diol-epoxide. *Carcinogenesis*, **1**, 33–6.

Vigny, P., Kindts, M., Cooper, C. S., Grover, P. L. & Sims, P. (1981). Fluorescence spectral of nucleoside–hydrocarbon adducts formed in mouse skin treated with 7,12-dimethylbenz[a]anthracene. *Carcinogenesis*, **2**, 115–19.

Vigny, P., Brunissen, A., Phillips, D. H., Cooper, C. S., Hewer, A., Grover, P. L. & Sims, P. (1985). Metabolic activation of 7,12-dimethylbenz[a]anthracene in rat mammary tissue: fluorescence spectral characteristics of hydrocarbon–DNA adducts. *Cancer Lett.*, **26**, 51–9.

Vogel, K., Bentley, P., Glatt, K. & Oesch, F. (1980). Rat liver cytoplasmic dihydrodiol dehydrogenase, purification to apparent homogeneity and properties. *J. Biol. Chem.*, **225**, 9621–5.

Vyas, K. P., Van Bladeren, P. J., Thakker, D. R., Yagi, H., Sayer, J. M., Levin, W. & Jerina, D. M. (1983). Regioselectivity and stereoselectivity in the metabolism of *trans*-1,2-dihydroxy-1,2-dihydrobenz[a]anthracene by rat liver microsomes. *Molec. Pharmacol.*, **24**, 115–23.

Wagner, D. A., Naylor, P. H., Kim, U., Shea, W., Ip, C. & Ip, M. M. (1982). Interaction of dietary fat and the thymus in the induction of mammary tumours by 7,12-dimethyl-benz[a]anthracene. *Cancer Res.*, **42**, 1266–73.

Walaszek, Z., Hanausek-Walaszek, M. & Webb, T. E. (1984). Inhibition of 7,12-dimethylbenzanthracene-induced rat mammary tumorigenesis by 2,5-di-*O*-acetyl-D-glucaro-1,4:6,3-dilactone, an *in vivo* β-glucuronidase inhibitor. *Carcinogenesis*, **5**, 767–72.

Walters, M. A. (1966). The induction of lung tumours by the injection of 9,10-dimethyl-1,2-benz[a]anthracene (DMBA) into newborn suckling and young adult mice. *Br. J. Cancer*, **20**, 148–60.

Watabe, T., Ishizuka, T., Isobe, M. & Ozawa, N. (1982). A 7-hydroxymethyl sulphate ester as an active metabolite of 7,12-dimethylbenz[a]anthracene. *Science*, **215**, 403–5.

Watabe, T., Hiratsuka, A., Ogura, K. & Endoh, K. (1985). A reactive hydroxymethyl sulphate ester formed regioselectively from the carcinogen, 7,12-dihydroxymethyl-benz[a]anthracene by rat liver sulfotransferase. *Biochem. Biophys. Res. Commun.*, **131**, 694–9.

Wattenberg, L. W. (1980). Inhibition of polycyclic aromatic hydrocarbon-induced neoplasia by sodium cyanate. *Cancer Res.*, **40**, 232–4.

Wattenberg, L. W. (1983). Inhibition of neoplasia by minor dietary constituents. *Cancer Res.*, **43**, 2448s–53s.

Weems, H. B., Mushtaq, M. & Yang, S. K. (1985). Resolution of epoxide enantiomers of PAH by chiral stationary-phase HPLC. *Anal. Biochem.*, **148**, 328–38.

Welsh, C., Smith, M., Brown, C., Greene, H. & Hamel, E. J. (1981). Selenium and the genesis of murine mammary tumours. *Carcinogenesis*, **2**, 519–22.

Welsch, C. W. & Aylsworth, C. F. (1983). Enhancement of murine mammary tumorigenesis by feeding high levels of dietary fat: a hormonal mechanism. *J. Nat. Cancer Inst.*, **70**, 215–21.

Weston, A., Grover, P. L. & Sims, P. (1983). Formation of the 1,2-diol as a metabolite of 7,12-dimethylbenz[a]anthracene by rodent and human skin. *Carcinogenesis*, **4**, 1307–11.

Wettstein, J. G., Chien, M. T. & Flesher, J. W. (1979). DNA binding and mutagenicity of 7-substituted derivatives of benz[a]anthracene. *Drug and Chemical Toxicol.*, **2**, 383–96.

Wheatley, D. N., Hamilton, A. G., Currie, A. R., Boyland, E. & Sims, P. (1966*a*). Adrenal necrosis induced by 7-hydroxymethyl-12-methylbenz[a]anthracene and its prevention. *Nature*, **211**, 1311–12.

Wheatley, D. N., Kernohan, I. R. & Currie, A. R. (1966*b*). Liver injury and the prevention of massive adrenal necrosis from 9,10-dimethyl-1,2-benzanthracene in rats. *Nature*, **211**, 387–9.

Wheatley, D. N. & Inglis, M. S. (1968). Mammary tumours induced in Sprague–Dawley female rats by 7,12-dimethylbenz[a]anthracene and its hydroxymethyl derivatives. *Br. J. Cancer*, **22**, 122–7.

White, F. R. & Eschenbrenner, A. B. (1945). Note on the occurrence of hepatomas in rats following the ingestion of 1,2-benzanthracene. *J. Nat. Cancer Inst.*, **6**, 19–23.

White, G. L., Fu, P. P. & Heflich, A. (1985). Effect of nitro substitution on the light-mediated mutagenicity of polycyclic aromatic hydrocarbons in *Salmonella typhimurium* TA98. *Mutation Res.*, **144**, 1–7.

Williams, M. G. (1958). The response of the human epidermis to the application of carcinogenic hydrocarbons. *J. Invest. Dermatology*, **30**, 13–20.

Wilson, N. M., Christou, M., Turner, C. R., Wrighton, S. A. & Jefcoate, C. R. (1984). Binding and metabolism of benzo[a]pyrene and 7,12-dimethylbenz[a]anthracene by seven purified forms of cytochrome P-450. *Carcinogenesis*, **5**, 1475–83.

Wislocki, P. G., Chang, R. L., Wood, A. W., Levin, W., Yagi, H., Hernandez, O., Mah, H. D., Dansette, P. M., Jerina, D. M. & Conney, A. H. (1977). High carcinogenicity of 2-hydroxybenzo[a]pyrene on mouse skin. *Cancer Res.*, **37**, 2608–11.

Wislocki, P. G., Kapitulnik, J., Levin, W., Lehr, R., Schaefer-Ridder, M., Karle, J. M., Jerina, D. M. & Conney, A. H. (1978). Exceptional carcinogenic activity of benz[a]anthracene 3,4-dihydrodiol in the newborn mouse and the bay region theory. *Cancer Res.*, **38**, 693–6.

Wislocki, P. G., Buening, M. K., Levin, W., Lehr, R. E., Thakker, D. R., Jerina, D. M. & Conney, A. H. (1979). Tumorigenicity of the diastereomeric benz[a]anthracene 3,4-diol 1,2-epoxide and the (+) and (−) enantiomers of benz[a]anthracene 3,4-dihydrodiol in newborn mice. *J. Nat. Cancer Inst.*, **63**, 201–4.

Wislocki, P. G., Gadek, K. M., Chou, M. W., Yang, S. K. & Lu, A. Y. H. (1980). Carcinogenicity and mutagenicity of the 3,4-dihydrodiols and other metabolites of 7,12-dimethylbenz[a]anthracene and its hydroxymethyl derivatives. *Cancer Res.*, **40**, 3661–4.

Wislocki, P. G., Fiorentini, K. M., Fu, P. P., Chou, M. W., Yang, S. K. & Lu, A. Y. H. (1981*a*). Tumor-initiating activity of the dihydrodiols of 8-methylbenz[a]anthracene and 8-hydroxymethylbenz[a]anthracene. *Carcinogenesis*, **2**, 507–9.

Wislocki, P. G., Juliana, M. M., MacDonald, J. S., Chou, M. W., Yang, S. K. & Lu, A. Y. H. (1981*b*). Tumorigenicity of 7,12-dimethylbenz[a]anthracene, its hydroxy-methylated derivatives and selected dihydrodiols in the newborn mouse. *Carcinogenesis*, **2**, 511–14.

Wislocki, P. G., Fiorentini, K. M., Fu, P. P., Yang, S. K. & Lu, A. Y. H. (1982). Tumour-initiating ability of the twelve monomethylbenz[a]anthracenes. *Carcinogenesis*, **3**, 215–17.

Wood, A. W., Levin, W., Lu, A. Y. H., Ryan, D., West, S. B., Lehr, R. E., Schaefer-Ridder, M., Jerina, D. M. & Conney, A. H. (1976). Mutagenicity of metabolically activated benz[a]anthracene 3,4-dihydrodiol: evidence for bay region activation of carcinogenic polycyclic hydrocarbons. *Biochem. Biophys. Res. Commun.*, **72**, 680–6.

Wood, A. W., Chang, R. L., Levin, W., Lehr, R. E., Schaefer-Ridder, M., Karle, J. M., Jerina, D. M. & Conney, A. H. (1977*a*). Mutagenicity and cytotoxicity of benz[a]anthracene diol epoxides and tetrahydro-epoxides: exceptional activity of the bay region 1,2-epoxides. *Proc. Nat. Acad. Sci. U.S.A.*, **74**, 2746–50.

Wood, A. W., Levin, W., Chang, R. L., Lehr, R. E., Schaefer-Ridder, M., Karle, J. M., Jerina, D. M. & Conney, A. H. (1977b). Tumorigenicity of five dihydrodiols of benz[a]anthracene on mouse skin: exceptional activity of benz[a]anthracene 3,4-dihydrodiol. *Proc. Nat. Acad. Sci.*, 74, 3176–9.

Wood, A. W., Lehr, R. E., Thakker, D. R., Yagi, H., Chang, R. L., Ryan, D. E., Thomas, P. E., Dansette, D. M., Whittaker, N., Turnjman, S., Lehr, R. E., Kumar, S., Conney, A. H. & Jerina, D. M. (1979). Biological activity of B[e]P. An assessment based on mutagenic activity and metabolic profiles of the polycyclic hydrocarbon and its derivatives. *J. Biol. Chem.*, 254, 4408–15.

Wood, A. W., Levin, W., Chang, R. L., Conney, A. H., Slaga, T. J., O'Malley, R. F., Newman, M. S., Buhler, D. R. & Jerina, D. M. (1982). Mouse skin tumour initiating activity of 5-, 7- and 12-methyl and fluorine-substituted benz[a]anthracenes. *J. Nat. Cancer Inst.*, 69, 725–8.

Wood, A. W., Chang, R. L., Levin, W., Yagi, H., Thakker, D. R., Van Bladeren, P. J., Jerina, D. M. & Conney, A. H. (1983). Mutagenicity of the enantiomers of the diastereomeric bay-region benz[a]anthracene 3,4-diol-1,2-epoxides in bacterial and mammalian cells. *Cancer Res.*, 43, 5821–5.

Yang, S. K. & Dower, W. V. (1975). Metabolic pathways of 7,12-dimethyl-benz[a]anthracene in hepatic microsomes. *Proc. Nat. Acad. Sci. U.S.A.*, 72, 2601–5.

Yang, S. K., Chou, M. W., Weems, H. B. & Fu, P. P. (1979a). Enzymatic formation of an 8,9-diol from 8-methylbenz[a]anthracene. *Biochem. Biophys. Res. Commun.*, 90, 1136–41.

Yang, S. K., Chou, M. W., Weems, H. B. & Roller, P. P. (1979b). Potential proximate carcinogens of 7,12-dimethylbenz[a]anthracene: characterisation of two metabolically formed *trans*-3,4-dihydrodiols. *J. Am. Chem. Soc.*, 101, 237–9.

Yang, S. K. & Chou, M. W. (1980a). Metabolism of the bay-region *trans*-1,2-dihydrodiol of benz[a]anthracene in rat liver microsomes occurs primarily at the 3,4-double bond. *Carcinogenesis*, 1, 803–6.

Yang, S. K., Chou, M. W. & Fu, P. P. (1980b). Metabolism of 6-, 7-, 8- and 12-methyl-benz[a]anthracenes and hydroxymethylbenz[a]anthracenes. In *Polynuclear Aromatic Hydrocarbons: Chemistry and Biological Effects*, ed. A. Bjorseth & A. J. Dennis, pp. 645–62. Columbus, Ohio: Battelle Press.

Yang, S. K., Chou, M. W., Wislocki, P. G. & Lu, A. H. Y. (1980c). Metabolism of 7,12-dimethylbenz[a]anthracene: quantitation of metabolite formation in rat liver microsomes and a reconstituted enzyme system containing highly purified cytochrome P-450 or P-448. In *Polycyclic Aromatic Hydrocarbons: Chemistry and Biological Effects*, ed. A. Bjorseth & A. J. Dennis, pp. 733–51. Columbus, Ohio: Battelle Press.

Yang, S. K. (1982a). The absolute stereochemistry of the major *trans*-dihydrodiol enantiomers formed from 11-methylbenz[a]anthracene by rat liver microsomes. *Drug Met. Dispos.*, 10, 205–11.

Yang, S. K., Chou, M. W., Fu, P. P., Wislocki, P. G. & Lu, A. H. Y. (1982b). Epoxidation reactions catalysed by rat liver cytochromes P-450 and P-448 occur at different faces of the 8,9-double bond of 8-methylbenz[a]anthracene. *Proc. Nat. Acad. Sci. U.S.A.*, 79, 6802–6.

Yang, S. K. & Fu, P. P. (1984a). Stereoselective metabolism of 7-methyl-benz[a]anthracene: absolute configuration of five dihydrodiol metabolites and the effect of dihydrodiol conformation on circular dichroism spectra. *Chem. Biol. Interact.*, 49, 71–8.

Yang, S. K. & Fu, P. P. (1984b). The effect of the bay-region 12-methyl group on the stereoselective metabolism of the K-region of 7,12-dimethylbenz[a]anthracene by rat liver microsomes. *Biochem. J.*, 223, 775–82.

Yang, S. K. & Chiu, P. (1985). Cytochrome P-450 catalysed stereoselective epoxidation

at the K-region of benz[a]anthracene and benzo[a]pyrene. *Arch. Biochem. Biophys.*,
240, 546–52.
Yuasa, Y., Srivastava, S., Dunn, C., Rhim, J. S., Reddy, E. & Aaronson, S. (1983).
Acquisition of transforming properties by alternative point mutations within C-*bas*/*has*
human proto-oncogene. *Nature*, **303**, 775–9.
Zarbl, H., Sukumar, S., Authur, A. V., Zanca, D. M. & Barbacid, M. (1985). Direct
mutagenesis of Ha-*ras*-1 oncogenes by N-nitroso-N-methylurea during initiation of
mammary carcinogenesis in rats. *Nature*, **315**, 382–5.
Zieger, S. B., Salmons, R., Konoshita, N. & Peacock, A. C. (1972). The binding of
9,10-dimethyl-1,2-benzanthracene to mouse epidermal satellite DNA *in vivo*. *Cancer
Res.*, **32**, 643–7.
Zijlstra, J. A. & Vogel, E. W. (1984). Mutagenicity of 7,12-dimethylbenz[a]anthracene
and some other aromatic mutagens in *Drosophila melanogaster*. *Mutation Res.*, **125**,
243–61.

Index

The abbreviations BA, MBA and DMBA have been used for benz[a]anthracene, methylbenz[a]anthracene and dimethyl-benz[a]anthracene respectively.

228   *Index*

Stobbe condensation, 38—9
Stromal cells, 111
Styrenes, use of in synthesis, 31
7-Substituted BAs, metabolism 97—9
Sulphate conjugates, 88, 90
7-SulphydrylBA
    synthesis, 18—19
Superoxide dismutase, 152
Syrian hamster embryo cells, malignant
    transformation of, 145

Tampons, use of in promotion, 174
Testes, effect of 7,12-DMBA on, 109, 180
Tetraugulol
    synthesis, 46
2,3,7,8-Tetrachlorodibenzo-*p*-dioxin,
    141—2, 174
12-*O*-Tetradecanoylphorbol-13-acetate, 173
1,2,3,4-TetrahydroBA, DNA interactions
    of, 116—17
8,9,10,11-TetrahydroBA, DNA interactions
    of, 116—17
1,2,3,4-TetrahydroBA quinone,
    synthesis, 31
1,2,3,4-Tetrahydro-7,12-DMBA
    carcinogenicity, 179
    mutagenicity, 154—6
TetraMBA
    syntheses of, references to, 52
7,8,9,12-TetraMBA
    carcinogenicity, 186
    synthesis, 6
Tetrasubstituted BAs, carcinogenicity, 186
Tetrol, from diol epoxide, 88
Thiol containing BAs, carcinogenicity,
    169
Transplacental carcinogenicity, 176
Trialkyl BA
    carcinogenicity, 183—5
    syntheses of, references to, 52
1,1,1-Trichloropropene-2,3-oxide, 133
9-Trifluoromethyl-7,12-DMBA
    carcinogenicity, 185
    synthesis, 13
10-Trifluoromethyl-7,12-DMBA
    carcinogenicity, 185
    synthesis, 13
TriMBA
    carcinogenicity, comparison of, 183—
    5
    syntheses of, references to, 52
1,7,12-TriMBA

carcinogenicity, 183—5
synthesis, 33
2,7,12-TriMBA
    carcinogenicity, 183—5
    synthesis, difficulties in, 6
3,7,12-TriMBA
    carcinogenicity, 183—5
4,7,12-TriMBA
    carcinogenicity, 183—5
5,7,12-TriMBA
    carcinogenicity, 183—5
6,7,8-TriMBA
    carcinogenicity, 183—5
    synthesis, 9
6,7,12-TriMBA
    carcinogenicity, 183—5
6,8,11-TriMBA
    synthesis, 40—1
6,8,12-TriMBA
    carcinogenicity, 183—5
7,8,12-TriMBA
    carcinogenicity, 183—5
7,9,12-TriMBA
    carcinogenicity, 183—5
7,10,12-TriMBA
    carcinogenicity, 183—5
7,11,12-TriMBA
    carcinogenicity, 183—5
    synthesis, 6
8,9,11-TriMBA
    synthesis, 29—30
Trisubstituted BAs
    carcinogenicity, 183—5
    DNA binding, 140—1
    metabolism, 112
    mutagenicity, 157—9
Tumour progression, model for, 168

Urine metabolite, 85

Vilsmeier reaction, 42
Vinyl cyclohexanes, use of in synthesis,
    31
Vinylene carbonate, use of in synthesis,
    11
Wagner-Meerwein rearrangement, 43—4
Wistar-Furth rat, 157
Wittig reaction, 42

X-ray crystallography, 140

Zona fasciculato, 109
Zona reticularis, 109